Chinese Life Sciences

Introductory Readings in Classical Chinese Medicine

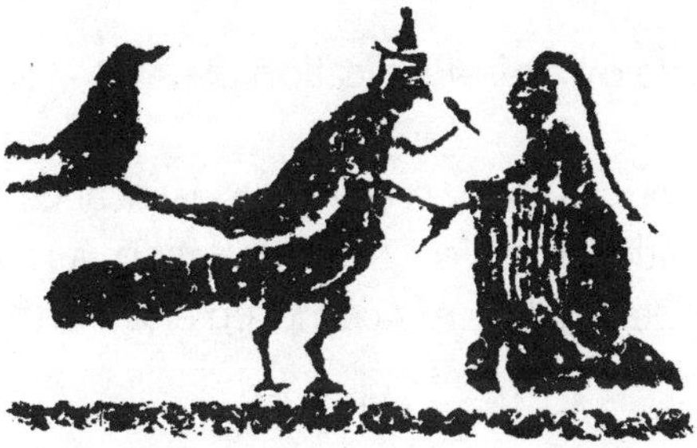

Sixty Texts with Vocabulary and Translation, a Guide to Research Aids and a General Glossary

Compiled and translated by

Paul U. Unschuld

Paradigm Publications

Taos, New Mexico 2005

Chinese Life Sciences
Introductory Readings in Classical Chinese Medicine

Sixty Texts with Vocabulary and Translation,
a Guide to Research Aids and a General Glossary

Compiled and translated by
Paul U. Unschuld

202 Bendix Drive, Taos, NM 87571
www.paradigm-pubs.com
Distributed by Redwing Book Company
www.redwingbooks.com

Library of Congress Cataloging-in-Publication Data

Chinese life sciences : introductory readings in classical Chinese medicine : sixty texts with vocabulary and translation, a guide to research aids, and a general glossary / compiled and translated by Paul U. Unschuld.-- 2nd ed.
p. ; cm.
Rev. ed. of: Introductory readings in classical Chinese medicine / compiled and translated by Paul U. Unschuld. Dordrecht ; Boston : Kluwer Academic Publishers, 1988.
Includes bibliographical references.
Text in Chinese and English.
ISBN 0-912111-81-X (notch pbk. : alk. paper)
1. Chinese language--Readers--Medicine, Chinese. 2. Medicine, Chinese. I. Unschuld, Paul U. (Paul Ulrich), 1943- II. Introductory readings in classical Chinese medicine.
PL1117.5.M43C42 2005
495.1'86421'02461--dc22

2005015687

Library of Congress Number: 2005015687
International Standard Book Number (ISBN): 0-912111-81-X
Printed in the United States of America

Table of Contents

Council of Oriental Medical Publishers Designation

This volume is a translation of excerpts from classical Chinese medical works. English terminology is included in the text.

Introductory Remarks

Chinese traditional life sciences no longer appeal only to practitioners on the fringes of Western medicine who believe so-called Traditional Chinese Medicine to offer a better alternative to so-called biomedicine, and the latter is no longer solely the focus of attention of politicians and health planners impressed by Chinese attempts at integrating indigenous and Westerns modes of prevention and therapy within one health care delivery system. Chinese traditional life sciences have turned into a serious subject of academic research, and of inquiries directed at their origins and development, their links with sociocultural characteristics of Chinese civilisation, and their place in the common intellectual heritage of mankind. Hence, an increasing number of students appears to be interested in mastering the Chinese language to the extent that they will no longer have to depend on secondary sources but will be capable of utilizing primary sources as well when they wish to familiarize themselves with the history, concepts, and practices of Chinese traditional life sciences.

Hitherto available textbooks, and the language training offered by Asian departments, have focussed with success on Chinese philosophy and religion, politics and economics, as well as general Chinese philology or history, but are still unprepared to instruct a student in one of the most important aspects of any culture and civilization: the reaction to illness and disease as existential problems confronting individuals and entire societies alike.

Although an impression is widespread in the West that medicine is separated, by a deep gulf, from the rest of culture, and follows, guided by science, its own path, medical thought and intervention have never ceased to be legitimated by general currents of thought and everyday life, and to reflect basic attitudes of the time. To leave the study of concepts of health care aside in one's study of any foreign (or domestic) culture and society means to disregard a most important key to the understanding of value-systems and world views. A growing awareness of these links has led medical anthropologists and political economists, historians of religion and philosophy as well as scholars from many more disciplines to take a closer look at health care, and a concern with Chinese traditional life sciences has grown into an integral aspect of Chinese studies per se.

This book has resulted from the need to develop a program for the teaching of classical Chinese medical thought and terminology to students from a variety of disciplines, including those with purely academic intentions and others with an interest in clinical application. Some of the students who entered the program had gone through Chinese language classes already, others had never before attempted to write even a single Chinese character. The texts collected in this primer reflect some of the experiences I have gathered over the past decades. Selected from a wider range of primary sources used as teaching materials at one time or another, they have proven to be suitable introductory readings for all the students who have come to us, despite diverging backgrounds and motives. Graduates from Chinese studies have of course finished this collection of texts in a much shorter time than, for instance, young M.D.s who had decided to venture into Chinese medicine. But they all alike benefitted from a selection of literature excerpts that combined a gradual increase of sophistication with a thematic structure that served well as an initial guide through the maze of classical Chinese ideas of the origin, nature, prevention, and treatment of illness and disease. For students with no prior knowledge of Chinese, a vocabulary explaining the meaning of every new character was added to each of the sixty texts; students with extensive expertise in classical Chinese did not need this vocabulary; they concentrated, instead, on a concise list of key medical terms and phrases compiled, in addition, with each of the ten lessons.

The methodology of rendering Chinese medical terminology applied in this program coincides with the approach developed in the various volumes of my *Medicine in China* series, published by University of California Press. Chinese medicine has never known a terminology as abstract and stringent as is the terminology of modern science; rather the situation in traditional Chinese medicine may be compared to a time in the history of European medicine when Greek was both the vernacular of the population and the scholarly idiom used by physicians and scientists. Different levels of folk language and well-defined terminology penetrated each other. It was only after Greek and Latin had ceased to be living languages that countless attempts at reform provided Greek and Latin terms, particularly in the realm of anatomy, with that kind of precision and unambiguity that we tend to associate with scientific terminology in general; it should not be overlooked, though, that Western clinical terminology, in contrast to anatomy, is laden, even today, with a mixture of scientific terms and folk expressions that may not be too different from earlier times.

In China, traditional medical terminology includes a number of designations that appear to have no counterpart in current Western languages. The rendering of these terms poses difficulties reminiscent of those that confronted scholars intending, almost a millennium ago, to translate classic European medicine from Arabic sources into Latin. Many of the terms coined by Arabian authors remained incomprehensible; they were simply written down in Latin letters, and have lost their foreignness, through continuous usage, only after many centuries. For the most part, however, Chinese medical terminology, as is characteristic of a system of thought that is based on analogies rather than analysis, consists of terms and phrases that convey images and meanings linking anatomical entities, physiological functions, and pathological processes, as well as concepts and modes of therapeutic interventions to phenomena of the human environment, be they natural or man-made.

Earlier attempts at creating an artificial Greco-Latin nomenclature to render these terms and phrases have proven to support a misunderstanding of the conceptual basis of traditional Chinese medicine. A terminology, in contrast to a nomenclature, is always a historical product resulting from the convergence of different streams of language and thought. Traditional Chinese medical terminology is no exception from this rule, and it is quite legitimate to apply a complex approach when rendering it into our own language. Such an approach includes the literal or etymological translation of images, as well as a rendering of unambiguous terms, for instance from anatomy, with their exact Western vernacular (or, if such are not available, even scientific) counterparts, and it includes also a mere transliteration of terms conveying unclear concepts, or new ideas hitherto unknown to us.

The sixty texts of this primer were selected from thirty-two sources, covering a time-span from 90 BCE through CE 1891. An alphabetical list of these sources, with their authors and years of publication, follows these introductory remarks. The texts grouped together in each of the ten lessons are introduced by a short survey of their common theme. It was my intention to confront students through this selection not only with a wide range of topics related to diverging arenas of theory and clinical practice in Chinese classical medicine, but also with different types of texts. Thus, readers will find excerpts from the classics compiled by anonymous authors two millennia ago, and from more recent texts written in the Ming and Qing dynasties by well-known physicians or scientists. Some of the texts include short commentaries interspersed in the original texts by unknown copyists; others carry lengthy explications informing students of the nature of scientific argumentation in pre-modern China.

In general, the texts offer a good mixture of types of sources students may encounter when they approach primary Chinese traditional medical literature for further research.

This book was written for independent usage but its readers will find it beneficial to consult the aforementioned volumes of the *Medicine in China* series and, published by University of California Press more recently, the title *Huang Di Nei Jing Su Wen, Nature, Knowledge, Imagery in an Ancient Chinese Medical Text.* Traditional Chinese medicine is far too complex to point out all its subtleties in but a few pages, and many of the concepts that appear in the texts of the present collection are discussed in more detail, and within their broader historical context, in those monographs. Hence only the most essential notes have been added to the texts here.

A guide to 'Special Research Aids' listing dictionaries, bibliographies, biographies, philologically sound translations of seminal texts, and a few other works specifically pertaining to Chinese traditional medicine was added to this book as an appendix to facilitate further independent studies by its readers.

This book was first published by Kluwer Academic Publishers in 1988. That edition, I was happy to state at the end of the original preface, had greatly benefitted from many questions raised by our students; individual texts had been discussed with Dr. Akira Akahori, Dr. Hermann Kogelschatz, Rupprecht Mayer, Dr. Jürgen Kovacs, Prof. Zheng Jinsheng, Dr. Hwang Shen-chang, and Prof. Ma Kanwen. The entire manuscript had been read by Dr. Paul Zmiewski (+), who offered many suggestions how to adapt my renderings to a rising level of standardized terminology applied in English translations of current and ancient Chinese medical texts.

Fifteen years have passed since this first edition was published, and I am happy to see a second edition prepared by Paradigm Publications. In its basic structure and intention, the book has remained identical with the first edition. I have changed romanization of Chinese characters from the Wade-Giles system to pinyin, and I have expanded, with the help of Prof. Zheng Jinsheng, the section on special research aids to include valuable titles published in the meantime. Also, the many years of using this primer in university classes as well as the continuing development of Chinese medical philology has led to some adaptations in the English rendering of the texts. I am particularly grateful to Dr. Hermann Tessenow for his suggestions to this effect. Finally, I should like to thank Prof. Zheng Jinsheng for his technical support in rewriting this volume.

Munich, August 2004 Paul U. Unschuld

List of Sources Quoted
(With year of publication)

Běn cǎo cóng xīn 本草從新
by Wú Yíluò 吳儀洛 1757
Běn cǎo gāng mù 本草綱目
by Lǐ Shízhēn 李時珍 1596
Běn cǎo qiú zhēn 本草求真
by Huāng Gōngxiù 黃宮綉 1769
Cháng shā fāng gē kuò 長沙方歌括
by Chén Niànzǔ 陳念祖 1820
Chóng xiū zhèng hé jīng shǐ zhèng lèi bèi yòng běn cǎo 重修政和經史證類備用本草
by Táng Shènwēi 唐慎微 1249
Dú yī suí bǐ 讀醫隨筆
by Zhōu Xuéhǎi 周學海 1891
Gǔ jīn yī tǒng dà quán 古今醫統大全
by Xú Chūnfǔ 徐春甫 1556
Huáng dì nèi jīng, Líng shū 黃帝內經·靈樞
author unknown 2nd c. BCE to 8th c. CE
Huáng dì nèi jīng, Sù wèn 黃帝內經·素問
author unknown 2nd c. BCE to 8th c. CE
Huáng dì nèi jīng, Tài sù 黃帝內經·太素
author unknown 2nd c. BCE to 7th c. CE
Huí xī mài xué 洄溪脉學
by Xú Dàchūn 徐大椿 ca. 1764
Jiě wéi yuán sǒu 解圍元藪
by Shěn Zhīwèn 沈之問 1550
Nàn jīng 難經
author unknown 2nd c. BCE to 1st/2nd c. CE

Pí wèi lùn 脾胃論
by Lǐ Gǎo 李杲 1249
Rú mén shì qīn 儒門事親
by Zhāng Cóngzhèng 張從正 ca. 1228
Sān yīn jí yī bìng zhèng fāng lùn 三因極一病證方論
by Chén Yán 陳言 1174
Shèn jí chú yán 慎疾芻言
by Xú Dàchūn 徐大椿 1767
Shǐ jì 史記
by Sīmǎ Qiān 司馬遷 90 BCE
Shí wù běn cǎo yuē yán 食物本草約言
by Xuē Jǐ 薛己 1550
Shòu shì bǎo yuán 壽世保元
by Gōng Tíngxián 龔廷賢 1616
Tāng yè běn cǎo 湯液本草
by Wáng Hàogǔ 王好古 ca. 1248
Tú shū biān 圖書編
by Zhāng Huáng 章潢 16th c.
Tú zhù bā shí yī nàn jīng 圖註八十一難經
by Zhāng Shìxián 張世賢 1510
Xīn xiū běn cǎo 新修本草
by Sū Jìng 蘇敬 et al. 659
Yī shuō 醫說
by Zhāng Gǎo 張杲 1224
Yī xué jí chéng 醫學集成
by Fù Zī 傅滋 1516
Yī xué liù yào 醫學六要
by Zhāng Sānxī 张三锡 1609
Yī xué shí zài yì 醫學實在易
by Chén Niànzǔ 陳念祖 1808
Yī xué yuán liú lùn 醫學源流論
by Xú Dàchūn 徐大椿 1757
Yù jiàn zá shū 玉澗雜書
by Yè Mèngdé 葉夢德 12th c.
Zhāng shì yī tōng 張氏醫通
by Zhāng Lù 張潞 1695
Zhū bìng yuán hòu lùn 諸病源候論
by Cháo Yuánfāng 巢元方 610
Zhù jiě shāng hán lùn 註解傷寒論
by Chéng Wújǐ 成無已 11th c.

Lesson One

General Values

Similar to other conceptual systems of health care based on the paradigms of systematic correspondence (e.g., Indian ayurveda, and Greek medicine of humoral pathology), classic Chinese medicine placed particular emphasis on prevention through adherence to a specific lifestyle. Where it was known that human life and the functioning of the human organism are but an integral aspect of the all-embracing workings of some fundamental laws of nature, it was only logical to formulate and pursue a way of life that was thought to ensure continuing harmony with those all-pervasive laws, a harmony that meant health. Illness was conceptualized as a departure from the norms found in nature and society, and, in general, it was considered to be reversible only if one found that harmony again. On the basis of such a therapeutic optimism it is understandable that the treatment advocated by classic Chinese medicine of systematic correspondence did not emphasize means to attack an inner enemy, or to chase away, by means of violent poisons or drastic remedies (such as purgatives, emetics, or sudorifics) some evil intruder or unwanted pathogenic agent from the organism. Rather, a soft stimulus appeared preferable to help the organism or its affected parts to return to a normal functioning, and to re-establish a healthy correspondence to the eternal reality of the universe.

Drugs, although known and applied in China to attack and eliminate pathogens in the body, and to cause various physiological changes, since times immemorial, were not part of the classical medicine of systematic correspondence. They were integrated into the paradigms of yinyang and of the five agents only beginning with the thirteenth century, when external circumstances of a sociopolitical nature suggested such a change.

Key Terms Introduced in Lesson One

陰陽	yīn yáng	yin and yang, the two categories of all phenomena.
生	shēng	life
逆	nì	to oppose

死	sǐ	death
治	zhì	order; to put in order; to treat
亂	luàn	disorder; chaos
病	bìng	disease; illness; to be ill
藥	yào	pharmaceutical drug; to employ drugs
藏	zàng	a "depot" storage unit in the body
疾	jí	illness
針	zhēn	a needle
府	fǔ	a "palace" processing unit in the body
表	biǎo	outside; exterior
裏	lǐ	inside; interior
刺	cì	to pierce
灸	jiǔ	to cauterize by burning moxa
砭	biān	a pointed stone
毒	dú	poison; toxic
八正	bā zhèng	the eight cardinal [turning points]
九候	jiǔ hòu	the nine indicators (where the movement in the vessels can be felt)
診	zhěn	to examine; diagnosis
醫	yī	medicine
寒	hán	cold
熱	rè	hot; heat
虛	xū	depletion; depleted
實	shí	repletion
證	zhèng	evidence; symptoms
命	mìng	life; fate
禀	bǐng	natural endowment
厚	hòu	substantial; generous
薄	bó	poor; shabby
經	jīng	a conduit
絡	luò	a network (vessel)
氣	qì	Qi
血	xuě	blood
傷	shāng	harm; to harm

七情	qī qíng	the seven emotions/affects
方	fāng	prescription; recipe
緩	huǎn	slow
急	jí	urgent; fast
色	sè	color; complexion
脉	mài	vessel
微	wēi	weak; minor
形	xíng	physical appearance
身	shēn	the body
心	xīn	the mind
患	huàn	to suffer; suffering
服	fú	to ingest (pharmaceutical substances); to take (medicine)
痲	má	numb; numbness
散	sǎn	powder
腹	fù	the abdomen
背	bèi	the back
割	gé	to cut
腸	cháng	the intestines
胃	wèi	the stomach
傅	fū	to apply (an ointment)
膏	gāo	ointment
創	chuāng	wound
愈	yù	to heal
平	píng	normal
湯	tāng	hot liquid; decoction
撟引	jiǎo yǐn	massage
皮	pí	the skin
肌	jī	the flesh under the skin
抉	jué	to take out; to tear out
衇 (脉, 脈)	mài	the blood vessels
筋	jīn	the sinews
壽	shòu	longevity
夭	yāo	to die young

1.a *Huáng dì nèi jīng, Sù-wèn* 2
黃帝內經 · 素問
Sì qì tiáo shén dà lùn 四氣調神大論
Comprehensive Treatise on the Regulation of the Spirit in Accord with the Four Seasons

---

從陰陽則生。逆之則死。從之則治。逆之則亂。反順爲逆。是謂內格。是故聖人不治已病治未病。不治已亂治未亂。此之謂也。夫病已成而後藥之。亂已成而後治之。譬猶渴而穿井。鬪而鑄錐。不亦晚乎。

從	cóng	to follow; to comply with
陰陽	yīn yáng	yin and yang, the two categories of all phenomena. The term yin yang refers here to natural law in general; it stands for the processes of generation and decline, of balance and mutual interdependence of virtually all aspects of existence
則	zé	a particle indicating consequence or result; translated here as "then … results"
生	shēng	life
逆	nì	to oppose
之	zhī	pronoun, referring here to the laws of yin and yang
死	sǐ	death
治	zhì	order; to put in order; to regulate. This term is applied to the treatment or management of both

		individual and social crisis.The present paragraph combines both these meanings
亂	luàn	disorder; chaos
反	fǎn	to oppose
順	shùn	to be appropriate; to act appropriately
爲	wéi	to be; to represent
是	shì	this; that
謂	wèi	to say; to call; to express the meaning of
內	nèi	inner
格	gé	to resist; to obstruct
內格	nèigé	inner obstruction
是故	shì gù	hence
聖人	shèng rén	a sage
不	bù	not
已	yǐ	already
病	bìng	disease; illness; to be ill
未	wèi	not yet
此之謂也	cǐ zhī wèi yě	this expresses the meaning of that [what was said above]
夫	fū	now
成	chéng	to be fully developed; to complete
後	hòu	after
藥	yào	pharmaceutical drug; to employ drugs
譬	pì	to compare; to be comparable
猶	yóu	like; similar to
渴	kě	to be thirsty; thirst
而	ér	and; and yet
穿	chuān	to bore; to dig a hole
井	jǐng	a well
鬪	dòu	to fight; battle
鑄	zhù	to cast metals
錐	zhuī	a pointed weapon, used here in the sense of "weapon" in general
亦	yì	also; likewise

晚	wǎn	late
乎	hū	interrogative/exclamatory particle

Cóng yīn yáng zé shēng. nì zhī zé sǐ. cóng zhī zé zhì. nì zhī zé luàn. fǎn shùn wéi nì. shì wèi nèi gé. shī gù shèng rén bù zhì yǐ bìng zhì wèi bìng. bù zhì yǐ luàn zhì wèi luàn. cǐ zhī wèi yě. fū bìng yǐ chéng ér hòu yào zhī. luàn yǐ chéng ér hòu zhì zhī. pì yóu kě ér chuān jǐng. dòu ér zhù zhuī. bù yì wǎn hū.

If one follows yin and yang, then life results; if one opposes them, then death results. If one follows them, then order results; if one opposes them, then disorder results. To act contrary to what is appropriate, this is opposition. This is called inner obstruction.[1] Hence, [when it is said] "the sages did not treat those already ill, but treated those not yet ill;[2] they did not regulate what was already in disorder, but regulated what was not yet in disorder," then this expresses the meaning of that [what was said above]. Now, when drugs are employed for therapy only after a disease has become fully developed, when [attempts at] restoring order are initiated only after disorder has fully developed, this is as if a well were dug when one is thirsty, and as if weapons were cast when the fight is on. Would this not be too late, too?

Notes

[1] These two sentences ("To act ... obstruction") constitute a more recent textual layer of the *Su wen* that was added, presumably, in the first half of the first millennium CE by an anonymous commentator.

[2] Chinese physicians have distinguished between signs of a disease (i.e. pathological changes noted by a patient himself or by a third person) and diseases (i.e. the conceptual identification of the health problem underlying these signs) for the past two millennia. Still, similar to English vernacular language, Chinese medical terminology did not clearly distinguish between these two levels. Thus, in the following translations, the term *bìng* 病 (and also the term *jí* 疾, see 1.b) will be translated as "disease" whenever the Chinese author appears to have hinted at a conceptual construct. A translation as "illness" seemed more appropriate where the term may have been used to designate the ailment(s) resulting from a disease. Still, a clear-cut differentiation of what the Chinese authors may have had in mind is not possible. Hence individual interpretations of such passages may vary.

1.b *Huáng dì nèi jīng, Líng shū* 1
黃帝內經・靈樞
Jiǔ zhēn shí èr yuán 九針十二原
The Nine Needles and the Twelve Origins

今夫五藏之有疾也。譬猶刺也。猶污也。猶結也。猶閉也。刺雖久猶可拔也。污雖久猶可雪也。結雖久猶可解也。閉雖久猶可決也。或言久疾之不可取者。非其說也。夫善用針者。取其疾也。猶拔刺也。猶雪污也。猶解結也。猶決閉也。疾雖久猶可畢也。言不可治者。未得其術也。

今	jīn	now
五	wǔ	five
藏	zàng	a "depot" storage unit in the body, i.e. liver, heart, spleen, lung, and kidneys
有	yǒu	to have
疾	jí	illness
也	yě	final particle
刺	cì	a thorn
污	wū	filthy; soiled
結	jié	to tie knots; to bind
閉	bì	to close; be closed
猶	yóu	still
雖	suī	even if; although
久	jiǔ	a long time
可	kě	can; be able

拔	bá	to pluck up; to pull out
雪	xuě	snow; here: to whiten; to cleanse
解	jiě	to untie
決	jué	to clear a water-way; to open
或	huò	sometimes; in some cases; someone
言	yán	to speak; to state
之	zhī	a possessive pronoun
取	qǔ	to take hold of; to take away
者	zhě	those who
非	fēi	to be not; to be wrong; to regard as wrong; condemn
其	qí	this; a demonstrative and possessive pronoun
說	shuō	to explain; an explanation; a statement; a doctrine
善	shàn	good; to be good in; to be an expert in
用	yòng	to use
針	zhēn	a needle
畢	bì	to finish
得	dé	to acquire
術	shù	art; technique; skills

Jīn fū wǔ zàng zhī yǒu jí yě. pì yóu cì yě. yóu wū yě. yóu jié yě. yóu bì yě. cì suī jiǔ yóu kě bá yě. wū suī jiǔ yóu kě xuě yě. jié suī jiǔ yóu kě jiě yě. bì suī jiǔ yóu kě jué yě. huò yán jiǔ jí zhī bù kě qǔ zhě. fēi qí shuō yě. fū shàn yòng zhēn zhě. qǔ qí jí yě. yóu bá cì yě. yóu xuě wū yě. yóu jiě jié yě. yóu jué bì yě. jí suī jiǔ yóu kě bì yě. yán bù kě zhì zhě. wèi dé qí shù yě.

Now, when the five depots are affected by a disease, that is as if a thorn [stuck in one's skin], as if [something was] soiled, as if [a rope was] knotted, or as if [a passageway was] blocked. Although that thorn [stuck in one's skin] for a long time, it could still be pulled out. Although [something was] soiled for a long time, it could still be cleansed [again]. Although [a rope was] knotted for a long time, it could still be untied [again; and] although [a passageway was] blocked for a long time, it could still be opened [again]. There are those who say that a disease which has persisted for a long time cannot be removed.

[That] is not this (i.e. our) doctrine. When someone who is an expert in utilizing the needles, removes such a disease, it is as if he pulled out a thorn, as if he cleansed what is soiled, as if he untied what is knotted, and as if he opened what is blocked. Although a disease has persisted for a long time, it can likewise be brought to an end. Those who state [that such illnesses] cannot be cured have not yet acquired the respective skills.

I.c. *Huáng dì nèi jīng, Sù wèn* 77
黃帝內經 · 素問
Shū wǔ guò lùn 疏五過論
On the Five Errors

聖人之治病也。必知天地陰陽。四時經紀。五藏六府。雌雄表裏。刺灸砭石、毒藥所主。從容人事。以明經道。貴賤貧富。各異品理。問年少長勇怯之理。審於分部。知病本始。八正九候。診必副矣。

必	bì	certainly; definitely; must
知	zhī	to know; to be aware of
天	tiān	heaven
地	dì	the earth
四	sì	four
時	shí	a season
經	jīng	a warp; to pass through; invariable rule; a standard
紀	jì	a skein; to regulate; a principle
經紀	jīng jì	ordering principle; invariable rule
六	liù	six
府	fŭ	a "palace" processing unit in the body, i.e. gall bladder, small intestine, triple burner, stomach, large intestine, urinary bladder
雌	cí	female
雄	xióng	male
表	biǎo	outside; exterior

裏	lǐ	inside; interior
刺	cì	to pierce
灸	jiǔ	to cauterize, mostly by burning moxa
砭	biān	a pointed stone
石	shí	a stone
毒	dú	poison; toxic
所	suǒ	(preceding a verb; usually replacing its object:) that which; whom; etc.
主	zhǔ	to master
從容	cóng róng	to approach naturally
事	shì	an affair
以	yǐ	so as to; in order to; thereby
明	míng	clear; to understand
經	jīng	classic (scripture; containing standards of knowledge)
道	dào	a way; a path
貴	guì	high-class; noble
賤	jiàn	low; common
貧	pín	poor
富	fù	wealthy
各	gè	each; every; all
異	yì	different
品	pǐn	class; rank
理	lǐ	to structure; to arrange; an order; structure
問	wèn	to inquire
年	nián	a year; age
少	shào	young
長	zhǎng	to grow; senior
勇	yǒng	brave; courage
怯	qiè	to be afraid; timidity
審	shěn	to conduct an examination; to investigate
於	yú	with reference to
分	fēn	a part
部	bù	a section

本	běn	a root
始	shǐ	the beginning
八	bā	eight
八正	bā zhèng	the eight cardinal [turning points]
九	jiǔ	nine
候	hòu	indicator
九候	jiǔ hòu	the nine indicators (where the movement in the vessels can be felt)
診	zhěn	to examine; diagnosis
副	fù	to assist
矣	yǐ	a final particle

Shèng rén zhī zhì bìng yě. bì zhī tiān dì yīn yáng. sì shí jīng jì. wǔ zàng liù fǔ. cí xióng biǎo lǐ. cì jiǔ biān shí、 dú yào suǒ zhǔ. cóng róng rén shì. yǐ míng jīng dào. guì jiàn pín fù. gè yì pǐn lǐ. wèn nián shào zhǎng yǒng qiè zhī lǐ. shěn yú fēn bù. zhī bìng běn shǐ. bā zhèng jiǔ hòu. zhěn bì fù yǐ.

When the sages treated a disease, they certainly knew the yin and yang [qi] of heaven and earth and the invariable rules followed by the four seasons; the five depots and six palaces,[1] female and male, exterior and interior, [as well as] piercing, cauterization, pointed stones, and toxic drugs with all [the diseases] they master. Their approach to the human affairs was natural, thereby understanding the Way laid down in the classics. The noble and the common, the poor and the wealthy, they all [represent] a structure of different ranks, [and the sages] inquired [from the patients] whether they [belonged to] the order of youth or adulthood, of courage or timidity. They investigated [all the] parts and sections [of the human body] and they knew the root and the beginning of the diseases [to be treated]. As for the eight cardinal [turning points][2] and the nine indicators,[3] in their examinations they were of definite help [too].

Notes

[1] The acknowledgment of the yinyang dualism as one of the pervasive structuring principles of all existence required the identification of two types of organs. The designations chosen were metaphors borrowed from the realm of social institutions, i. e. *fu* 府 in the sense of a storage unit where items are kept only temporarily before being emitted again, and *zang* 藏 in the sense of an innermost storage unit where items are kept for a long time, if not forever. The former, including small

and large intestines, urinary bladder, gallbladder, stomach, and heart enclosure, were identified as yang, signifying notions such as "outer" and "passage", the latter, including lung, heart, spleen, liver, and kidneys, were identified as yin, signifying notions such as "interior" and "tranquillity". However, a second metaphorical usage of *fu* 府 identified small and large intestines, urinary bladder, gallbladder, stomach, and heart enclosure as "palaces" housing the *zhu* 主, "rulers", lung, heart, spleen, liver, and kidneys, respectively. Thus, in ancient Chinese medical literature, the term *fu* 府 is encountered in two different social metaphorical contents. In my translations of the terms *zang* 藏 and *fu* 府, I render the former as "depot", thereby referring to the storage unit metaphor, and the latter as "palace", thereby referring to the ruler-palace metaphor. A clear identification of each usage of the term *fu* 府 as either "palace" or "short-term storage unit" appears impracticable.

[2] A reference to the qi at "the eight seasonal turning points", i.e. the two solstices, the two equinoxes, and the four first days of the four seasons. These are critical terms in the course of each year.

[3] For the "nine indicators", see below text 6.b, "On the Three Sections and Nine Indicators".

1.d *Yī xué jí chéng* 醫學集成
(Gǔ jīn tú shū jí chéng yī bù quán lù 古今圖書集成醫部全錄 503; Yī bù zǒng lùn 醫部總論 3)

Yī xué xū huì qún shū zhī cháng
醫學須會羣書之長
Medical Learning Must Combine the Best from All Writings

醫之爲道。非精不能明其理。非博不能至其約。是故前人立教。必使之先讀儒書。明易理。素。難。本草。脈經。而不少略者。何也。蓋非四書無以通義理之精微。非易無以知陰陽之消長。非素問無以識病。非本草無以識藥。非脈經無以從診候而知寒熱虛實之證。故前此數者。缺一不可且人之生命至重。病之變化無窮。年有老幼。禀有厚薄。治分五方。令別四時。表裏陰陽寒熱須辯。臟腑經絡氣血宜分。六氣之交傷。七情之妄發。運氣變遷不常。製方緩急尤異。更復合其色脉。問其起居。證有相似。治實不同。聖賢示人。略舉其端而已。後學必須會羣書之長。參所見而施治之。然後爲可。

醫	yī	medicine
道	dào	a doctrine
非	fēi	(is) not
非…不…	fēi…bù…	if .. is not, then …does not
精	jīng	subtleties
能	néng	to be able; can
理	lǐ	principle; structure
博	bó	extensive; broad
至	zhì	to reach; to arrive at
約	yuē	concise
故	gù	cause; reason
前	qián	former; earlier
立	lì	to establish
教	jiào	teachings
使	shǐ	to send; to let
先	xiān	before; at first
讀	dú	to study; to read
儒	rú	Confucian
書	shū	books; writings
易	yì	to change; here: short title for *Yi jing* 易經, "Book of Changes"
素	sù	pure; basic; here: short title for *Huang Di nei jing, Su wen* 黃帝內經素問, "Huang Di's Inner Classic, Basic Questions", a medical classic first compiled probably during the Han dynasty but lost in the original version and recompiled between the Han and Tang dynasties.
難	nàn	difficulty; here: short title for *Nan jing* 難經, "Classic of Difficult Issues", a medical classic compiled about the 1st or 2nd c. CE
本草	běn cǎo	"Materia medica"; here: short title of *Shen nong ben cao jing* 神農本草經; "Shennong's Classic on Materia Medica", a pharmaceutical classic compiled about the 1st c. CE

脈經	mài jīng	*Mài jīng* 脈經 ; "Classic on [Movements in] the Vessels." Classic on vessel diagnosis by Wang Shuhe 王叔和 of the 3rd c. CE
少略	shǎo lüè	to diminish; to leave out
何	hé	what?
也	yě	is
蓋	gài	initial particle: namely; for; now; the fact is …
無	wú	to be without; to have not
無以	wú yǐ	there is nothing to rely on to ...; there is no way to ...
通	tōng	to penetrate; to understand
義	yì	moral standards; moral behavior; principle; meaning; interpretation
義理	yì lǐ	moral standards; moral order; principles
微	wēi	subtle; minute
消	xiāo	to wane
識	shí	to know
從	cóng	to originate from; to start from
寒	hán	cold
熱	rè	hot; heat
虛	xū	depletion; depleted
實	shí	repletion
證	zhèng	evidence; symptoms
數	shù	to enumerate
缺	quē	deficiency; to be lacking
一	yī	one
且	qiě	moreover
命	mìng	life; fate
至	zhì	extremely; very
重	zhòng	important
變	biàn	to change; to transform
化	huà	to transform
窮	qióng	exhausted
無窮	wú qióng	inexhaustible

老	lǎo	old; aged
幼	yòu	young; immature
禀	bǐng	to receive from above; natural endowment
厚	hòu	thick; substantial; generous
薄	bó	thin; poor; shabby
分	fēn	to divide; to distinguish
方	fāng	direction; region
五方	wǔ fāng	the five cardinal points, including North, South, West, East, and Center
令	lìng	[monthly] commands [i.e. ancient rules guiding appropriate behavior in conformity with the seasons]; to cause; to let;
別	bié	to divide; to distinguish
須	xū	necessary; must
辯	biàn	to discuss; to distinguish
經	jīng	a conduit
絡	luò	a network (vessel)
氣	qì	qi; vapor; breath; finest matter (forming the entire world and circulating in the body)
血	xuě	blood
宜	yí	suitable; fitting
交	jiāo	to interact; to change; to deliver
傷	shāng	harm; to harm
七	qī	seven
情	qíng	emotion; affect
妄	wàng	wildly; incoherently; disorderly
發	fā	to rise; to erupt; to develop
運	yùn	to revolve; time period
遷	qiān	to shift
常	cháng	normal; regular
製	zhì	to make; to construct
方	fāng	prescription; recipe
緩	huǎn	slow
急	jí	urgent; fast

尤	yóu	more; particularly; especially
更	gèng	more; furthermore
復	fù	to return; again
合	hé	to join; to pair
色	sè	color; complexion
脉	mài	a vessel; a blood vessel; a movement in the vessels
起	qǐ	to rise
居	jū	to dwell; to rest
相	xiāng	reciprocal; each other
似	sì	like; resembling
實	shí	really
同	tóng	identical; alike
賢	xián	virtuous; exemplary (man)
示	shì	to proclaim; to instruct
略	lüè	summary; outline
舉	jǔ	to raise; to recommend
端	duān	a point of departure; a principle
已	yǐ	finished
而已	ér yǐ	and nothing else
後	hòu	afterwards; later
學	xué	to study
會	huì	to combine; to bring together
羣	qún	all
長	cháng	profitable; excelling
參	cān	to consider; to compare
見	jiàn	to see
施	shī	to act; to do; used to strengthen the verb which it precedes
然	rán	to be like this
然後	ránhòu	thereafter; this way

Yī zhī wéi dào. fēi jīng bù néng míng qí lǐ. fēi bó bù néng zhì qí yuē. shī gù qián rén lì jiào. bì shǐ zhī xiān dú rú shū. míng yì lǐ. sù. nàn. běn cǎo. mài jīng. ér bù shǎo lüè zhě. hé yě. gài fēi sì shū wú yǐ tōng yì lǐ zhī jīng wēi. fēi yì wú yǐ zhī yīn yáng zhī xiāo zhǎng. fēi sù- nàn wú yǐ shí bìng. fēi běn cǎo wú yǐ shí yào. fēi mài jīng wú yǐ cóng zhěn hòu ér zhī hán rè xū shí zhī zhèng. gù qián cǐ shù zhě. quē yī bù kě. qiě rén zhī shēng mìng zhì zhòng. bìng zhī biàn huà wú qióng. nián yǒu lǎo yòu. bǐng yǒu hòu bó. zhì fēn wǔ fāng. lìng bié sì shí. biǎo lǐ yīn yáng hán rè xū biàn. zàng fǔ jīng luò qì xuě yí fēn. liù qì zhī jiāo shāng. qī qíng zhī wàng fā. yùn qì biàn qiān bù cháng. zhì fāng huǎn jí yóu yì. gèng fù hé qí sè mài. wèn qí qǐ jū. zhèng yǒu xiāng sì. zhì shí bù tóng. shèng xián shì rén. lüè jǔ qí duān ér yǐ. hòu xué bì xū huì qún shū zhī cháng. cān suǒ jiàn ér shī zhì zhī. rán hòu wéi kě.

Medicine is a doctrine whose [general] principles can only be understood if [one concentrates on its most] subtle aspects, and whose essential points can only be grasped after extensive [studies]. When, therefore, the people of former times established their teachings, inevitably they let their [students] first of all read the Confucian writings, have them understand the principles of [the Book of] Changes, [and also let them study] the *Su* [*wen*], the *Nan* [*jing*], the *Ben cao*, and the *Mai jing*. Not [a single text] was to be left out. Why is this so? Now, if it were not for the Four Books, there would be no way to penetrate the subtleties in the moral standards [of medical treatment]; if it were not for the Book of Changes, there would be no way to know about the waning and waxing of yin and yang; if it were not for the *Su wen*, there would be no way to know the illnesses; if it were not for the *Ben cao*, there would be no way to know the drugs; and if it were not for the *Mai jing*, there would be no way to know the symptoms of cold and heat, and of depletion and repletion following an examination of the indicators [revealing the movements in the vessels]. Hence, one must not leave out even one of the [writings] enumerated above. Moreover, human life is extremely valuable. The illnesses may appear in countless variations. [A person] may be old or young in age, and his natural endowment may be strong or weak. In treating [patients], one distinguishes the five cardinal points [where they come from]; in the [monthly] commands, one distinguishes the four seasons, and one must distinguish whether [a disease is located in the] interior or exterior, in the yin or yang [regions of the organism], and whether it is [an affliction caused by] cold or heat. [Similarly,] one should distinguish [in which of the] depots and palaces, main conduits and network [vessels a disease may have settled], and whether it is [an affliction of] the qi or the blood. The causation of harm through any of the six qi[1], the disorderly rise of any of the seven emotions, and abnormalities [caused by] the [annual] changing and shifting of the [five] Periods and [six] Qi,[2] as well as the designing of prescriptions with slow or fast [effects] – [all of these should be] differentiated with particular [care]. In addition, [one must] pair a [patient's facial] coloring with [the movement in his] vessels; [one must] ask when he gets up and when he goes to rest. The symptoms [displayed by different diseases] may be identical, but the treatment must, in fact, be different. When the sages and the exemplary [men of the past] instructed the people, they offered them only general principles. Ever since, those who study [medicine] have to take the best from all the many books [available], combine it with what they see with their own eyes, and apply it in medical practice. This way [their learning and their therapies] will be all right.

Notes

[1] The "six qi" are defined as wind, fire, summerheat, cold, dryness, and dampness

[2] A reference to a theory developed during the Han era pointing out that each year differs from others in its climatic conditions. The theory of the "five periods and six qi" offers explanations for these differences and permits to predict the climatic pecularities of any future year. At the same time, it predicts possible health risks and suggests appropriate ways of behavior to prevent disease. The theory is based on a specific version of the five agents doctrine and the notion of a cyclical recurrence of certain years within a 60-years cycle.

1.e *Gŭ jīn yī tŏng dà quán* 3
古今醫統大全
Shèn jí shèn yī 慎疾慎醫
Take Care in Regard of Disease! Take Care in Regard of Physicians!

聖人治未病。不治已病。非謂已病而不治。亦非謂已病而不能治也。蓋謂治未病。在謹厥始。防厥微。以治之。則成功多而受害少也。惟治於始微之際。則不至於已著而後治之。亦自無已病而後治也。今人治已病。不治未病。蓋謂病形未著。不加愼防。直待病勢已著。而後求醫以治之。則其微之不謹。以至於著。斯可見矣。聖人起居動履。罔不攝養有方。間有幾微隱晦之疾。必加意以防之。用藥以治之。聖人之治未病不治已病有如此。論語曰。子之所愼。齊。戰。疾。釋云。齊所以交神明。誠至而神格。疾爲身之生死所關。戰爲國家存亡所係。然此三愼誠爲最大。而疾與乎其中。得非以身爲至重耶。康子饋藥。則曰。未達。不敢嘗。可見聖人愼疾愼醫之心至且盡矣。世之人非惟不知治未病。及至已病。尙不知謹。始初微略。恣意無忌。釀成大患。方急而求醫。曾不加擇。惟以其風聞。或憑

其吹薦委之。狂愚卒以自壞。皆其平日慢不究心於醫。至於倉卒。不暇擇請。殊不知醫藥人人所必用。雖聖人有所不免。顧在平昔講求。稔知其爲明醫。偶有微疾。則速求之。以藥治如反掌。

愼	shèn	to act with care
謂	wèi	to say; that is to say
在	zài	at; in; with reference to
謹	jĭn	attentive; carefully
厥	jué	a personal pronoun; he, his, theirs
防	fáng	to protect from
微	wēi	weak; minor
成	chéng	merit; good results
成功	chéng gōng	to achieve success
多	duō	many
受	shòu	to receive; to absorb
害	hài	to injure; injury
惟	wéi	only; here; initial particle
於	yú	at
際	jì	a time; while
著	zhù	to manifest
自	zì	from; from itself; naturally
自 ..而後	zì .. ér hòu	from (a certain point of time) on
形	xíng	physical appearance
加	jiā	to add; to apply
直	zhí	only; merely
待	dài	to wait for
勢	shì	strength
求	qiú	to seek after
斯	sī	this
動	dòng	to move; to take action
履	lǚ	to walk; to proceed

動履	dòng lǚ	daily activities
罔	wǎng	to have not; there is no ...
罔不	wǎng bù	there is nothing which not ..; in all cases; always
攝	shè	to assist; to preserve
養	yǎng	to support; to nourish
方	fāng	method
間	jiàn	among; in; occasionally
幾	jǐ	subtle; hidden; some
隱	yǐn	hidden
晦	huì	obscure
意	yì	a thought
如	rú	just as; like
論語	lún yǔ	*Lun yu*, the *Confucian Analects*
曰	yuē	to say; it is said
子	zǐ	the Master
齊	qí	to fast (used for 齋 *zhāi*)
戰	zhàn	war
釋	shì	to explain
云	yún	to say
交	jiāo	to exchange; to communicate; to join
神	shén	spirit
明	míng	brilliance; brilliant
誠	chéng	sincerity
格	gé	to come or go to; to reach
身	shēn	the body
關	guān	a pass; to close; to be closely linked
國家	guó jiā	country; the state
存	cún	to be in existence; to exist
亡	wáng	to perish
係	xì	to belong to; to depend on
然	rán	however
三	sān	three
最	zuì	very; most; extreme
大	dà	great; extensive

與	yǔ	to take part in; together with; to give
乎	hū	in; at (used for 於 *yú* and 于 *yú*)
與乎其中	yǔ hū qí zhōng	[this] is part of them; [this] one of them
中	zhōng	middle
得	dé	ought; should
得非	dé fēi	is is not that …?
耶	yé	a final interrogative particle
康子	kāng zǐ	Kang zi, a statesman, contemporary of Confucius
饋	kuì	to offer food to a superior
達	dá	to apprehend; to penetrate
敢	gǎn	to dare
嘗	cháng	to taste; to try
心	xīn	the heart; the mind
盡	jìn	entirely; all; wholly
世	shì	an age
及	jí	to reach; and
尙	shàng	still
初	chū	the beginning
恣	zī	to throw off restraint
恣意	zī yì	at random; careless
忌	jì	to avoid
無忌	wú jì	reckless
釀	niáng	to cause
釀成	niáng chéng	to bring about
患	huàn	to suffer; suffering
方	fāng	just in this moment; just then
曾	cēng	already; past
擇	zé	to select
風	fēng	fame; reputation
聞	wén	reputation
或	huò	or else; perhaps
憑	píng	to rely on
吹	chuī	to praise; to brag
薦	jiàn	to recommend; to introduce

委	wěi	to commission; to engage someone; to give up
狂	kuáng	mad; reckless
愚	yú	stupid
卒	zú	finally; eventually; as a result
自	zì	self
壞	huài	ruined
皆	jiē	all
平	píng	peaceful; even
日	rì	a day
慢	màn	neglectful
究	jiū	to examine into
究心	jiū xīn	to conduct thorough inquiries
倉	cāng	hasty
卒	cù	suddenly; urgent
暇	xiá	leisure
請	qǐng	to ask
殊	shū	really
免	miǎn	to avoid
顧	gù	used here for 故 *gù*; therefore
平昔	píng xī	in former times; beforehand
講	jiǎng	to investigate
稔	rěn	to be familiar with
偶	ǒu	unexpectedly
速	sù	hurried
反	fǎn	to turn over
掌	zhǎng	the palm of the hand
反掌	fǎn zhǎng	to turn the hand; very easily done

Shèng rén zhì wèi bìng. bù zhì yǐ bìng. fēi wèi yǐ bìng ér bù zhì. yì fēi wèi yǐ bìng ér bù néng zhì yě. gài wèi zhì wèi bìng. zài jǐn jué shǐ. fáng jué wēi. yǐ zhì zhī. zé chéng gōng duō ér shòu hài shǎo yě. wéi zhì yú shǐ wēi zhī jì. zé bù zhì yú yǐ zhù ér hòu zhì zhī. yì zì wú yǐ bìng ér hòu zhì yě. jīn rén zhì yǐ bìng. bù zhì wèi bìng. gài wèi bìng xíng wèi zhù. bù jiā shèn fáng. zhí dài bìng shì yǐ zhù. ér hòu qiú yī yǐ zhì zhī. zé qí wēi zhī bù jǐn. yǐ zhì yú zhù. sī kě jiàn yǐ. shèng rén qǐ jū dòng lǚ. wǎng bù shè yǎng yǒu fāng. jiàn yǒu jī wēi yǐn huì zhī jí. bì jiā yì yǐ fáng zhī. yòng yào yǐ zhì zhī. shèng rén zhī zhì wèi bìng bù zhì yǐ bìng yǒu rú cǐ. lún-yǔ yuē. zǐ zhī suǒ shèn. qí. zhàn. jí. shì yún. qí suǒ yǐ jiāo shén míng. chéng zhì ér shén gé. jí wéi shēn zhī shēng sǐ suǒ guān. zhàn wéi guó jiā cún wáng suǒ xì. rán cǐ sān shèn chéng wéi zuì dà. ér jí yǔ hū qí zhōng. dé fēi yǐ shēn wéi zhì zhòng yé. kāng zǐ kuì yào. zé yuē. wèi dá. bù gǎn cháng. kě jiàn shèng rén shèn jí shèn yī zhī xīn zhì qiě jìn yǐ. shì zhī rén fēi wéi bù zhī zhì wèi bìng. jí zhì yǐ bìng. shàng bù zhī jǐn. shǐ chū wēi lüè. zī yì wú jì. niáng chéng dà huàn. fāng jí ér qiú yī. cēng bù jiā zé. wéi yǐ qí fēng wén. huò píng qí chuī jiàn wěi zhī . kuáng yú zú yǐ zì huài. jiē qí píng rì màn bù jiū xīn yú yī. zhì yú cāng cù. bù xiá zé qǐng. shū bù zhī yī yào rén rén suǒ bì yòng. suī shèng rén yǒu suǒ bù miǎn. gù zài píng xī jiǎng qiú. rěn zhī qí wéi míng yī. ǒu yǒu wēi jí. zé sù qiú zhī. yǐ yàozhì rú fǎn zhǎng.

[When it is said] "the Sages treated those not yet ill; they did not treat those who were already ill," this does not mean that if anybody was ill they would not treat him, and it does not mean that if anybody was ill they were not able to treat him. In fact, this is to say that to treat those who are not yet ill consists in treating by paying great attention to a [disease's] very beginning and in applying protective measures when it is still very weak! Consequently, they achieved many successes, and seldom suffered from any harm. Only if one treats [a disease] at the moment of its onset, and when it is still very weak, then it will never happen that one has to treat it after it has already become manifest. In other words, one conducts the treatment from [a point in time] on when the disease is not yet manifest. [In obvious contrast to this], the people of today treat those who are ill; they do not treat those who are not yet ill. That is to say, as long as a disease has not yet become physically manifest, they do not pay attention to protective measures. They simply wait until a disease has become manifest with full vigor, and only then do they seek a physician to treat it. Hence, it is obvious that they pay no attention [to a disease] as long as it is still weak, and therefore it becomes manifest. In getting up and in going to rest, as well as in all their daily activities, the Sages always followed [specific] methods to support and nourish [their health]. When they encountered some very minor and hardly perceivable disease, they took great care to prevent [its further spreading], and they employed drugs to treat it. This is how the Sages treated those who were not yet ill, but did not treat those who were already ill. In the *Lun yu* it is stated: "The Master is careful with respect to fasting, wars, and disease." And the commentary states: "Through fasting one may join the spirit-brilliance. [A state of] sincerity comes upon one and the spirits contact [him]. Disease is the [point] where a body's life and death border at each other. War is that on which depends a country's existence or doom." Now, among these three [issues to be] careful about, [the state] of sincerity [reached through fasting] is [listed as] the most important, but does not [the fact that] disease is listed as one of them [indicate that] the body is of extreme importance [too]? When Kang zi offered drugs [to Confucius, the latter] replied: "I am not yet familiar [with such things]; I do not dare to ingest them." From this it is obvious that the careful attitude exhibited by the Sages with regard both to disease and healers was extreme and all-encompassing. The people of [our] generation do not only fail to know how to treat [themselves] before they are ill; even when a disease has emerged already, they still do not know how to be careful. As long as [a disease] is at its beginning, and as long as it is still quite weak, [the people] continue their unrestrained way of life and follow no limitations whatsoever. It is when the moment has come that [their diseases] have developed into severe suffering, that they are in great haste to seek a physician. Since they have not selected one before, they are forced now to engage someone only because they have heard of him, or because they rely on his self-advertisement. It is because of their own negligence and foolishness that they eventually destroy themselves. All of this [happens because] they are neglectful in healthy days and do not pay attention to [the selection of a skilled] physician until a situation emerges where they have to pick [a physician] in great haste and without leisure. They all do – obviously – not know that everybody is bound to make use of a physician and drugs [at some time or other]. Even the Sages could not avoid [physicians and drugs] entirely. Hence, one should start one's search and become acquainted with brilliant physicians beforehand. If a minor disease happens to occur, then one should call for that [physician whom one had selected before]. He will apply his drugs, and within a short time will have conducted a successful treatment.

1.f *Yù jiàn zá shū* 玉澗雜書

(Gǔ jīn tú shū jí chéng yī bù quán lù, 古今圖書集成醫部全錄 501; Yī bù zǒng lùn 醫部總論1)

Yī bù néng qǐ sǐ rén 醫不能起死人

Physicians are Unable to Raise Dead People [to Life Again]

華佗固神醫也。然范曄。陳壽。記其治疾。皆言若發結於內。針藥所不能及者。乃先令以酒服麻沸散。既醉無所覺。因刳破腹背。抽割積聚。若在腸胃。則斷裂湔洗。除去疾穢。既而縫合。傅以神膏。四五日創愈。一月之間皆平復。此决無之理。人之所以爲人者以形。而形之所以生者以氣也。佗之藥能使人醉無所覺。可以受其刳割。與能完養。使毀者復合。則吾所不能知。然腹背腸胃既已破裂斷壞。則氣何由舍。安有如是而復生者乎。審佗能此。則凡受支解之刑者。皆可使生。王者之刑。亦無所復施矣。太史公扁鵲傳。記虢庶子之論。以爲治病不以湯液醴酒。鑱石撟引。而割皮解肌。抉脈結筋。湔洗腸胃。漱滌五臟者。言古俞跗有是術耳。非謂扁鵲能之也。而世遂以附會於佗。凡人壽夭死生。豈一醫工所

能增損。不幸疾未必死。而爲庸醫所殺者。或有之矣。未有不可爲之疾而醫可活也。方書之設。本以備可治之疾。使無至於傷人而已。扁鵲亦自言。越人非能生死人也。彼當生者。越人能起之耳。故人與其因循疾病而受欺於庸醫好奇無驗之害。不若稍知治身攝生於安樂無事之時。以自養其天年也。

起	qǐ	to raise
華佗	huà tuó	Hua Tuo, physician and medical author (110-207)
固	gù	definitely
范曄	fàn yè	Fan Ye, compiler of the *History of the Eastern Han Dynasty* (died 445)
陳壽	chén shòu	Chen Shou, editor of the *History of the Three Kingdoms* (233-297)
若	ruò	if; when
結	jié	to clot; clotting
乃	nǎi	then
先	xiān	first; foremost
酒	jiǔ	wine
服	fú	to ingest (pharmaceutical substances); to take (medicine)
痲	má	numb; numbness
沸	fèi	to bubble up; to boil
散	sǎn	powder
既	jì	after
既而	jì ér	afterwards
醉	zuì	intoxicated; drunk
覺	jué	to perceive; to feel
因	yīn	hence; consequently

刳	kū	to cut open
破	pò	to break
腹	fù	the abdomen
背	bèi	the back
抽	chōu	to pull open; to draw out
割	gé	to cut
積	jī	to gather; to store up
聚	jù	to gather
腸	cháng	the intestines
胃	wèi	the stomach
斷	duàn	to break off; to cut off
裂	liè	to rip open; to open
湔	jiān	to wash
洗	xǐ	to wash; to cleanse
除	chú	to exclude; to remove
去	qù	to remove
穢	huì	foul; spoiled
縫	féng	to seam; to sew
傅	fū	to apply (an ointment)
膏	gāo	ointment
創	chuāng	wound
愈	yù	to heal
月	yuè	month
平	píng	normal
决	jué	decidedly; before a negative adds strong emphasis
所以	suǒ yǐ	that which (someone) takes; that which (someone) relies on
者	zhě	that which
使	shǐ	to cause
與	yǔ	and
完	wán	to finish; to complete
毀	huǐ	to destroy
吾	wū	I; me
由	yóu	origin

舍	shě	to release; to bestow
安	ān	an interrogative; how?
審	shěn	to examine; truly; really
凡	fán	all
支(肢)	zhī	a branch
支解	zhī jiě	dismemberment
刑	xíng	punishment
王	wáng	king; royal
太史公	tài shǐ gōng	lit.: Great Historiographer. Title of Sima Qian 司馬遷 (145 - ca. 80 BCE), the compiler of the *Shi ji* 史記
傳	zhuàn	a biography
虢	Guó	name of an ancient feudal state
庶子	shù zǐ	tutor to the heir apparent
論	lùn	to discuss; discourse
扁鵲	biǎn què	Bian Que, a legendary physician of the sixth or fifth c. BCE
以爲	yǐ wéi	to hold; to believe
湯	tāng	hot liquid; decoction
液	yè	juices; extract
醴	lǐ	sweet wine
鑱	chán	chisel
撟	jiǎo	to stretch
引	yǐn	to pull
撟引	jiǎo yǐn	massage
皮	pí	the skin
肌	jī	the flesh under the skin
抉	jué	to take out; to tear out
衇 (脉, 脈)	mài	the blood vessels; the vessels
筋	jīn	the sinews
漱	shù	to rinse out
滌	dí	to wash
古	gǔ	ancient
俞跗	yú fū	Yu Fu, a legendary physician

耳	ěr	a final particle
遂	suí	to follow; consequently
附	fù	to attribute; to add to
會	huì	to meet; to associate with
壽	shòu	longevity
夭	yāo	to die young
工	gōng	a practitioner
增	zēng	to add to; to increase
損	sǔn	to injure; to damage
幸	xìng	lucky; fortunate
庸	yōng	ordinary; common
殺	shā	to kill
爲	wéi	to manage; to cure
活	huó	alive; to keep alive
設	shè	to establish; to arrange
本	běn	basically; fundamental
備	bèi	to provide; to prepare
越人	yuè rén	Yueren, personal name of Bian Que
生	shēng	to give life to
彼	bǐ	those
當	dāng	ought; should
生	shēng	to live
因	yīn	to follow
循	xún	to follow; because
欺	qī	to cheat
好	hào	to love
奇	qí	strange; rare
驗	yàn	to examine; to experience; success
與(A)- yú .. bù ruò		(A) is not as good as (B); in comparsion to (A)
不若(B)		it is better that (B)
稍	shāo	a little
安	ān	peace; tranquil
樂	lè	joy; to rejoice
無事	wú shì	nothing to worry about; no problems
時	shí	time

Huà tuó gù shén yī yě. rán Fàn yè. Chén shòu. jì qí zhì jí. jiē yán ruò fā jié yú nèi. zhēn yào suǒ bù néng jí zhě. nǎi xiān lìng yǐ jiǔ fú má fèi sǎn. jì zuì wú suǒ jué. yīn kū pò fù bèi. chōu gé jī jù. ruò zài cháng wèi. zé duàn liè jiān xǐ. chú qù jí huì. jì ér féng hé. fū yǐ shén gāo. sì wǔ rì chuāng yù. yí yuè zhī jiān jiē píng fù. cǐ jué wú zhī lǐ. rén zhī suǒ yǐ wéi rén zhě yǐ xíng. ér xíng zhī suǒ yǐ shēng zhě yǐ qì yě. tuó zhī yào néng shǐ rén zuì wú suǒ jué. kě yǐ shòu qí kū gé. yǔ néng wán yǎng. shǐ huǐ zhě fù hé. zé wū suǒ bù néng zhī. rán fù bèi cháng wèi jì yǐ pò liè duàn huài. zé qì hé yóu shě. ān yǒu rú shī ér fù shēng zhě hū. shěn tuó néng cǐ. zé fán shòu zhī jiě zhī xíng zhě. jiē kě shǐ shēng. wáng zhě zhī xíng. yì wú suǒ fù shī yǐ. tài shǐ gōng biǎn què zhuàn. jì guó shù zǐ zhī lùn. yǐ wéi zhì bìng bù yǐ tāng yè lǐ jiǔ. chán shí jiǎo yǐn. ér gé pí jiě jī. jué mài jié jīn. jiān xǐ cháng wèi. shù dí wǔ zàng zhě. yán gǔ yú fū yǒu shī shù ěr. fēi wèi biǎn què néng zhī yě. ér shì suí yǐ fù huì yú tuó. fán rén shòu yāo sǐ shēng. qǐ yī yī gōng suǒ néng zēng sǔn. bù xìng jí wèi bì sǐ. ér wéi yōng yī suǒ shā zhě. huò yǒu zhī yǐ. wèi yǒu bù kě wéi zhī jí ér yī kě huó yě. fāng shū zhī shè. běn yǐ bèi kě zhì zhī jí. ér yī kě huó yě. fāng shū zhī shè. běn yǐ bèi kě zhì zhī jí. shǐ wú zhì yú shāng rén ér yǐ. biǎn què yì zì yán. yuè rén fēi néng shēng sǐ rén yě. bǐ dāng shēng zhě. yuè rén néng qǐ zhī ěr. gù rén yǔ qí yīn xún jí bìng ér shòu qī yú yōng yī hào qí wú yàn zhī hài. bù ruò shāo zhī zhì shēn shè shēng yú ān lè wú shì zhī shí. yǐ zì yǎng qí tiān nián yě.

Hua Tuo was certainly a spirit[-like] physician! However, when it is stated, in both Fan Ye's and Chen Shou's reports on how [Hua Tuo] treated illnesses, that whenever some clotting had formed in a [patient's] interior – where needles or drugs could not reach – [Hua Tuo] would first let [the patient] consume a *ma fei* powder with wine, and after [that person] had become intoxicated and would not feel anything, then [Hua Tuo] would cut open [the patient's] abdomen or back to cut away any accumulations [that had formed internally]; if these were in the intestines or in the stomach, he would dissect them, wash and rinse them, and discard what was sick or spoiled, and afterwards sew them together again, smear some spirit-ointment on them so that the wound would heal within four to five days, and the patients had fully recovered within one month - these are principles which definitely do not exist! Humans are humans because of their physical appearance; and this physical appearance has life because of qi. I do not know whether [Hua] Tuo's drugs were indeed able to render a person intoxicated so that he would not feel anything, and hence was able to endure to be cut open. [And I do not know whether Hua Tuo] was able to bring [such persons] back to a complete state of health and let that what he had destroyed grow together again. However, once the abdomen, the back, the intestines, or the stomach have been ripped open and cut apart – wherefrom shall any qi be released? How could such a state result in life again? If [Hua] Tuo was in fact able to do this, then all those who have been subjected to the punishment of dismemberment could be brought back to life again! And, likewise, there would be no [reason] for applying mutilating punishments[1] any longer. When Tai shi gong in his biography of Bian Que quotes the argumentation of the tutor to the heir-apparent of the state of Guo implying that in treating illnesses [one had] not [necessarily] to rely on hot liquids or juices, on medicinal wines, on pointed stones, or a massage, and that instead [in treating illnesses one could] cut open the skin and separate the flesh, take out the vessels and tie the sinews, and that [one could] wash the intestines and the stomach, and rinse out the five depots, he mentions only that Yu Fu was capable of this technique in ancient times. [The text] does not state that Bian Que was able to do this. But generations in the [times] to follow attributed [this capability to Hua] Tuo! How could it be that a single physician were able to add to or take away from man's long life or short existence, [and decide about a person's] life or death! There are unfortunate cases in which common physicians kill someone whose illness would not necessarily have resulted in death. Never has there been a case [though] in which a physician could keep [someone] alive [who suffered from] a disease that could not be overcome! The fundamental design of prescription books is such that they provide [knowledge how to deal] with illnesses that can be cured so that they do not reach [a point] where they harm the people. Also, Bian Que himself has stated that [he himself, i.e.] Yueren, was unable to raise dead persons back to life again. Yueren could raise only those who ought to stay alive [anyway]. Hence, if someone, in the course of a disease, receives the harm of being cheated by common physicians who love strange [remedies] but do not achieve any results, [these people] would fare better if they had [at least] a little knowledge [themselves] how to treat their body, and how to maintain their lives in times when they are [still] happy and have not encountered any problem yet. This way they could support themselves throughout the years [allotted to them by] heaven.

Note

1 In ancient China, a mutilating punishment required special consent by the ruler. Hence, the text speaks of "royal punishment".

Lesson Two

On the Structure and Functions of the Organism

When approximately during the third and second centuries BCE the first theories concerning structure and functions of the human organism were thought of in China, it was assumed that it is the basic function of the organism to receive nourishment from outside, mainly through food and beverages, to digest the essence qi needed for the continuation of life from such nourishment, and to discharge the remainder. The distribution of the essence qi within the body through a complex network of conduits, the absorption of these qi by a number of units responsible for the maintenance of all the body's external and internal functions, as well as the relationships and exchanges among these units themselves and among them and the outside world represent a sophisticated system of ideas, based on the doctrines of yinyang and the five agents. The medicine of systematic correspondence gained its understanding of the structure and functions of the human organism from images observed and from facts experienced in the natural and social environment. However, it would be quite inaccurate to assume that the interior of the human body remained entirely unknown to the authors of ancient and medieval Chinese medical literature. Ancient Chinese physicians were quite familiar with the basic elements of the actual morphological structure of the human body, and when an author spoke of heart, lung, spleen, and liver, he had anatomical entities in mind, even though the terms he used implied a lot more than just a designation of some tangible piece of tissue. Some of the entities described in ancient texts as constituting the human organism cannot be verified by anatomical evidence; and it may well be that they were but projections of an external reality. The fact that such concepts, as for instance the "triple burner" and the "gate of life", remained controversial topics of discussions continuing throughout the history of Chinese medicine (in contrast to such concepts as heart or uterus) demonstrates a persistent tendency to associate assumed functions with tangible substrata.

Key Terms Introduced in Lesson Two

頭	tóu	the head
足	zú	foot
目	mù	eye
竅	qiào	hole; opening; orifice
喜	xǐ	joy
怒	nù	anger; rage
肢	zhī	limb
手	shǒu	hand
指	zhǐ	finger; toe
莖	jìng	stalk; the penis
垂	chuí	the scrotum
足	zú	enough
肩	jiān	shoulder
膝	xī	knee
腋	yè	armpit
膕	guó	the hollow behind the knee
毫毛	háo máo	the fine hair on the body
牙	yá	tooth
齒	chǐ	tooth
骨	gǔ	bone
募	mù	membrane (used here for 膜 *mò*)
䐃	jùn	lump; accumulation of flesh
精	jīng	semen; essence
胞	bāo	the womb
胎	tāi	the fetus
胚	pī	embryo
腎	shèn	the kidneys
脾	pí	the spleen
肝	gān	the liver
肺	fèi	the lung
小腸	xiǎo cháng	the small intestine
大腸	dà cháng	the large intestine

膽	dǎn	the gallbladder
膀胱	páng guāng	the bladder
三焦	sān jiāo	the triple burner
八脈	bā mài	the eight single conduit vessels; short for 奇經八脈 *qī jīng bā mài*
孫	sūn	grandchild; tertiary
穴	xuè	hole (insertion point for needles in acupuncture)
耳	ěr	ear
口	kǒu	the mouth
鼻	bí	the nose
骸	hái	the human bones
髮	fà	the hair on the head
味	wèi	flavor
營	yíng	camp [qi]
衛	wèi	protective [qi]
精	jīng	essence
胸	xiōng	the breast; the chest
喉嚨	hóu lóng	the wind-pipe
呼	hū	to exhale
吸	xī	to inhale
命門	mìng mén	the gate of life
督脈	dū mài	the supervisor (conduit) vessel
椎	zhuī	vertebra; backbone section
腧穴	shū xuè	transport point (where a needle is inserted in acupuncture to affect the passage of qi)
幽門	yōu mén	the dark gate
臍	qí	the navel
産	chǎn	to give birth
泄	xiè	to discharge
飛門	fēi mén	the flying gate
唇	chún	the lips
戶門	hù mén	the door-gate
吸門	xī mén	the inhalation-gate
會厭	huì yàn	the epiglottis

賁門	bēn mén	the strong-gate
太倉	tài cāng	the big granary; the stomach
闌門	lán mén	the screen-gate
魄門	pò mén	the *po*-gate
肛門	gāng mén	the rectum-gate
溺	niào	urine
氣門	qì mén	the qi-gate
胎元	tāi yuán	the fetus
膈	gé	the diaphragm
乳	rǔ	the breasts
陷	xiàn	a fold
脘	wǎn	a duct in the body
喉嚨	hóu lóng	the throat
脊	jí	the spine; the back
脅	xié	the ribs
任脉	rèn mài	the controller [conduit] vessel
衝脉	chōng mài	the through-way [conduit] vessel
喉管	hóu guǎn	the wind-pipe
葉	yè	a lobe
眼	yǎn	eye
喘	chuǎn	to pant
嗽	sòu	to cough
皺	zhòu	wrinkled
膜	mó	membrane

2.a *Huáng dì nèi jīng, Líng shū* 71

黃帝內經·靈樞
Xié kè邪客
Evil Visitors

天圓地方。人頭圓足方以應之。天有日月。人有兩目。地有九州。人有九竅。天有風雨。人有喜怒。天有雷電。人有音聲。天有四時。人有四肢。天有五音。人有五臟。天有六律。人有六腑。天有冬夏。人有寒熱。天有十日。人有手十指。辰有十二。人有足十指。莖垂以應之。女子不足二節。以抱人形。天有陰陽。人有夫妻。歲有三百六十五日。人有三百六十節。地有高山。人有肩膝。地有深谷。人有腋膕。地有十二經水。人有十二經脈。地有泉脈。人有衛氣。地有草蓂。人有毫毛。天有晝夜。人有臥起。天有列星。人有牙齒。地有小山。人有小節。地有山石。人有高骨。地有林木。人有募筋。地有聚邑。人有䐃肉。歲有十二月。人有十二節。地有四時不生草。人有無子。此人與天地相應者也。

圓	yuán	round
方	fāng	square
頭	tóu	the head
足	zú	foot
應	yìng	to correspond

日	rì	the sun
月	yuè	the moon
兩	liǎng	two; a pair
目	mù	eye
州	zhōu	district
竅	qiào	hole; opening; orifice
風	fēng	wind
雨	yǔ	rain
喜	xǐ	joy
怒	nù	anger; rage
雷	léi	thunder
電	diàn	lightning
音	yīn	sound;tone
聲	shēng	voice; sound
肢	zhī	limb
律	lǜ	the yang sounds among the twelve pitch-pipes
冬	dōng	winter
夏	xià	summer
手	shǒu	hand
十	shí	ten
指	zhǐ	finger; toe
辰	chén	one of the twelve divisions of daytime
莖	jìng	stalk; the penis
垂	chuí	to hang down; the scrotum
女	nǚ	female; woman
子	zǐ	noun-ending
足	zú	enough
二	èr	two
節	jié	section
抱	bào	to hold in one's arms; to hatch, to encompass
夫	fū	husband
妻	qī	wife
歲	suì	year
百	bǎi	hundred
高	gāo	high

山	shān	mountain
肩	jiān	shoulder
膝	xī	knee
深	shēn	deep
谷	gǔ	valley
腋	yè	armpit
膕	guó	the hollow behind the knee
經	jīng	a big river; stream
水	shuǐ	water
泉	quán	spring
衛	wèi	protective; to guard
草	cǎo	grass; plant
蓂	míng	a creeping plant
毫	háo	fine; minute
毛	máo	body hair
晝	zhòu	daytime; daylight
夜	yè	night; darkness
臥	wò	to lie down
列	liè	to arrange in order
星	xīng	star
牙	yá	tooth
齒	chǐ	tooth
小	xiǎo	small
小節	xiǎo jié	small section; i.e. the end sections of fingers and toes
骨	gǔ	bone
林	lín	forest
木	mù	wood; tree
募	mù	membrane (used here for 膜 *mò*)
邑	yí	a city; town
䐃	jùn	lump; accumulation of flesh
肉	ròu	flesh
十二節	shí èr ji	the twelve limb-sections; i.e. hands, lower arms, upper arms, feet, lower legs, upper legs
子	zǐ	child

Tiān yuán dì fāng. rén tóu yuán zú fāng yǐ yìng zhī. tiān yǒu rì yuè. rén yǒu liǎng mù. dì yǒu jiǔ zhōu. rén yǒu jiǔ qiào. tiān yǒu fēng yǔ. rén yǒu xǐ nù. tiān yǒu léi diàn. rén yǒu yīn shēng. tiān yǒu sì shí. rén yǒu sì zhī. tiān yǒu wǔ yīn. rén yǒu wǔ zàng. tiān yǒu liù lǜ. rén yǒu liù fǔ. tiān yǒu dōng xià. rén yǒu hán rè. tiān yǒu shí rì. rén yǒu shǒu shí zhǐ. chén yǒu shí èr. rén yǒu zú shí zhǐ. jìng chuí yǐ yìng zhī. nǚ zǐ bù zú èr jié. yǐ bào rén xíng. tiān yǒu yīn yáng. rén yǒu fū qī. suì yǒu sān bǎi liù shí wǔ rì. rén yǒu sān bǎi liù shí jié. dì yǒu gāo shān. rén yǒu jiān xī. dì yǒu shēn gǔ. rén yǒu yè guó. dì yǒu shí èr jīng shuǐ. rén yǒu shí èr jīng mài. dì yǒu quán mài. rén yǒu wèi qì. dì yǒu cǎo míng. rén yǒu háo máo. tiān yǒu zhòu yè. rén yǒu wò qǐ. tiān yǒu liè xīng. rén yǒu yá chǐ. dì yǒu xiǎo shān. rén yǒu xiǎo jié. dì yǒu shān shí. rén yǒu gāo gǔ. dì yǒu lín mù. rén yǒu mù jīn. dì yǒu jù yí. rén yǒu jùn ròu. suì yǒu shí èr yuè. rén yǒu shí èr jié. dì yǒu sì shí bù shēng cǎo. rén yǒu wú zǐ. cǐ rén yǔ tiān dì xiāng yìng zhě yě.

Heaven is round; the earth is square. Man's head is round; his feet are square so as to correspond to the [shape of heaven and earth]. Heaven has sun and moon; man has a pair of eyes. The earth has the nine districts; man has the nine orifices. Heaven has wind and rain; man has joy and anger. Heaven has thunder and lightning; man has the sounds of [his] voice. Heaven has the four seasons; man has the four limbs. Heaven has the five tones; man has the five depots. Heaven has the six pitch-pipes; man has the six palaces. Heaven has winter and summer; man has cold and heat. Heaven has the [cycle of] ten days; man has, at his hands, ten fingers. There are twelve divisions of daytime; man has, at his feet, ten toes and he has a penis and a scrotum so as to correspond to this [number of twelve]. Females lack [the latter] two sections so that they can hatch a human appearance. Heaven has yin and yang; man has husband and wife. A year has 365 days; the human [skeleton] has 365 sections. The earth has high mountains; man has shoulders and knees. The earth has deep valleys; man has armpits and the hollows behind the knees. The earth has the water of the twelve streams; man has the twelve conduit-vessels. The earth has the vessels [supplying] the springs; man has guardian qi. The earth has the grasses and plants; man has his fine body hair. Heaven has day and night; man has [times] to rest and to rise. Heaven has an orderly arrangement of stars; man has his teeth. The earth has small mountains; the human [body] has its short sections. The earth has mountain rocks; man has high-rising bones. The earth has forests and woods; man has membranes and sinews. The earth has gatherings [of people] and towns; man has lumps of flesh. The year has the twelve months; man has the twelve sections [of his limbs]. The earth has [regions where] during all four seasons no grasses grow; among men are those who have no children. These are the mutual correspondences between man and heaven and earth.

2.b *Tú shū biān* 圖書編
Zàng fŭ shĭ shēng zŏng lùn
臓腑始生總論
General Survey of the Origins of the Depots and Palaces

夫人之有生也。禀天地之陰陽。假父母之精血。交感凝結。以爲胞胎也。乾道成男。坤道成女。始自襁褓。以至髫齔。迨其成童與夫壯年。豈易言哉。故一月之孕。有白露之稱。二月之胚。有桃花之譬。及其三月。先生右腎則爲男。先生左腎則爲女。其次腎生脾。脾生肝。肝生肺。肺生心。以生其勝己者。腎屬水。故五臓由是爲陰。其次心生小腸。小腸生大腸。大腸生膽。膽生胃。胃生膀胱。膀胱生三焦。以生其己勝者。小腸屬火。六腑由是爲陽。其次三焦生八脈。八脈生十二經。十二經生十二絡。十二絡生一百八十系絡。系絡生一百八十纏絡。纏絡生三萬四千孫絡。孫絡生三百六十五骨節。骨節生三百六十五大穴。大穴生八萬四千毛竅。則耳目口鼻。四肢百骸之身皆備矣。所謂四月形像具。五月筋骨成。六月毛髮生。正謂此也。至七月則游其魂而能動左手。八月游其魄而能動右手。九月三轉

身。十月滿足。母子分解。其有過月生者。必係富貴之子。不足月生者。必爲貧薄之人。

假	jiǎ	to receive
父	fù	father
母	mǔ	mother
精	jīng	semen; essence
交	jiāo	to meet each other; to exchange
感	gǎn	to affect; to touch
凝	níng	to congeal; to freeze; to coagulate
結	jié	to unite
胞	bāo	the womb
胎	tāi	the fetus
乾	qián	heaven; male
男	nán	male
坤	kūn	the earth; female
始	shǐ	to begin
襁	qiǎng	the cloth in which children are carried on the back
褓	bǎo	a swaddling cloth
以至	yǐ zhì	until; up to
髫	tiáo	the tufts of hair on the head of little children
齔	chēn	the period when the milk teeth are shed
迨	dài	until
成	chéng	to become
童	tóng	boy
壯	zhuàng	strong; robust
易	yì	easy
哉	zāi	an exclamation
孕	yùn	to be pregnant
白	bái	white
露	lù	dew
稱	chēng	name; designation
胚	pī	embryo

桃	táo	the peach
花	huā	flower
生	shēng	to grow
右	yòu	right
腎	shèn	the kidneys
左	zuǒ	left
次	cì	next
生	shēng	to generate
脾	pí	the spleen
肝	gān	the liver
肺	fèi	the lung
勝	shèng	to overcome
己	jǐ	self
屬	shǔ	to belong to
由	yóu	from
小腸	xiǎo cháng	the small intestine
大腸	dà cháng	the large intestine
膽	dǎn	the gallbladder
膀胱	páng guāng	the bladder
三焦	sān jiāo	the triple burner
八脈	bā mài	the eight single conduit vessels; short for 奇經八脈 *qi jīng bā mài*
系	xì	link; connection
纏	chán	to entwine
萬	wàn	ten thousand; myriad
千	qiān	thousand
孫	sūn	grandchild; tertiary
穴	xuè	hole (insertion point for needles in acupuncture)
耳	ěr	ear
口	kǒu	the mouth
鼻	bí	the nose
骸	hái	the human bones
矣	yǐ	particle indicating completion of a development
形像	xíng xiǎng	figure; form

具	jù	prepared
成	chéng	to create
髮	fà	the hair on the head
遊	yóu	to travel; to arrive
魂	hún	the *hun*-soul (believed to continue existing after a person's physical death)
魄	pò	the *po*-soul (believed to cease to exist after a person's physical death)
轉	zhuǎn	to revolve; to turn over
滿	mǎn	full; entire
分	fēn	to divide; to separate
解	jiě	to separate
過	guò	to exceed

Fū rén zhī yǒu shēng yě. bǐng tiān dì zhī yīn yáng. jiǎ fù mǔ zhī jīng xuě. jiāo gǎn níng jié. yǐ wéi bāo tāi yě. qián dào chéng nán. kūn dào chéng nǚ. shǐ zì qiǎng bǎo. yǐ zhì tiáochēn. dài qí chéng tóng yǔ fū zhuàng nián. qǐ yì yán zāi. gù yí yuè zhī yùn. yǒu bái lù zhī chēng. èr yuè zhī pī. yǒu táo huā zhī pì. jí qí sān yuè. xiān sheng yòu shèn zé wéi nán. xiān sheng zuǒ shèn zé wéi nǚ. qí cì shèn shēng pí. pí shēng gān. gān shēng fèi. fèi shēng xīn. yǐ shēng qí shèng jǐ zhě. shèn shǔ shuǐ. gù wǔ zàng yóu shī wéi yīn. qí cì xīn shēng xiǎo cháng. xiǎo cháng shēng dà cháng. dà cháng shēng dǎn. dǎn shēng wèi. wèi shēng páng guāng. páng guāng shēng sān jiāo. yǐ shēng qí jǐ shèng zhě. xiǎo cháng shǔ huǒ. liù fǔ yóu shī wéi yáng. qí cì sān jiāo shēng bā mài. bā mài shēng shí èr jīng. shí èr jīng shēng shí èr luò. shí èr luò shēng yī bǎi bā shí xì luò. xì luò shēng yī bǎi bā shí chán luò. chán luò shēng sān wàn sì qiān sūn luò. sūn luò shēng sān bǎi liù shí wǔ gǔ jié. gǔ jié shēng sān bǎi liù shí wǔ dà xuè. dà xuè shēng bā wàn sì qiān máo qiào. zé ěr mù kǒu bí. sì zhī bǎi hái zhī shēn jiē bèi yǐ. suǒ wèi sì yuè xíng xiǎng jù. wǔ yuè jīn gǔ chéng. liù yuè máo fà shēng. zhèng wèi cǐ yě. zhì qī yuè zé yóu qí hún ér néng dòng zuǒ shǒu. bā yuè yóu qí pò ér néng dòng yòu shǒu. jiǔ yuè sān zhuǎn shēn. shí yuè mǎn zú. mǔ zǐ fēn jiě. qí yǒu guò yuè shēng zhě. bì xì fù guì zhī zǐ. bù zú yuè shēng zhě. bì wéi pín bó zhī rén.

Man has life because he is endowed with the yin and yang [qi] of heaven and earth, and has received from his father and mother semen and blood. When [the latter two] contact each other, they unite and congeal to become a fetus in the womb. If it takes the way of heaven, a male is generated; if it takes the way of the earth, a female is generated. In the beginning, [the children are] carried on the back and need a swaddling cloth. [Life continues to the time when they wear] tufts of hair on their heads and when they shed their milk teeth, until they become boys and [adults] in their strongest age. How could anybody speak [of this process] lightheartedly! Thus, the [state of] pregnancy of the first month is called "white dew". The embryo of the second month is compared to peach blossoms. When, in the third month, the right kidney grows first, [the child] will be a male; if the left kidney grows first, it will be a girl. Next, the kidneys generate the spleen, the spleen generates the liver, the liver generates the lung, the lung generates the heart, because each [depot] generates [the depot] by which itself can be overcome.[1] The kidneys belong to [the agent] water. Hence the five depots are yin. Next, the heart generates the small intestine, the small intestine generates the large intestine, the large intestine generates the gallbladder, the gallbladder generates the stomach, the stomach generates the urinary bladder, and the urinary bladder generates the triple burner, because each [palace] generates [the palace] it can overcome. The small intestine belongs to [the agent] fire. Hence the six palaces are yang. Next, the triple burner generates the eight [single conduit] vessels, the eight [single conduit] vessels generate the twelve conduits, the twelve conduits generate the twelve network [vessels], the twelve network [vessels] generate the one hundred eighty linking network [vessels], the linking network [vessels] generate the one hundred eighty entwining network [vessels], the entwining network [vessels] generate the thirty-four thousand tertiary network [vessels], the tertiary network [vessels] generate the three hundred sixty-five bone-sections, the bone-sections generate the three hundred sixty-five large holes [on the conduits],[2] the large holes generate the eighty-four thousand pores with hair. Finally, the body with all its ears, eyes, mouth, four limbs, and hundreds of bones is completed. When it is said that during the fourth month the physical appearance is prepared, that during the fifth month sinews and bones are generated, and that during the sixth month the body hair and the hair on the head grow, this refers exactly to this [process outlined above]. During the seventh month, then, its *hun*-soul is set into motion so that [the fetus] is able to move its left hand. During the eighth month, its *po*-soul is set into motion and [the fetus] is able to move its right hand. During the ninth month, the body [of the fetus] turns over three times. After ten months are full, mother and child separate. Those children who exceed this [number of] months belong to the rich and have a noble status; those who are born short of [this number of] months belong to the poor and needy.

Notes

[1] According to the five-agents doctrine, the following correspondences exist among the body's functional units and the five agents: kidney/water; spleen/soil; liver/wood; lung/metal; heart/fire; small intestine/fire; large intestine/metal; gallbladder/wood; stomach/soil; urinary bladder/water; triple burner/fire. Water is blocked by soil (i.e. dikes); soil is weakened by wood (i.e. penetrated by the roots of trees); wood is cut by metal; metal is melted by fire; fire is extinguished by water.

[2] Originally, the term *xuè* 穴denoted the "caves" from where the winds were thought to emanate and affect humans. With the supplementation of wind etiology by an etiology based on the concept of vapor qi, the term *xuè* was redefined to denote those "holes" on the surface of the body where needles could be inserted to permit qi to enter or leave the body.

2.c *Huáng dì nèi jīng, Tài sù* 2
黃帝內經·太素
Tiáo shí 調食
To Balance Nourishment

黃帝曰。願聞穀氣有五味。其入五藏。分別奈何。伯高曰。胃者。五藏六府之海也。水穀皆入於胃。五藏六府皆稟於胃。胃受水穀。變化以滋五藏六府。五味各走其所喜。穀味酸。先走肝。穀味苦。先走心。穀味甘。先走脾。穀味辛。先走肺。穀味鹹。先走腎。穀氣津液已行。營衛大通。乃化糟粕。以次傳下。水穀化爲津液。清氣猶如霧露。名營衛。行脈內外。無所滯礙。故曰大通。其沉濁者。名爲糟粕。泌別汁入於膀胱。故曰以次傳下也。黃帝曰。營衛之行奈何。伯高曰。穀始入於胃。其精微者。先出於胃之兩焦。以既五臟。別出兩行於營衛之道。精微。津液也。津液資五藏已。衛氣出胃上口。營氣出於中焦之後。故曰兩行道也。其大氣之摶而不行者。積於胸中。命曰氣海。出於肺。循喉嚨。故呼則出。吸則入。摶。聚也。穀化爲氣。計有四道。精微營衛。以爲二道。化爲糟粕及濁氣幷尿。其與精下傳。復爲一道。摶而不行。積於胸中。名氣海。以爲呼吸。復爲一道。合爲四道也。

黃帝	huáng dì	Huang Di, The Yellow Thearch; legendary ruler whose dialogues with his advisers constitute major parts of the classical Chinese medical texts
願	yuàn	to desire; to wish
聞	wén	to hear
穀	gǔ	grain
味	wèi	flavor
入	rù	to enter; into
奈何	nài hé	how can one? How is it?
伯高	bó gāo	Bo Gao, one of the legendary advisers of Huang Di
者	zhě	a particle indicating that the preceding word is to be read as a noun
海	hǎi	sea; ocean
於	yú	in; into
稟	bǐng	to receive supplies
於	yú	indicating passive: by/from someone or something
滋	zī	to nourish; to supply
走	zǒu	to depart; to go
喜	xǐ	to enjoy; to prefer
酸	suān	sour
苦	kǔ	bitter
甘	gān	sweet
辛	xīn	acrid
鹹	xián	salty
津液	jīn yè	liquid
行	xíng	to move
營	yíng	camp [qi][1]
糟粕	zāo pò	waste; dregs
以次	yǐ cì	consecutively; step by step
次	cì	a series
傳	chuán	to transmit
下	xià	downwards

清	qīng	clear
霧	wù	fog; mist
名	míng	name; to name
滯	zhì	to obstruct
礙	ài	to obstruct; to hinder
沉	chén	to sink down
濁	zhuó	turbid
泌	mì	to gush forth
汁	zhī	juice; sap
精	jīng	essence; essential
出	chū	to go out; to leave
焦	jiāo	a burner
既	jì	to supply with; to nourish
別	bié	separate
資	zī	to help; to provide; to nourish
上	shàng	upper
口	kǒu	opening
後	hòu	behind
大氣	dà qì	the important qi (refers here to the qi of the universe that enter the body through inhalation)
搏	bó	to seize
胸	xiōng	the breast; the chest
中	zhōng	in
喉嚨	hóu lóng	the wind-pipe
呼	hū	to exhale
吸	xī	to inhale
計	jì	to count
幷	bìng	and; also
尿	niào	urine
與	yǔ	with
合	hé	together

Huáng dì yuē. yuàn wén gǔ qì yǒu wǔ wèi. qí rù wǔ zàng. fēn bié nài hé. bó gāo yuē. wèi zhě. wǔ zàng liù fǔ zhī hǎi yě. shuǐ gǔ jiē rù yú wèi. wǔ zàng liù fǔ jiē bǐng yú wèi. wèi shòu shuǐ gǔ. biàn huà yǐ zī wǔ zàng liù fǔ. wǔ wèi gè zǒu qí suǒ xǐ. gǔ wèi suān. xiān zǒu gān. gǔ wèi kǔ. xiān zǒu xīn. gǔ wèi gān. xiān zǒu pí. gǔ wèi xīn. xiān zǒu fèi. gǔ wèi xián. xiān zǒu shèn. gǔ qì jīn yè yǐ xíng. yíng wèi dà tōng. nǎi huà zāo pò. yǐ cì chuán xià. shuǐ gǔ huà wéi jīn yè. qīng qì yóu rú wù lù. míng yíng wèi. xíng mài nèi wài. wú suǒ zhì ài. gù yuē dà tōng. qí chén zhuó zhě. míng wéi zāo pò. mì bié zhī rù yú páng guāng. gù yuē yǐ cì chuán xià yě. Huáng dì yuē. yíng wèi zhī xíng nài hé. bó gāo yuē. gǔ shǐ rù yú wèi. qí jīng wēi zhě. xiān chū yú wèi zhī liǎng jiāo. yǐ jì wǔ zàng. bié chū liǎng xíng yú yíng wèi zhī dào. jīng wēi. jīn yè yě. jīn yè zī wǔ zàng yǐ. wèi qì chū wèi shàng kǒu. yíng qì chū yú zhōng jiāo zhī hòu. gù yuē liǎng xíng dào yě. qí dà qì zhī bó ér bù xíng zhě. jī yú xiōng zhōng. mìng yuē qì hǎi. chū yú fèi. xūn hóu lóng. gù hū zé chū. xī zé rù. bó. jù yě. gǔ huà wéi qì. jì yǒu sì dào. jīng wēi yíng wèi. yǐ wéi èr dào. huà wéi zāo pò jí zhuó qì bìng niào. qí yǔ jīng xià chuán. fù wéi yí dào. bó ér bù xíng. jī yú xiōng zhōng. míng qì hǎi. yǐ wéi hū xī. fù wéi yí dào. hé wéi sì dào yě.

Huang Di: I should like to hear [about the following].[2] The qi of the grains have five flavors. When they enter the five depots – according to what [kind of criteria] are they separated?
Bo Gao: The stomach is the sea for the five depots and six palaces. All the water and the grains [that man consumes] enter the stomach. The five depots and six palaces receive all their supplies from the stomach. The stomach receives the water and the grains; it transforms them to nourish the five depots and six palaces. The five flavors move each to [the one depot] which they prefer. The sour flavor of the grains moves first into the liver. The bitter flavor of the grains moves first into the heart. The sweet flavor of the grains moves first into the spleen. The acrid flavor of the grains moves first into the lung. The salty flavor of the grains moves first into the kidneys. As soon as the qi of the grains and all the liquids have begun their passage [through the organism], and when the camp and the guardian [qi] penetrate the entire [body], dregs result from transformations and are transmitted downward step by step. The water and the grains are transformed into liquids. There are clear qi resembling mist and dew; they are called camp and guardian [qi], and they proceed inside and outside the vessels. There is nothing that could obstruct [their flow]. Hence, [the text] states "penetrate the entire [body]." Those that sink down and are turbid are called dregs. They gush, as separate juices, into the urinary bladder. Hence, [the text] states: "are transmitted downward, step by step."
Huang Di: How do the camp and the guardian [qi] move [through the body]?
Bo Gao: The grain first enter the stomach. Their essential and subtle [compo-

nents] leave the stomach first through two of its burners[3] [before] they nourish[4] the five depots. They leave [the stomach through two] separate [openings], and proceed through the two paths of the camp and guardian [qi, respectively]. The essential and subtle [components] are the liquids. After the liquids have nourished the five depots, the guardian qi leave through the upper opening of the stomach; the camp qi leave from behind the central burner. Hence, the text states "proceed through two paths". Those major [portions of] the qi which are seized and do not move on, they are collected in the chest, and this is called "sea of qi"; its outlet is through the lung, via the wind-pipe. Hence, to exhale [causes the qi] to leave; to inhale [causes them] to enter [the body]. "Are seized" stands for "are accumulated." The grains are transformed into qi. Altogether, there are four paths [for the qi to enter and leave the body, and pass through it]. The essential and the subtle [components, i.e. the] camp and guardian [qi] occupy two paths. The transformation into dregs and turbid qi, and also urine, and the passage downwards together with the semen, that constitutes yet another path. [Those qi that are] seized and do not move on, and which are accumulated in the chest, they are called "sea of qi". From this originates exhalation and inhalation, which constitutes yet another path. Together these are four paths.

Notes

[1] Once the dualism of yin and yang had been acknowledged as one of the basic structuring principles of all existence, the juxtaposition of a "camp" qi, *ying* 營, and a "guardian" qi, *wei* 衛 , was one of the results of a determination of ancient Chinese naturalists to identify yin and yang correspondences for all phenomena. *Ying* 營 and *wei* 衛 are images borrowed from the military to describe the defense system of the human organism. A "camp" may be moved but is a more sedentary entity, and therefore yin. A "guardian" should be constantly on the move, and is therefore yang. Modern Western texts on so-called Traditional Chinese Medicine, disregarding many of the ancient metaphors, often erroneously translate *ying* 營 qi as "constructive qi".

[2] The text reproduced here in large characters appears also in *Huang Di Nei Jing, Ling Shu*, treatise 56, Wu wei 五味. Small print in the Chinese texts and in the English translation refer to commentaries inserted into the text by Yang Shangshan 楊上善 of the seventh century.

[3] The term 兩焦 *liǎng jiāo* has been the source of differing interpretations. Various authors have seen this term as indicating the upper and the lower burner, or the upper and the central burner. Also, 兩焦 *liǎng jiāo* has been interpreted as "the second burner", referring to the stomach itself. My rendering is based on *Tai Su*, treatise 12, "Camp and Guardian Qi", 營衛氣 Ying wei qi, where the upper opening of the stomach is identified as the location where the upper burner leaves: 上焦出於胃上口 *shàng jiāo chū yú wèi shàng kou.* Similarly, the Ying wei qi states: "the central burner leaves from behind the upper burner": 中焦出上焦之後 *zhōng jiāo chū shàng jiāo zhī hòu.* The third burner is the lower burner, *xìa jiāo* 下焦 which is identified by the Ying wei qi as the exit, from the stomach, into the intestines.

[4] *Ling Shu*, treatise 56, has 漑 *gài* ("to flood", "to flow") instead of 既.

2.d *Chén xiū yuán yī shū wǔ shí zhǒng*
陳修園醫書五十種
(Yī xué shí zài yì 醫學實在易 1)
Mìng mén shuō命門說
On the Gate of Life

人之强弱壽夭。全係命門。命門不是右腎。亦非兩腎中間。更非督脈十四椎下命門之腧穴。考之內經。太陽根於至陰。結於命門。命門者。目也。靈樞根結篇。衛氣篇。素問陰陽離合論。三說俱同。後讀黃庭經云。上有黃庭下關元。後有幽門前命門。方悟其處。凡人受生之初。先天精氣。聚於臍下。當關元氣海之間。其在女者。可以手捫而得。俗名產門。其在男者。于泄精之時。自有關闌知覺。此北門鎖鑰之司。人之生命處也。又考越人七衝門之說。謂飛門。唇也。戶門。齒也。吸門。會厭也。賁門。胃之上口也。幽門。太倉下口也。闌門。小腸下口也。魄門。肛門也。便溺由氣化而出。又增溺竅爲氣門。凡稱之曰門。蓋指出入之處而言也。況身形未生之初。父母交會之際。男之施由此門而出。女之受由此門而入。及胎元既足。復由此門而生。故於八門之外。重之曰命門也。

强	qiáng	strong
弱	ruò	weak
全	quán	all
門	mén	gate; door
命門	mìng mén	the gate of life
是	shì	to be; is; are
間	jiān	space between
督脈	dū mài	the supervisor vessel
椎	zhuī	vertebra; backbone section
下	xià	below
腧穴	shū xuè	transport point (where a needle is inserted in acupuncture to affect the passage of qi)
考	kǎo	to examine
內經	nèi jīng	*Nei jing*, abbreviation of *Huang Di nei jing*, "Huang Di's Inner Classic"
根	gēn	origin; root
至陰	zhì yīn	the *zhi yin* ("extreme yin") (insertion point)
結	jié	to finish
靈樞	líng shū	*Ling shu*, abbreviation of the *Huang Di nei jing ling shu*, "Huang Di's Inner Classic, Magic Pivot"
篇	piān	a book; a section of a book
離	lí	to part; to separate
說	shuō	to say
俱	jù	all; every
黃庭經	huáng tíng jīng	*Huang ting jing*, the "Classic of the Yellow Court"; in its nuclear parts a late Han text on human meditative physiology
黃庭	huáng tíng	the "yellow court"; a Daoist term referring to the center of the body, and to the navel
元	yuán	origin; original
關元	guān yuán	the *guan yuan* (needle insertion point; located three inches below the navel)
幽門	yōu mén	the dark gate

前	qián	in front of; prior to; before
悟	wù	to apprehend
處	chù	place
先天	xiān tiān	previous to one's existence; transmitted by one's parents
臍	qí	the navel
當	dāng	exactly
捫	mén	to feel; to lay the hand on
俗	sú	vulgar; common
產	chǎn	to give birth
泄	xiè	to discharge
自	zì	since; because
關	guān	a gate
闌	lán	a barrier
北	běi	north
鎖	suǒ	a lock; to lock
鑰	yuè; yào	a key
司	sī	to control
又	yòu	again; in turn; moreover
衝	chōng	a thoroughfare
衝門	chōng mén	the through-gates
飛	fēi	to fly
飛門	fēi mén	the flying gate
唇	chún	the lips
戶	hù	door
戶門	hù mén	the door-gate
吸門	xī mén	the inhalation-gate
會厭	huì yàn	the epiglottis
賁門	fén mén	the big gate
太倉	tài cāng	the big granary; the stomach
闌門	lán mén	the screen-gate
魄門	pò mén	the *po*-gate
肛	gāng	the rectum
肛門	gāng mén	the rectum-gate

便	biàn	convenience; stool
溺	niào	urine
氣門	qì mén	the qi-gate
指	zhǐ	to refer; to point to
况	kuàng	further; moreover
施	shī	to discharge
胎元	tāi yuán	the fetus
既	jì	if; when
外	wài	outside; extra
重	chóng	to add

Rén zhī qiáng ruò shòu yāo. quán xì mìng mén. mìng mén bù shì yòu shèn. yì fēi liǎng shèn zhōng jiān. gèng fēi dū mài shí sì zhuī xià mìng mén zhī shū xuè. kǎo zhī nèi-jīng. tài yáng gēn yú zhì yīn. jié yú mìng mén. mìng mén zhě. mù yě. líng-shū gēn jié piān. wèi qì piān. sù-wèn yīn yáng lí hé lùn. sān shuō jù tóng. hòu dú huáng tíng jīng yún. shàng yǒu huáng tíng xià guān yuán. hòu yǒu yōu mén qián mìng mén. fāng wù qí chù. fán rén shòu shēng zhī chū. xiān tiān jīng qì. jù yú qí xià. dāng guān yuán qì hǎi zhī jiān. qí zài nǚ zhě. kě yǐ shǒu mén ér dé. sú míng chǎn mén. qí zài nán zhě. yú xiè jīng zhī shí. zì yǒu guān lán zhī jué. cǐ běi mén suǒ yuè zhī sī. rén zhī shēng mìng chù yě. yòu kǎo yuè rén qī chōng mén zhī shuō. wèi fēi mén. chún yě. hù mén. chǐ yě. xī mén. huì yàn yě. fén mén. wèi zhī shàng kǒu yě. yōu mén. tài cāng xià kǒu yě. lán mén. xiǎo cháng xià kǒu yě. pò mén. gāng mén yě. biàn niào yóu qì huà ér chū. yòu zēng niào qiào wéi qì mén. fán chēng zhī yuē mén. gài zhǐ chū rù zhī chù ér yán yě. kuàng shēn xíng wèi shēng zhī chū. fù mǔ jiāo huì zhī jì. nán zhī shī yóu cǐ mén ér chū. nǚ zhī shòu yóu cǐ mén ér rù. jí tāi yuán jì zú. fù yóu cǐ mén ér shēng. gù yú bā mén zhī wài. chóng zhī yuē mìng mén yě.

Whether a man is strong or weak, [enjoys] longevity or [succumbs to] a premature death, all this is related to the gate of life. The gate of life is not the right kidney, it is not situated between the two kidneys, and it is certainly not the transportation hole [called] "gate of life" on the supervisor vessel below the fourteenth vertebra. Examining the *Nei jing* for this [issue, one finds the statement]: "The major yang [conduit] emerges from the *zhi yin* [hole] and ends at the gate of life." The [term] "gate of life" [refers to] the eyes [here]. The Gen jie and the Wei qi sections of the *Ling shu*, and the treatise Yin yang li he of the *Su wen*, all three of them have identical statements. Later, I read the *Huang ting jing* where it says: "Above is the yellow court; below is the *guan yuan* [hole]. In the back is the dark gate; in the front is the gate of life." Only then I understood its position. At the beginning of man's getting his life, the seminal qi from previous to his existence collect below the navel exactly between the *guan yuan* [hole] and the sea of qi. In females one can lay one's hand [on this place] and feel it; it is commonly called birth gate. Its position in males can be felt at the moment of the discharge of semen because of a gate's barrier [that opens at that moment]. This is [the place] where the closing mechanism of the Northern Gate[1] is controlled; this is the place where man's life and existence [commence]. In addition, [I] examined what Yueren said on the seven through-gates. He stated: the flying-gate are the lips; the door-gate are the teeth; the inhalation-gate is the epiglottis; the big gate is the upper opening of the stomach; the dark-gate is the lower opening of the big granary; the screen gate is the lower opening of the small intestine; and the *po*-gate is the rectum-gate. Stool and urine result from transformed qi, and the urine hole is to be added which is the qi-gate. Everything that is designated with the name "gate" is called so because it is a place where [something] moves in or out. Moreover, at the beginning, before the physical appearance of a human being has emerged, when father and mother cohabitate, the discharge of the male leaves through this gate, and the female conceives through this gate. And when the fetus is complete, once again it is born from this gate. Hence in addition to the eight gates [named above] one speaks of an extra gate of life.

Note

[1] "Northern Gates" stands for "back door"; a metaphor for a strategically very sensitive position.

2.e *Nàn jīng* 難經
Sān shí yī nàn 三十一難
The Thirty-First Difficult Issue

三焦者。何稟何生。何始何終。其治常在何許。可曉以不。然。三焦者。水穀之道路。氣之所終始也。上焦者。在心下。下膈。在胃上口。主內而不出。其治在膻中。玉堂下一寸六分。直兩乳間陷者是。中焦者。在胃中脘。不上不下。主腐熟水穀。其治在齊傍。下焦者。當膀胱上口。主分別清濁。主出而不內。以傳導也。其治在齊下一寸。故名曰三焦。其府在氣街。一本曰衝。

終	zhōng	end
許	xǔ	place; to allow
曉	xiǎo	to know
以	yǐ	or
路	lù	road; way; path
下	xià	to descend
膈	gé	the diaphragm
內	nèi	to take in
膻中	dàn zhōng	the *dan zhong* (insertion point)
玉堂	yù táng	the *yu tang* (insertion point)
寸	cùn	inch
分	fēn	section; one tenth of an inch; fen
直	zhí	exactly
乳	rǔ	the breasts
陷	xiàn	a fold

脘	wǎn	a duct in the body
腐	fǔ	rotten; to spoil
熟	shú	cooked; to process
齊	qí	the navel
傍	páng	side; side-wise
導	dǎo	to lead
府	fǔ	collecting point
氣街	qì jiē	the qi street; *qi jie* (insertion point)
一	yì	another

Sān jiāo zhě. hé bǐng hé shēng. hé shǐ hé zhōng. qí zhì cháng zài hé xǔ. kě xiǎo yǐ bù. rán. sān jiāo zhě. shuǐ gǔ zhī dào lù. qì zhī suǒ zhōng shǐ yě. shàng jiāo zhě. zài xīn xià. xià gé. zài wèi shàng kǒu. zhǔ nèi ér bù chū. qí zhì zài shān zhōng. yù táng xià yí cùn liù fēn. zhí liǎng rǔ jiān xiàn zhě shī. zhōng jiāo zhě. zài wèi zhōng wǎn. bù shàng bù xià. zhǔ fǔ shú shuǐ gǔ. qí zhì zài qí páng. xià jiāo zhě. dāng páng guāng shàng kǒu. zhǔ fēn bié qīng zhuó. zhǔ chū ér bù nèi. yǐ chuán dǎo yě. qí zhì zài qí xià yí cùn. gù míng yuē sān jiāo. qí fǔ zài qì jiē. yì běn yuē chōng.

The triple burner: how is it supplied and what does it generate? Where does it start, and where does it end? And where, in general, [are its disorders] regulated? Can that be known? It is like this. The triple burner encompasses the passage ways of water and grains [in the organism]. It represents the conclusion and the start of [the course of] qi. The upper [section of the triple] burner extends from below the heart downwards through the diaphragm [and ends] at the upper opening of the stomach. It is responsible for intake but not for discharge. [Disorders in this section are] regulated at the *dan zhong* [hole, located] one inch and six fen below the *yu tang* [hole], exactly in the fold between the two breasts. The central [section of the triple] burner is located in the central duct of the stomach; it does not extend further upwards or downwards. It is responsible for the spoiling and processing of water and grains. [Disorders in this section are] regulated sidewards of the navel. The lower [section of the triple] burner is located exactly at the upper opening of the bladder. It is responsible for separating the clear from the turbid [portions]. It masters discharge but not intake, and it serves as transmitter. [Disorders in this section are] regulated one inch below the navel. Hence one speaks of a triple burner. This palace is situated[1] at the qi street. Another copy [of this text] calls it the [qi] thoroughfare.

Note

[1] This reading is suggested by ancient commentators. See Paul U. Unschuld, *Nan-ching. The Classic of Difficult Issues*, Berkeley-Los Angeles-London, 1986, p.351 f. The term *fŭ* 府 could also be read as a verb in the sense of "to collect". In this case, this passage has the meaning of "Its collecting [point] is at the qi street".

2.f *Tú shū biān* 圖書編
Zàng fŭ quán tú shuō 臟腑全圖說
Completely Illustrated Discourse on the Depots and Palaces

崇寧五年。梁少保知大名府。有群盜起。內一强寇楊宗。以計擒之。案首惡論死。臨刑命醫官幷畫工畫之。適徐州歐希範作惡。當刑三十人。亦送來刑。命畫工於法場割開諸人胸腹。詳視畫之。見喉嚨中排三竅。曰水。曰食。曰氣。相推惟水食同一竅。走胸中。入胃上口。一竅通肺。循腹。抵脊脅。轉臍。下兩腎。與任衝督三脉會丹田者。氣海也。喉管下有肺兩葉。爲華蓋。蓋諸臟腑。肺下有心。外有黄脂裹之。其色赤黄。割視其心。箇箇不同。有竅無竅。有毛無毛。尖者長者。心下有羅膈。羅膈下有胃。積曲。可容一斗物。外有黄脂。如旗燄。左有肝。一二三四五葉者。亦各不同。內歐患眼。肝有白黑子兩張。氣喘而且嗽。其肺皺而黑。所謂表裏相應也。其肝短葉上有膽。右胃。左脾。與胃同膜。狀如馬蹄。肝赤紫。下有小腸。盤十六曲。極瑩淨。化物通行。右有大腸。亦十六曲。內有所出糟粕之路。外有黄脂。粘作一塊。下有膀胱。居

脬。亦瑩淨。外無所入穴。全借氣施行津液。入胞爲尿。此君子小人之體。各異如此。

崇寧	chóng níng	the *chong ning* ("reverence of peace") reign period (1102-1106 CE)
梁	liáng	a family name
少保	shào bǎo	Junior Guardian (of the heir apparent); honorary title conferred upon high officials
知	zhī	to administer
大名	dà míng	name of a prefecture
府	fǔ	a prefecture
群	qún	a multitude
盜	dào	robber
內	nèi	among
寇	kòu	bandit
楊宗	yáng zōng	Yang Zong; name of a bandit
計	jì	to plan; to scheme
擒	qín	to arrest
案	àn	a law-case; a trial
首	shǒu	chief
惡	è	vicious; bad; malevolent
首惡	shǒu è	chief culprit
論	lùn	to sentence
臨	lín	just before
刑	xíng	the death-penalty; execution
命	mìng	to order
官	guān	officer; official
畫	huà	to draw a picture; picture
適	shì	to happen; just now
徐	xú	Xu, name of a district
歐希範	ōu xī fàn	Ou Xifan; name of a criminal
作	zuò	to do
當	dāng	to bear

送	sòng	to send
來	lái	to receive
法場	fă chăng	the place of execution
開	kāi	to open
諸	zhū	all; every
詳	xiáng	detail
視	shì	to look
喉嚨	hóu lóng	the throat
排	pái	to arrange; arranged
食	shí	food
相推	xiāng tuī	to look at and conclude; to study
同一	tóng yī	the same
抵	dĭ	to arrive
脊	jí	the spine; the back
脅	xié	the ribs
任脉	rèn mài	the controller [conduit] vessel
衝脉	chōng mài	the through-way [conduit] vessel
丹田	dān tián	the cinnabar field; an anatomically nonverifiable area in the body conceptualized in the context of alchemistic-macrobiotic reasoning
管	guăn	a tube
喉管	hóu guăn	the wind-pipe
葉	yè	a lobe
華蓋	huá gài	a canopy
蓋	gài	to cover
脂	zhī	fat
裹	guŏ	to wrap
赤	chì	red
箇	gè	classifier
箇箇	gè gè	one by one; each
尖	jiān	pointed
長	cháng	long
羅	luó	net; spread out
曲	qū	crooked; bent

積曲	jī qū	to have [many] bends [inside]; coiled
容	róng	to contain
斗	dǒu	a peck
物	wù	matter; substance
旗燄	qí yàn	blazing flag
眼	yǎn	eye
黑	hēi	black
子	zǐ	spot
張	zhāng	a classifier of flat objects
喘	chuǎn	to pant
嗽	sòu	to cough
皺	zhòu	wrinkled
短	duǎn	short
膜	mó	membrane
狀	zhuàng	appearance; form
馬蹄	mǎ tí	the hoof of a horse
紫	zǐ	dark red; purplish
盤	pán	to coil up; to wind around
極	jí	very
瑩	yíng	bright; pure
淨	jìng	pure; clean
粘	zhān	to adhere; to stick to
作	zuò	to make; to be
塊	kuài	lump; piece
居	jū	to be
脬	pāo	a bladder; a balloon
借	jiè	to borrow; to depend upon
施	shī	to bestow
施行	shī xíng	to provide with
胞	bāo	the bladder
君	jūn	gentleman; noble
小人	xiǎo rén	petty person
體	tǐ	the body

Chóng níng wǔ nián. liáng shào bǎo zhī dà míng fǔ. yǒu qún dào qǐ. nèi yī qiáng kòu yáng zōng. yǐ jì qín zhī. àn shǒu è lùn sǐ. lín xíng mìng yī guān bìng huà gōng huà zhī. shì xú zhōu Ōu xī fàn zuò è. dāng xíng sān shí rén. yì sòng lái xíng. mìng huà gōng yú fǎ chǎng gé kāi zhū rén xiōng fù. xiáng shì huà zhī. jiàn hóu lóng zhōng pái sān qiào. yuē shuǐ. yuē shí. yuē qì. xiāng tuī wéi shuǐ shí tóng yī qiào. zǒu xiōng zhōng. rù wèi shàng kǒu. yí qiào tōng fèi. xūn fù. dǐ jí xié. zhuǎn qí . xià liǎng shèn. yǔ rèn chōng dū sān mài huì dān tián zhě. qì hǎi yě. hóu guǎn xià yǒu fèi liǎng yè. wéi huá gài. gài zhū zàng fǔ. fèi xià yǒu xīn. wài yǒu huáng zhī guǒ zhī. qí sè chì huáng. gé shì qí xīn. gè gè bù tóng. yǒu qiào wú qiào. yǒu máo wú máo. jiān zhě cháng zhě. xīn xià yǒu luó gé. luó gé xià yǒu wèi. jī qū. kě róng yì dǒu wù. wài yǒu huáng zhī. rú qí yàn. zuǒ yǒu gān. yī èr sān sì wǔ yè zhě. yì gè bù tóng. nèi ōu huàn yǎn. gān yǒu bái hēi zǐ liǎng zhāng. qì chuǎn ér qiě sòu. qí fèi zhòu ér hēi. suǒ wèi biǎo lǐ xiāng yìng yě. qí gān duǎn yè shàng yǒu dǎn. yòu wèi. zuǒ pí. yǔ wèi tóng mó . zhuàng rú mǎ tí. gān chì zǐ. xià yǒu xiǎo cháng. pán shí liù qū. jí yíng jìng. huà wù tōng xíng. yòu yǒu dà cháng. yì shí liù qū. nèi yǒu suǒ chū zāo pò zhī lù. wài yǒu huáng zhī. nián zuò yí kuài. xià yǒu páng guāng. jū pāo. yì yíng jìng. wài wú suǒ rù xuè. quán jiè qì shī xíng jīn yè. rù bāo wéi niào. cǐ jūn zǐ xiǎo rén zhī tǐ. gè yì rú cǐ.

In the fifth year of the *chong ning* period of reign, Junior Guardian Liang was Prefect of Daming. At that time, a number of robbers emerged among whom was a strong bandit [with the name of] Yang Zong. [Liang] managed to capture him, and during the [following] trial [Yang Zong was identified as] chief culprit and sentenced to death. As he faced his execution, [the prefect] ordered a medical official and an artist to draw pictures of him. At about the same time, in the district of Xu, Ou Xifan committed crimes. [Altogether] thirty men were to receive capital punishment, and they too were sent [to Daming] to be executed. [Liang] ordered an artist on the execution grounds to cut open the chest and abdomen of all these persons, take a close look, and draw pictures of them. He observed three holes in the throat, and identified them as [the passage-ways of] water, food, and qi. Further studies revealed, though, that there is only one common hole for water and food together [serving as a starting-point of a passage-way] that proceeds through the chest and enters the stomach through its upper opening. Another hole serves as a passage-way into the lung, whence its path proceeds further through the abdomen to reach the back and the ribs. [This path, then,] turns around the navel and descends to the "cinnabar field" where the two kidneys meet with the three vessels of the controller, through-way, and supervisor [conduits. This] is the sea of qi.

Below the wind-pipe [the artist observed] the lung with its two lobes, forming a canopy that covered all depots and palaces. Below the lung was the heart. It was wrapped by yellow fat, and its color was red-yellow. When [the criminals] were cut open to expose their hearts, the [latter] were all different. [Some] had holes, [others] had no holes; [some] had hairs, [others] had no hairs. There were pointed ones and long ones. Below the heart was a net[-like] diaphragm, and below this net[-like] diaphragm was the stomach. [The stomach] had many bends [inside] and could hold one peck of substances. It was wrapped by yellow fat, resembling a blazing flag. To the left was the liver with one, two, three, four, or five lobes – they too were all different. Among [all these criminals], Ou [Xifan] suffered from an eye affliction, and his liver had two lobes with black and white spots. He panted his breath and, moreover, [he suffered from] cough. His lung was wrinkled and black. That was [an example of] the so-called mutual correspondence of outside [symptoms] and inside [conditions]. His liver was short. Above its lobes was the gallbladder. To the right was the stomach; to the left was the spleen, sharing one membrane with the stomach. Its shape resembled that of the hoof of a horse[1]; the liver was red-purplish. Below was the small intestine, coiled up in sixteen bends. It was very clean. – It transforms substances [and causes them] to pass on. – To the right was the large intestine, coiled up sixteen times too. – Inside [the large intestine] is the path where the dregs are emitted. – Outside was yellow fat that stuck to it as a lump. Below was the urinary bladder which was [shaped like] a balloon. It, too, was clean, and it had no hole [for anything] to enter from the outside. – It relies solely on qi for activating the body fluids to enter the bladder[2] where they become urine. – This is how the bodies of the noble and of petty people differ from each other.

Notes

[1] This is perhaps an allusion to a part or fruit of various plants called "horse's hoof", as, for instance, the water-chestnut.

[2] The term *bāo* 胞 refers to organs serving as "enclosures", i.e. the womb, the urinary bladder, and the eyelids. In the sentence here it refers to the urinary bladder but may have been employed instead of the preceding and synonymous *páng guāng* 膀胱 not only for stylistic reasons but also to emphasize a notion of a balloon-like organ shut off from the outside.

Lesson Three

General Pathology

Numerous diverging, sometimes contradictory ideas were developed to apply the fundamental tenet of the medicine of systematic correspondence concerning the causation of illness, that is, a belief in the loss of harmony with the basic laws of nature, to the actual process of falling ill. Prior to the emergence of the medicine of correspondence, an awareness of the power of ancestors and spirit-demons had dominated the explanation of illness in Chinese society, and this awareness did by no means fade into non-existence after the first purely this-wordly, non-metaphysical system of concepts concerning the origins and nature of illness had emerged in China. The question whether demons existed or not, and whether they had a hand in the onset of illness, was discussed in medical texts until recent centuries because the majority of the population remained firmly convinced of their important role. Still, the basic idea of the medicine of systematic correspondence (whose founders argued vehemently against any vestiges of the concepts of demonology) was to distinguish between a proper (*zhèng*正) behavior resulting in a proper state of health, and the dominance of proper qi in the organism, on the one side, and a deviant or heterodox or evil (all three concepts covered by the term *xié*邪) mode of behavior permitting something deviant or evil either to happen within the organism or to enter the organism from outside. General pathology included the consequences of such evil developments, as are the ceasing of proper functioning of the functional units constituting the organism, resulting in an impairment of secondary functions (such as vision or hearing), and the blockage of transportation channels/conduits, leaving one or more functional units unsupplied.

Key Terms Introduced in Lesson Three

邪	xié	evil; abnormal
因	yīn	cause
暑	shǔ	summer-heat

濕	shī	humidity; dampness
饑	jī	hunger
飽	bǎo	fullness
勞	láo	taxation
鬼	guǐ	demon
疫	yì	epidemic
癘	lì	a serious illness affecting many
瘦	shòu	thin; emaciated
療	liáo	to heal; to cure
丸	wán	a pill
膏	gāo	below the heart
肓	huāng	above the diaphragm
皮膚	pí fū	the skin
急	jí	tense; taut
腠理	còu lǐ	skin structures
緩	huǎn	relaxed
賊風	zèi fēng	the robber wind
八正	bā zhèng	the eight seasonal turning points (s.a. 1.c.)
病	bìng	to make ill; to cause a disease
濕	shī	humidity; moisture
榮	róng	used here for 營 *yíng*, military camp
血脈	xuě mài	the blood vessels
湯	tāng	hot water; hot baths
熨	yùn	to iron; to apply hot pressure
醪	láo	the lees of wine; wine
髓	suǐ	marrow
五行	wǔ xíng	the five agents; five interrelated categories of all phenomena in existence
舌	shé	the tongue
志	zhì	the mind
意	yì	the sentiments
憂	yōu	mourning
燥	zào	dry; dryness
悲	bēi	grief

驚	jìng	fright; terror
症	zhèng	illness; complaints
饑	jī	hunger
疲	pí	tired; weary; exhausted
瘡	chuāng	a wound
踒	wō	to slip; to sprain
疰	zhù	possession (by demons)
附著	fù zhuó	possession (by demons)
痎	jiē	*jie*, an ancient term for a disease unidentifiable today
瘧	nüè	the *nüe* disease, malaria
痿	wěi	limpness
厥	jué	receding [qi]

3.a *Gŭ jīn yī tŏng dà quán* 3
古今醫統大全
(Yì yī tōng kăo 翼醫通考)
Bìng zhī suŏ yóu 病之所由
The Origins of Disease

夫病之所由來雖多端。而皆關於邪。邪者。不正之因。謂非人身之常理。風寒暑濕、饑飽勞逸。皆各是邪。非獨鬼氣疫癘者矣。人生氣中。如魚在水。水濁則魚瘦。氣昏則人病。邪氣之傷人。最爲深重。經絡既受此氣。傳入臟腑。臟腑隨其虛實冷熱。結以成病。病又相生。故流通遂廣。精神者。本宅身以爲用。身既受邪。精神亦亂。神既亂矣。則鬼靈斯入。鬼力漸強。神守漸弱。豈得不至於死乎。古人譬之植楊。斯理當矣。但病亦別有先從鬼神來者。則宜以祈禱祛之。雖曰可祛。猶因藥療致益。李子豫有赤丸之例是也。其藥療無益者。是則不可祛。晉景公膏肓之例是也。大都鬼神之害則多端。疾病之源種。蓋有輕重者爾。

來	lái	to come
由來	yóu lái	origin
端	duān	beginning; final cause

關於	guān yú	to be related to; to result from
邪	xié	evil; abnormal
正	zhèng	proper, regular
因	yīn	cause
謂	wèi	that is to say
人	rén	human
暑	shǔ	summer-heat
濕	shī	humidity; dampness
饑	jī	hunger
飽	bǎo	fullness
勞	láo	taxation
逸	yì	indulgence; idleness
獨	dú	only; alone
鬼	guǐ	demon
疫	yì	epidemic
癘	lì	a serious illness affecting many
中	zhōng	amidst; surrounded by
魚	yú	fish
瘦	shòu	thin; emaciated
昏	hūn	confused; irregular
深	shēn	intense; very
重	zhòng	grave
此	cǐ	these
隨	suí	to follow; in accordance with
冷	lěng	cool; cold
流	liú	to flow; to spread
通	tōng	throughout
遍	biàn	everywhere
遂	suí	to proceed to
廣	guǎng	extensive; broad
宅	zhái	to reside; lodging
用	yòng	application; tool
亂	luàn	disturbance; confused
靈	líng	spirits

力	lì	strength
漸	jiàn	gradually
守	shǒu	to guard; to protect
得	dé	to achieve; to be able
植	zhí	to plant
楊	yáng	the willow tree
當	dāng	appropriate; fitting
但	dàn	but
別	bié	other
祈	qí	to pray
禱	dǎo	to pray
祛	qū	to drive off
因	yīn	because of
療	liáo	to heal; to cure
致	zhì	to cause; to result in
益	yì	to benefit
李子豫	lǐ zǐ yù	Li Ziyu; name of a legendary healer of the Zhou era
丸	wán	a pill
例	lì	precedent; example
是	shì	in fact
晉景公	jìn jǐng gōng	Duke Jing of Jin
膏	gāo	below the heart
肓	huāng	above the diaphragm
都	dū	all; the whole
源	yuán	a source
種	zhǒng	seed; many; numerous
輕	qīng	minor; light
爾	ěr	only

Fū bìng zhī suǒ yóu lái suī duō duān. ér jiē guān yú xié. xié zhě. bù zhèng zhī yīn. wèi fēi rén shēn zhī cháng lǐ. fēng hán shǔ shī, jī bǎo láo yì. jiē gè shī xié. fēi dú guǐ qì yì lì zhě yǐ. rén shēng qì zhōng. rú yú zài shuǐ. shuǐ zhuó zé yú shòu. qì hūn zé rén bìng. xié qì zhī shāng rén. zuì wéi shēn zhòng. jīng luò jì shòu cǐ qì. chuán rù zàng fǔ. zàng fǔ suí qí xū shí lěng rè. jié yǐ chéng bìng. bìng yòu xiāng shēng. gù liú tōng suí guǎng. jīng shén zhě. běn zhái shēn yǐ wéi yòng. shēn jì shòu xié. jīng shén yì luàn. shén jì luàn yǐ. zé guǐ líng sī rù. guǐ lì jiàn qiáng. shén shǒu jiàn ruò. qǐ dé bù zhì yú sǐ hū. gǔ rén pì zhī zhí yáng. sī lǐ dāng yǐ. dàn bìng yì bié yǒu xiān cóng guǐ shén lái zhě. zé yí yǐ qí dǎo qū zhī. suī yuē kě qū. yóu yīn yào liáo zhì yì. Lǐ zǐ yù yǒu chì wán zhī lì shì yě. qí yào liáo wú yì zhě. shī zé bù kě qū. jìn jǐng gōng gāo huāng zhī lì shī yě. dà dū guǐ shén zhī hài zé duō duān. jí bìng zhī yuán zhǒng. gài yǒu qīng zhòng zhě ěr.

Although the origins of diseases are traceable to many causes, all of them result from [something] evil. Evil is the cause of [anything that is] not regular. That is to say, everything that is not part of the normal order in the human organism, [such as] wind, cold, dampness, hunger, fullness, taxation, and idleness, is evil – and not solely the qi of demons and epidemic illnesses [as some authors have claimed]. [1] Just as the fish exist in water, man lives surrounded by qi. If the water is turbid, the fish waste away. If the qi [to which man is exposed] are irregular, man falls ill. The most severe harm to man is caused by evil qi. Once the main conduits and the network [vessels] have absorbed such qi, they transmit them into the depots and palaces. In the depots and palaces, as a result of [already existing] depletion or repletion, or as a consequence of [irregular] heat or cold, [the evil qi] may accumulate, and diseases are generated. As these diseases, in turn, may cause further diseases, they spread in all directions throughout [the body]. The spirit uses the body as his residence. Now, if the body has absorbed evil [qi], the spirit will also be disturbed. When the spirit is disturbed, demons and [foreign] spirits will enter its [place]. This way, the strength of the demons increases gradually, while the protection provided by [one's own] spirit decreases continuously. How could death be avoided [in such a situation]! In ancient times, the people compared this to the planting of willow trees;[2] the underlying principle is precisely the same. However, among the diseases there are different [types]. Some result, in the first place, from demon-spirits. In these cases, then, it is suitable to expel [these creatures] by means of prayers. Although it is said that [demon-spirits] can be driven off [by means of prayers], it may well be that it is because of drugs that one achieves good results. Li Ziyu with his red pills is an example.[3] In cases where drugs are ineffective, an exorcism is impossible too. An example is the disease in the *gao huang* region of Duke Jing of Jin.[4] In general, injuries caused by demon-spirits may be manifold. The origins of diseases are numerous. It is simply such that there are diseases that may be considered minor, and others that are serious.

Notes

[1] In ancient Chinese medical literature, this is an example of a most precise definition of a key pathological concept in Chinese traditional medicine, expressed by means of the term 邪 *xié*, "evil", "irregular", as opposed to *zhèng*, "proper", "regular". The juxtaposition of "evil" and "proper" reflects a projection of moral categories on the causes of disease. A rendering of 邪 *xié* as "heteropathy", as has been introduced in some English renderings of Chinese traditional medical terminology, is to be avoided as it serves to obfuscate the political and moral background of pathological theory in the medicine of systematic correspondences.

[2] This sentence may be an allusion to a reference in Ge Hong's 葛洪 (281-341) *Bao pu zi, Nei pian* 抱樸子 內篇. Ge Hong states here that willows are quite sturdy but once they are really hurt, even the best care cannot keep them from dying. Man, in contrast, is weak and vulnerable by nature; hence he should care for his health all the more, beginning from his very youth.

[3] Li Ziyu is mentioned in the *Sou shen hou ji* 搜神後記 of the third or fourth century CE as successfully curing, with a red pill, a patient from the presence of two demons in his body.

[4] The 膏肓 *gāo huāng* case is recorded in the 左傳 *Zuo zhuan*, bk. 8, tenth year. In Marquis Jing of Jin, two demons had taken up a position in the region below the heart and above the diaphragm, inaccessible to any therapy.

3.b *Huáng dì nèi jīng, Tài sù* 28
黃帝內經·太素
Sān xū sān shí 三虛三實
The Three States of Depletion, and the Three States of Repletion

---

黃帝問少師曰。余聞四時八風之中人也。故有寒暑。寒則皮膚急而腠理閉。暑則皮膚緩而腠理開。賊風邪氣因以得入乎。將必須八正虛邪乃能傷人乎。少師答曰。不然。賊風邪氣之中人也。不得以時。然必因其開也。其入也深。其內極也疾。其病人卒暴。因其閉也。其入也淺以留。其病人也徐以持也。黃帝曰。有寒溫和適。腠理不開。然有卒病者。其故何也。少師曰。帝弗知邪入乎。雖平居。其腠理開閉緩急。固常有時也。黃帝曰。可得聞乎。少師曰。人與天地相參也。與日月相應也。故月滿則海水西盛。人血氣精。肌肉充。皮膚緻。毛髮堅。當是之時。雖遇賊風。其入淺。亦不深。至其月郭空。則海水東盛。人血氣虛。其衛氣去。形獨居。肌肉減。皮膚緩。腠理開。毛髮淺。當是之時。遇賊風。則其入也深。其病人也卒暴。

少師	shào shī	Shaoshi; one of the legendary advisers of Huang Di
余	yú	I; myself
中	zhòng	to hit; to strike
膚	fū	the skin
皮膚	pí fū	the skin
急	jí	tense; taut
腠理	còu lǐ	skin structures
緩	huǎn	relaxed
賊風	zèi fēng	the robber wind
將	jiāng	a particle indicating future; here: or (connecting two questions)
必須	bì xū	must
八正	bā zhèng	the eight seasonal turning points (s.a. 1.c.)
答	dá	to answer
疾	jí	fast
病	bìng	to make ill; to cause a disease
暴	bào	violent
淺	qiǎn	shallow; near the surface
留	liú	to keep; to remain
徐	xú	slow; sedate
持	chí	to control
溫	wēn	warm
和	hé	harmony with
適	shì	to suit; proper
帝	dì	Di; thearch (mythical); emperor (secular)
弗	fú	not
常	cháng	regular; a rule
參	cān	to take part; to be related
盛	shèng	abundant; flourishing
精	jīng	pure
充	chōng	to fill; filled
緻	zhì	fine; dense
堅	jiān	firm; hard

遇	yù	to meet
郭	guō	a rim
空	kōng	empty
月郭空	yuè guō kōng	new moon
减	jiǎn	to diminish; to reduce

Huáng dì wèn shào shī yuē. yú wén sì shí bā fēng zhī zhòng rén yě. gù yǒu hán shǔ. hán zé pí fū jí ér còu lǐ bì. shǔ zé pí fū huǎn ér còu lǐ kāi. zèi fēng xié qì yīn yǐ dé rù hū. jiāng bì xū bā zhèng xū xié nǎi néng shāng rén hū. shào shī dá yuē. bù rán. zèi fēng xié qì zhī zhōng rén yě. bù dé yǐ shí. rán bì yīn qí kāi yě. qí rù yě shēn. qí nèi jí yě jí. qí bìng rén cù bào. yīn qí bì yě. qí rù yě qiǎn yǐ liú. qí bìng rén yě xú yǐ chí yě. Huáng dì yuē. yǒu hán wēn hé shì. còu lǐ bù kāi. rán yǒu cù bìng zhě. qí gù hé yě. shào shī yuē. dì fú zhī xié rù hū. suī píng jū. qí còu lǐ kāi bì huǎn jí. gù cháng yǒu shí yě. Huáng dì yuē. kě dé wén hū. shào shī yuē. rén yǔ tiān dì xiāng cān yě. yǔ rì yuè xiāng yìng yě. gù yuè mǎn zé hǎi shuǐ xī shèng. rén xuě qì jīng. jī ròu chōng. pí fū zhì. máo fà jiān. dāng shī zhī shí. suī yù zèi fēng. qí rù qiǎn. yì bù shēn. zhì qí yuè guō kōng. zé hǎi shuǐ dōng shèng. rén xuě qì xū. qí wèi qì qù. xíng dú jū. jī ròu jiǎn. pí fū huǎn. còu lǐ kāi. máo fà qiǎn. dāng shī zhī shí. yù zèi fēng. zé qí rù yě shēn. qí bìng rén yě cù bào.

Huang Di asked Shaoshi: I have heard it said that cold and heat are responsible for whether someone is struck by the eight winds of the four seasons. When it is cold the skin is taut and the skin structures are closed. When it is hot the skin is relaxed and the skin structures are open. Could it be that this enables the evil qi of the robber wind to invade [the body]? Or must the depletion evil of the eight seasonal turning points also be present before man suffers harm?
Shaoshi replied: This is not the case. Whether or not the evil qi of a robber-wind strike someone does not depend on the seasons [of the year]. The necessary conditions are as follows. When [the skin structures] are open, the [evil qi] penetrate deep [into the body], quickly reaching the extreme interior and causing a sudden and violent illness in that person. When the [skin structures] are closed, the [evil qi] also penetrate [into the body], but they remain at the surface. The disease caused in that person will be slow and can be restrained.
Huang Di: What if someone is able to live in harmony with cold and warmth [and adapt himself to the requirements of the changes in the temperature] so that his skin structures are not open and yet [this person] nonetheless suddenly falls ill – what is the cause?

Shaoshi: [Huang] Di, are you then ignorant of the ways in which evil invades [the human body]? Even if a person conducts his life in an harmonious manner, it nonetheless depends on specific times whether or not his skin structures are open or closed [and his skin] is relaxed or taut.
Huang Di: Can I hear [more on this]?
Shaoshi: [The condition of] man and [the occurrences in] heaven and on earth are mutually related; [the condition of man] and [the status of the] sun and moon correspond to each other. Thus, when the moon is full, the waters of the sea are high in the west. At that time, man's blood and qi are pure and his muscles and flesh are filled. The skin is dense and the hair firm. Even if one encounters a robber-wind at this time, it will only penetrate the surface and is unable to invade deep into [the body]. During the new moon, however, the waters of the sea are hight in the east. At this time, man's blood and qi are depleted. The guardian qi leave [the body], the skin structures are open, the hair loses its deep roots. If at this time one should encounter a robber-wind, it will penetrate deep into the body, and that person will suffer from a sudden and violent illness.

3.c *Xú líng tāi xiān sheng yī shū quán jí* 1 徐靈胎先生醫書全集 (Yī xué yuán liú lùn 醫學源流論) Bìng yǒu guǐ shén lùn 病有鬼神論 On the Causation of Illnesses by Demons and Spirits

---

人之受邪也。必有受之之處。有以召之。則應者斯至矣。夫人精神完固。則外邪不敢犯。惟其所以禦之之具有虧。則侮之者斯集。凡疾病有爲鬼神所憑者。其愚魯者。以爲鬼神實能禍人。其明理者。以爲病情如此。必無鬼神。二者皆非也。夫鬼神。猶風寒暑濕之邪耳。衛氣虛。則受寒。榮氣虛。則受熱。神氣虛。則受鬼。蓋人之神屬陽。陽衰則鬼憑之。內經有五臟之病。則現五色之鬼。難經云。脫陽者見鬼。故經穴中有鬼牀、鬼室等穴。此諸穴者。皆賴神氣以充塞之。若神氣有虧。則鬼神得而憑之。猶之風寒之能傷人也。故治寒者。壯其陽。治熱者。養其陰。治鬼者。充其神而已。其或有因痰。因思。因驚者。則當求其本而治之。故明理之士。必事事窮其故。乃能無所惑而有據。否則執一端之見。而昧事理之實。均屬憒憒矣。其外更有觸犯鬼神之

病。則祈禱可愈。至於冤譴之鬼。則有數端。有自作之孽。深仇不可解者。有祖宗貽累者。有過誤害人者。其事皆鑿鑿可徵。似儒者所不道。然見於經史。如公子彭生。伯有之類甚多。目睹者亦不少。此則非藥石祈禱所能免矣。

召	zhāo	to call; to summon
固	gù	firm; strong
犯	fàn	to invade; to offend; to attack
禦	yù	to resist; to ward off
具	jù	tool; agent
虧	kuī	deficiency; fault
侮	wǔ	to insult; to attack
集	jí	to collect; to gather
憑	píng	to avail oneself of
魯	lǔ	stupid
禍	huò	calamity; to cause misery
情	qíng	facts; condition; feelings; emotions
榮	róng	used for 營 *yíng*, (military) camp
衰	shuāi	to decay; weak
現	xiàn	to manifest; become apparent
難經	Nàn-jīng	*Nan jing*; the "Classic of Difficult Issues" of the 1st c.CE
脫	tuō	to escape; to leave
牀	chuáng	a bed
室	shì	dwelling
等	děng	sign of plural
賴	lài	to rely upon; to need
塞	sāi	to stop up
猶	yóu	to compare
壯	zhuàng	to strengthen; to fill
痰	tán	phlegm

思	sī	to think; to ponder
驚	jìng	to startle; be terrified
本	běn	origin
士	shì	scholar
事事	shì shì	everything; in every respect
窮	qióng	to investigate thoroughly
惑	huò	to doubt
據	jù	to hold; according to; evidence
否	foǔ	if not
執	zhí	to hold
見	jiàn	view; perspective
昧	mèi	obscure; dark
均	jūn	all
憒憒	kuì kuì	confused
觸	chù	to run against; to offend; to attack
至於	zhì yú	as for
冤譴	yuān qiǎn	innocently blamed for some wrong
數	shù	numerous
自作孽	zì zuò niè	misfortune brought upon one by oneself
仇	chóu	to hate
解	jiě	to resolve
祖宗	zǔ zōng	ancestors
貽累	yí lèi	to involve
過	guò	error
誤	wù	to be mistaken
鑿鑿可徵	zuò zuò kě zhēng	indisputable evidence
似	sì	it seems
史	shǐ	history; historical accounts
公子彭生	gōng zǐ péng shēng	Gongzi Pengsheng; name of a courtier of Qi who was executed in 693 BCE and is said to have reappeared as a pig-shaped demon
伯有	bó yǒu	Bo You; another name of Liang Xiao, who was killed by Si Dai and returned as a demon to take revenge. The story is recorded in the Annals of the Spring and Autumn Period

類	lèi	class; sort; kind
甚	shèn	very
睹	dǔ	to observe
少	shǎo	few
免	miǎn	to expel

Rén zhī shòu xié yě. bì yǒu shòu zhī zhī chù. yǒu yǐ zhāo zhī. zé yìng zhě sī zhì yǐ. fū rén jīng shén wán gù. zé wài xié bù gǎn fàn. wéi qí suǒ yǐ yù zhī zhī jù yǒu kuī. zé wǔ zhī zhě sī jí. fán jí bìng yǒu wéi guǐ shén suǒ píng zhě. qí yú lǜ zhě. yǐ wéi guǐ shén shí néng huò rén. qí míng lǐ zhě. yǐ wéi bìng qíng rú cǐ. bì wú guǐ shén. èr zhě jiē fēi yě. fū guǐ shén. yóu fēng hán shǔ shī zhī xié ěr. wèi qì xū. zé shòu hán. róng qì xū. zé shòu rè. shén qì xū. zé shòu guǐ. gài rén zhī shén shǔ yáng. yáng shuāi zé guǐ píng zhī. nèi-jīng yǒu wǔ zàng zhī bìng. zé xiàn wǔ sè zhī guǐ. nàn-jīng yún. tuō yáng zhě jiàn guǐ. gù jīng xuè zhōng yǒu guǐ chuáng, guǐ shì děng xuè. cǐ zhū xuè zhě. jiē lài shén qì yǐ chōng sāi zhī. ruò shén qì yǒu kuī. zé guǐ shén dé ér píng zhī. yóu zhī fēng hán zhī néng shāng rén yě. gù zhì hán zhě. zhuàng qí yáng. zhì rè zhě. yǎng qí yīn. zhì guǐ zhě. chōng qí shén ér yǐ. qí huò yǒu yīn tán. yīn sī. yīn jìng zhě. zé dāng qiú qí běn ér zhì zhī. gù míng lǐ zhī shì. bì shì shì qióng qí gù. nǎi néng wú suǒ huò ér yǒu jù. foǔ zé zhí yì duān zhī jiàn. ér mèi shì lǐ zhī shí. jūn shǔ kuì kuì yǐ. qí wài gèng yǒu chù fàn guǐ shén zhī bìng. zé qí dǎo kě yù. zhì yú yuān qiān zhī guǐ. zé yǒu shù duān. yǒu zì zuò zhī niè. shēn chóu bù kě jiě zhě. yǒu zǔ zōng yí lèi zhě. yǒu guò wù hài rén zhě. qí shì jiē zuò zuò kě zhēng. sì rú zhě suǒ bù dào. rán jiàn yú jīng shǐ. rú gōng zǐ péng shēng bó yǒu zhī lèi shèn duō. mù dǔ zhě yì bù shǎo. cǐ zé fēi yào shí qí dǎo suǒ néng miǎn yǐ.

When a person receives evil [intruders in his body], there must be a place where they are granted entrance. [These evil intruders] have gone there because they responded to a summons! As long as a person's essence and spirits are complete and strong, no external evil will dare to offend [that person]. If, however, those agents that are responsible for warding off [evil intruders] fail to do so, those [intruders] attacking them will gather in their place. Whenever a disease can be traced to demon-spirits, ignorant [people] believe that demon-spirits are actually able to harm man, while those who understand the principles [of nature] believe that such diseases have definitely nothing to do with demon-spirits. Both are equally wrong. Demon-spirits are comparable to such evils as wind, cold, heat, and moisture. When the guardian qi are depleted, one absorbs cold. When the camp qi are depleted, one absorbs heat. When one's spirit-qi are depleted, one absorbs demons. Man's spirits belong to the yang [qi]. When one's yang [qi] are weak, demons avail themselves of [their location]. The *Nei jing* has [a passage stating that] in cases of diseases in the five depots, demons appear in the [respective] five colors. The *Nan jing* says: "Where the yang [qi] have left, one sees demons". Hence among the holes on the conduits are some bearing such [names] as "demons' bed" and "demons' dwelling". All these holes depend on [man's] spirit-qi to be stopped up and filled. Once there is a depletion of spirit-qi, the demon-spirits will be able to avail themselves [of the position of the spirit-qi]. That may be compared to the harm caused to man by wind or cold. In treating cases of cold, one strengthens the respective [patient's] yang [qi]. In treating cases of heat, one nourishes the respective [patient's] yin [qi]. In treating cases of demon [intrusion], one simply has to fill the respective [patient's] spirits. In cases where [a disease] is caused by phlegm or by [excessive] pondering or by someone's being terrified, one must search for the origin [of the affliction] and then treat it. Hence those scholars who understand the principles [of life] will take all circumstances into account and conduct a thorough investigation of the cause of a particular [illness]. Only then can they eliminate all doubt and have evidence [at their hands]. Those who fail [to conduct such thorough investigations] will stick to one-sided perspectives, and the reality of the facts and principles involved will remain obscure to them. All these cases belong to the category of confusion. In addition [to what I have outlined so far], there are illnesses [that result from one's own having] offended demon-spirits. [Such illnesses] can be cured by prayers. Furthermore, there are numerous reasons for demons [to seek revenge for] some wrong [they had been subjected to while they were still humans. Patients succumbing to illnesses caused by these demons] may have brought their misfortune upon themselves [by creating] hatred so deep [in someone else who is a demon now] that it cannot be dissolved. In other cases, [the original offense] may have been related to [the patient's] ancestors, and it may also be that oneself has inadvertently caused harm to someone else [who seeks revenge as a demon now]. For all such occurrences indisputable proof exists. It seems, though, as if the Confucians did not accept this as their doctrine. However, both in the [Confucian] classics and in the historical records one can see very many examples, such as those of Gongzi Pengsheng and of Bo You. Also, [I myself have] witnessed not a few such [occurrences] with [my own] eyes. These [demons] can be expelled neither by [herbal] drugs and minerals, nor by prayers.

3.d *Shǐ jì* 105 史記
Biǎn què cāng gōng liè zhuàn
扁鵲倉公列傳
The Biographies of Bian Que and Cang Gong

扁鵲過齊。齊桓侯客之。入朝見曰。君有疾。在腠理。不治將深。桓侯曰。寡人無疾。扁鵲出。桓侯謂左右曰。醫之好利也。欲以不疾者爲功。後五日。扁鵲復見。曰。君有疾。在血脈。不治恐深。桓侯曰。寡人無疾。扁鵲出。桓侯不悦。後五日。扁鵲復見。曰。君有疾。在腸胃間。不治將深。桓侯不應。扁鵲出。桓侯不悦。後五日。扁鵲復見。望見桓侯而退走。桓侯使人問其故。扁鵲曰。疾之居腠理也。湯熨之所及也。在血脈。鍼石之所及也。其在腸胃。酒醪之所及也。其在骨髓。雖司命無奈之何。今在骨髓。臣是以無請也。後五日。桓侯體病。使人召扁鵲。扁鵲已逃去。桓侯遂死。

過	guò	to pass by; to pass through
齊	qí	the state of Qi
桓侯	huán hōu	Marquis Huan
客	kè	visitor; guest
朝	cháo	the court

朝見	cháo jiàn	to have audience at the court
君	jūn	ruler; term to address a superior
寡	guǎ	a term of depreciation used by princes of themselves
左右	zuǒ yòu	those to the left and right; an entourage
利	lì	gain; profit
欲	yù	to desire; to wish
血脈	xuě mài	the blood vessels
恐	kǒng	to fear
悅	yuè	pleased; happy
應	yìng	to respond
望	wàng	to look at (from a distance)
退	tuì	to withdraw
湯	tāng	hot water; hot baths
熨	yùn	to iron; to apply hot pressure
醪	láo	the lees of wine; wine
髓	suǐ	marrow
無奈之何	wú nài zhī hé	nothing can be done
臣	chén	your subject; used for "I" when addressing a superior
是以	shì yǐ	therefore; same as 以是 *yǐ shì*
逃	táo	to flee; to escape
去	qù	to leave

Biǎn què guò qí. qí huán hōu kè zhī. rù cháo jiàn yuē. jūn yǒu jí. zài còu lǐ. bù zhì jiāng shēn. huán hōu yuē. guǎ rén wú jí. biǎn què chū. huán hōu wèi zuǒ yòu yuē. yī zhī hào lì yě. yù yǐ bù jí zhě wéi gōng. hòu wǔ rì. biǎn què fù jiàn. yuē. jūn yǒu jí. zài xuě mài. bù zhì kǒng shēn. huán hōu yuē. guǎ rén wú jí. biǎn què chū. huán hōu bù yuè. hòu wǔ rì. biǎn què fù jiàn. yuē. jūn yǒu jí. zài cháng wèi jiān. bù zhì jiāng shēn. huán hōu bù yìng. biǎn què chū. huán hōu bù yuè. hòu wǔ rì. biǎn què fù jiàn. wàng jiàn huán hōu ér tuì zǒu. huán hōu shǐ rén wèn qí gù. biǎn què yuē. jí zhī jū còu lǐ yě. tāng yùn zhī suǒ jí yě. zài xuě mài. zhēn shí zhī suǒ jí yě. qí zài cháng wèi. jiǔ láo zhī suǒ jí yě. qí zài gǔ suǐ. suī sī mìng wú nài zhī hé. jīn zài gǔ suǐ. chén shì yǐ wú qǐng yě. hòu wǔ rì. huán hōu tǐ bìng. shǐ rén zhāo biǎn què. biǎn què yǐ táo qù. huán hōu suí sǐ.

Bian Que passed through Qi, and Marquis Huan of Qi treated him as his guest. When [Bian Que] went to court to have an audience [with the Marquis], he said upon seeing him: "Sir, you have a disease which is located in the skin structures. If it is not cured now, it will penetrate more deeply." Marquis Huan replied: "I have no disease." After Bian Que had left, Marquis Huan said to those around him: "This is [an example of] the physicians' fondness of profits. They prefer to treat those who are not ill in order to achieve a success!" Five days later, Bian Que returned to see [the Marquis]. He told him: "Sir, your disease is in the blood vessels. If it is not cured now, it may penetrate more deeply." Marquis Huan replied: "I have no disease." After Bian Que had left, Marquis Huan felt unhappy. Five days later, Bian Que returned again to see [the Marquis], and he told him: "Sir, your disease is in the region of your intestines and stomach. If it is not cured now, it will penetrate more deeply." Marquis Huan did not respond. After Bian Que had left, Marquis Huang felt unhappy. Five days later, Bian Que returned another time to see [the Marquis]. He looked at him from a distance and went away. Marquis Huan sent someone after [Bian Que] to ask him for his reasons, and Bian Que told him: "When a disease is located in the skin structures, it can be reached by hot baths and hot pressure. When it is located in the blood vessels, it can be reached by needles and [pointed] stones. When it is located in the intestines or in the stomach, it can be reached with [medicinal] wines. But when it is located in the marrow of the bones, even [the spirit] who controls fate can no longer do anything about it. [In the case of Marquis Huan] now, [the disease] is located in the marrow of the bones. I preferred, therefore, not to ask [for an audience]." Five days later Marquis Huan's body became ill. He sent someone out to summon Bian Que. Bian Que had fled already. Subsequently, Marquis Huan died.

3.e *Sān yīn jí yī bìng zhèng fāng lùn* 2
三因極一病證方論
Sān yīn lùn 三因論
On the Three Causes [of Illness]

夫人稟天地陰陽而生者。蓋天有六氣。人以三陰三陽而上奉之。地有五行。人以五臟五腑而下應之。於是資生皮肉筋骨。精髓血脈。四肢九竅。毛髮齒牙唇舌。總而成體。外則氣血循環。流注經絡。喜傷六淫。內則精神魂魄。志意憂思。喜傷七情。六淫者。寒暑燥濕風熱是也。七情者。喜怒憂思悲恐驚是也。若將護得宜。怡然安泰。役冒非理。百痾生焉。病症既成。須尋所自。故前哲示教。謂之病源。經不云乎。治之極於一者因得之。閉戶塞牖。繫之病者。數問其經。以從其意。是欲知致病之本也。然六淫。天之常氣。冒之則先自經絡流入。內合于藏府。爲外所因。七情。人之常性。動之則先自藏府鬱發。外形於肢體。爲內所因。其如飲食饑飽。叫呼傷氣。盡神度量。疲極筋力。陰陽違逆。乃至虎狼毒蟲。金瘡踒折。疰忤附著。畏壓溺等。有背常理。爲不內外因。

奉	fèng	to receive; to pay tribute to; to support
五行	wǔ xíng	the five agents; five interrelated categories of all phenomena in existence
舌	shé	the tongue
總	zǒng	to sum up; all
成	chéng	to constitute
環	huán	a ring; to encircle
注	zhù	to flow
喜	xǐ	to tend to
淫	yín	excess; excessive
志	zhì	the mind
志意	zhìyì	thought
憂	yōu	grief
憂思	yōu sì	concern
燥	zào	dry; dryness
悲	bēi	mourning
驚	jìng	fright; terror
將	jiāng	to intend
護	hù	to protect; to preserve
怡然	yí rán	happy; harmonious
安泰	ān tài	peaceful; undisturbed
役	yì	to indulge in; to employ
冒	mào	risky; false; to neglect what is right
百	bǎi	hundred; many; all
痾	ē	ailment
焉	yān	final affirmative
症	zhèng	illness; evidence of disease
尋	xún	to search for
哲	zhé	wise
極	jí	to treat exhaustively
牖	yǒu	window
繫	jì	to bind; to be attached to
數	shuò	often; again and again
經	jīng	daily pursuits

意	yì	meaning
性	xìng	nature; disposition
動	dòng	to set in motion; to excite
鬱發	yù fā	to set free
形	xíng	to take shape
飲	yǐn	to drink; beverages
叫呼	jiào hū	to shout
盡	jìn	to exhaust
度量	dù liàng	capacity
疲	pí	tired; weary; exhausted
違逆	wéi nì	to oppose
虎	hǔ	tiger
狼	láng	wolf
蟲	chóng	worms; insects; bugs
金	jīn	metal
瘡	chuāng	a wound
踒	wō	to slip; to sprain
折	zhé	to break in two
疰	zhù	possession (by demons)
忤	wǔ	hostile
附著	fùzhuó	possession (by demons)
畏	wèi	to die a violent death
壓	yā	to be killed by a falling wall
溺	nì	to drown
背	bèi	to turn one's back against; to stand in contrast to

Fū rén bǐng tiān dì yīn yáng ér shēng zhě. gài tiān yǒu liù qì. rén yǐ sān yīn sān yáng ér shàng fèng zhī. dì yǒu wǔ xíng. rén yǐ wǔ zàng wǔ fǔ ér xià yìng zhī. yú shī zī shēng pí ròu jīn gǔ. jīng suǐ xuě mài. sì zhī jiǔ qiào. máo fà chǐ yá chún shé. zǒng ér chéng tǐ. wài zé qì xuě xūn huán. liú zhù jīng luò. xǐ shāng liù yín. nèi zé jīng shén hún pò. zhì yì yōu sī. xǐ shāng qī qíng. liù yín zhě. hán shǔ zào shī fēng rè shī yě. qī qíng zhě. xǐ nù yōu sī bēi kǒng jìng shī yě. ruò jiāng hù dé yí. yí rán ān tài. yì mào fēi lǐ. bǎi ē shēng yān. bìng zhèng jì chéng. xū xún suǒ zì. gù qián zhé shì jiào. wèi zhī bìng yuán. jīng bù yún hū. zhì zhī jí yú yī zhě yīn dé zhī. bì hù sāi yǒu. jì zhī bìng zhě. shuò wèn qí jīng. yǐ cóng qí yì. shī yù zhī zhì bìng zhī běn yě. rán liù yín. tiān zhī cháng qì. mào zhī zé xiān zì jīng luò liú rù. nèi hé yú zàng fǔ. wéi wài suǒ yīn. qī qíng. rén zhī cháng xìng. dòng zhī zé xiān zì zàng fǔ yù fā. wài xíng yú zhī tǐ. wéi nèi suǒ yīn. qí rú yǐn shí jī bǎo. jiào hū shāng qì. jìn shén dù liàng. pí jí jīn lì. yīn yáng wéi nì. nǎi zhì hǔ láng dú chóng. jīn chuāng wō zhé. zhù wǔ fù zhuó. wèi yā nì děng. yǒu bèi cháng lǐ. wéi bù nèi wài yīn.

[The fact] that man lives because he receives the yin and yang [qi] of heaven and earth [may be explained as follows]. Heaven has the six qi, and man with his three yin and yang [conduits] pays tribute to [heaven] above. The earth has the five agents, and man with his five depots and five palaces corresponds to them below. Based on these provisions grow his skin and his flesh, his sinews and his bones, his essence and his marrow, the blood vessels and the four extremities, the nine orifices, and the hair, the teeth, the lips, and the tongue. Together all of this constitutes the body. In the external [parts of the body], the [guardian] qi and the blood flow through the conduits and network [vessels] in a circulatory course. They tend to be harmed by the six excesses. In the interior [of the body reside] the essence and the spirit, the *hun* and the *po*, thought, and concern. They tend to be harmed by the seven affects. The six excesses are cold, summer-heat, dryness, moisture, wind, and heat. The seven affects are joy, anger, grief and pensiveness, mourning, fear, and fright. If one, in his efforts to preserve [his health], pursues a suitable [way of life, he will, as a result,] be happy and remain free from any disturbances. If, [however, one leads a] risky [life that] is not in accordance with the principles [of nature], all possible ailments may emerge as a consequence. Once the symptoms of a disease have become manifest, one must search for their origin. Hence the wise [men] of former times spoke, in their teachings, of the sources of diseases. And does not the classic state: "Those treatments that deal with one [disease] exhaustively will, therefore, be successful. Those who close the door and shut the windows, and tie themselves to the patients, they repeatedly consult his daily pursuits to follow his thoughts."[1] This is so because they wish to recognize in all respects the origin from which a [particular] disease has resulted! However, the six excesses are ordinary qi of heaven. If one fails to care about [their assimilation in correct proportions], they will flow into [the body] starting from the conduits and network [vessels, and, then,] unite internally in the depots and palaces. They are causes [of disease] that have come from outside. The seven affects are ordinary [attributes of] human nature. If one excites them, they will be set free first in the depots and palaces, and [then] they will take shape externally in [the appearance of man's] limbs and body. These are causes [of disease] that have come from inside. [Such factors contributing to disease as] food and beverages, hunger and overeating, shouting [to an extent that] harms the qi [of the lung], complete exhaustion of one's spirit, extreme fatigue of one's sinews, violations of [the correct ways of intercourse of] yin and yang, up to [injuries caused by] tigers, wolves, and poisonous bugs, wounds caused by metal [weapons], fractures resulting from falls, possession by hostile [forces], possession [by evil demons], death through violence, death through a falling wall, drowning, and further such [factors] in contrast to the normal principles [of life], they constitute neither internal nor external causes [of disease].

Note

[1] This is a quote from *Huang Di nei jing, Su wen*, 13.

3.f *Huáng dì nèi jīng, Sù wèn* 2
黃帝內經·素問
Sì qì tiáo shén dà lùn
四氣調神大論
Comprehensive Treatise on the Regulation of the Spirit in Accord with the Four Seasons

---

春三月。此謂發陳。天地俱生。萬物以榮。夜臥早起。廣步於庭。被髮緩形。以使志生。生而勿殺。予而勿奪。賞而勿罰。此春氣之應。養生之道也。逆之則傷肝。夏爲寒變。奉長者少。夏三月。此謂蕃秀。天地氣交。萬物華實。夜臥早起。無厭於日。使志無怒。使華英成秀。使氣得泄。若所愛在外。此夏氣之應。養長之道也。逆之則傷心。秋爲痎瘧。奉收者少。冬至重病。秋三月。此謂容平。天氣以急。地氣以明。早臥早起。與鷄俱興。使志安寧。以緩秋刑。收斂神氣。使秋氣平。無外其志。使肺氣清。此秋氣之應。養收之道也。逆之則傷肺。冬爲飧泄。奉藏者少。冬三月。此謂閉藏。水冰地坼。無擾乎陽。早臥晚起。必待日光。使志若伏若匿。若有私意。若已有得。去寒就溫。無泄皮膚。使氣亟

奪。此冬氣之應。養藏之道也。逆之則傷腎。春爲痿厥。奉生者少。

春	chūn	spring
陳	chén	to spread out
榮	róng	to flourish
早	zǎo	early
步	bù	a step; stride
庭	tíng	court; hall
被髮	pī fà	the hair hanging dishevelled down the back
勿	wù	a negative; not; do not
予	yǔ	to grant; to give
奪	duó	to take away
賞	shǎng	to reward; to praise
罰	fá	to punish
蕃	fán	opulence
秀	xiù	blossoming; luxuriance
華	huá	to bloom
厭	yàn	to be wearied with; satiated
華英	huá yīng	beauty; splendor
泄	xiè	to flow away
愛	ài	to love
秋	qiū	autumn
痎	jiē	*jie*, an ancient term for a disease unidentifiable today
瘧	nüè	malaria
冬至	dōng zhì	winter solstice
容	róng	to take in; to harvest; to gather
平	píng	balance
鷄	jī	chicken; fowl
俱	jù	together with
興	xīng	to rise
寧	níng	tranquil

緩	huǎn	to temper
收斂	shōu liàn	to collect
飧	sūn	a meal; food
藏	cáng	to store
冰	bīng	to freeze
坼	chè	to break open
擾	rǎo	to disturb
光	guāng	to shine
伏	fú	to hide; hidden
匿	nì	to shut in
私	sī	secret
就	jiù	to approach; to seek
亟	jí	fast; quickly
痿	wěi	limpness
厥	jué	receding [qi]

Chūn sān yuè. cǐ wèi fā chén. tiān dì jù shēng. wàn wù yǐ róng. yè wò zǎo qǐ. guǎng bù yú tíng. Pī fà huǎn xíng. yǐ shǐ zhì shēng. shēng ér wù shā. yǔ ér wù duó. shǎng ér wù fá. cǐ chūn qì zhī yìng. yǎng shēng zhī dào yě. nì zhī zé shāng gān. xià wéi hán biàn. fèng zhǎng zhě shǎo. xià sān yuè. cǐ wèi fán xiù. tiān dì qì jiāo. wàn wù huá shí. yè wò zǎo qǐ. wú yàn yú rì. shǐ zhì wú nù. shǐ huá yīng chéng xiù. shǐ qì dé xiè. ruò suǒ ài zài wài. cǐ xià qì zhī yìng. yǎng zhǎng zhī dào yě. nì zhī zé shāng xīn. qiū wéi jiē nüè. fèng shōu zhě shǎo. dōng zhì zhòng bìng. qiū sān yuè. cǐ wèi róng píng. tiān qì yǐ jí. dì qì yǐ míng. zǎo wò zǎo qǐ. yǔ jījù xīng. shǐ zhì ān níng. yǐ huǎn qiū xíng. shōu liàn shén qì. shǐ qiū qì píng. wú wài qí zhì. shǐ fèi qì qīng. cǐ qiū qì zhī yìng. yǎng shōu zhī dào yě. nì zhī zé shāng fèi. dōng wéi sūn xiè. fèng cáng zhě shǎo. dōng sān yuè. cǐ wèi bì cáng. shuǐ bīng dì chè. wú rǎo hū yáng. zǎo wò wǎn qǐ. bì dái rì guāng. shǐ zhì ruò fú ruò nì. ruò yǒu sī yì. ruò yǐ yǒu dé. qù hán jiù wēn. wú xiè pí fū. shǐ qì jí duó. cǐ dōng qì zhī yìng. yǎng cáng zhī dào yě. nì zhī zé shāng shèn. chūn wéi wěi jué. fèng shēng zhě shǎo.

The three months of spring, they denote effusion and spreading. In heaven and earth everything comes to life; the myriad beings flourish. Go to rest late at night and rise early. Move through the courtyard with long strides. Dishevel the hair and relax the physical appearance, thereby cause the mind to come to life. Generate and do not kill. Give and do not take. Reward and do not punish. This is the correspondence with the qi of spring and it is the Way to nourish life. Opposing it harms the liver. In summer, this causes changes to cold, and there is little to support growth.

The three months of summer, they denote opulence and blossoming. The qi of heaven and earth interact and the myriad beings bloom and bear fruit. Go to rest late at night and rise early. Never get enough of the sun. Let the mind have no anger. Stimulate beauty and have your elegance perfected. Cause the qi to flow away, as if that what you loved were located outside. This is correspondence with the qi of summer and it is the Way to nourish growth. Opposing it harms the heart. In autumn this causes *jie* and *malaria*, and there is little to support gathering. Multiple diseases [develop] at winter solstice.

The three months of autumn, they denote harvest and balance. The qi of heaven becomes tense. The qi of the earth becomes clear. Go to rest early and rise early, get up together with the chicken. Let the mind be peaceful and tranquil, so as to temper the punishment carried out in autumn. Collect the spirit qi and cause the autumn qi to be balanced. Do not direct your mind to the outside and cause the lung qi to be clear. This is correspondence with the qi of autumn and it is the Way to nourish gathering. Opposing it harms the lung. In winter this causes outflow of [undigested] food and there is little to support storage.

The three months of winter, they denote securing and storing. The water is frozen and the earth breaks open. Do not disturb the yang [qi]! Go to rest early and rise late. You must wait for the sun to shine. Let the mind enter a state as if hidden, as if shut in, as if you had secret intentions; as if you already had made a gain. Avoid cold and seek warmth and do not [allow sweat] to flow away through the skin. This would cause the qi to be carried away quickly. This is correspondence with the qi of winter and it is the Way of nourishing storage. Opposing it harms the kidneys. In spring this causes limpness with receding [qi], and there is little to support generation.

Lesson Four

Specific Illnesses and Diseases

For centuries if not millennia prior to the creation of the medicine of systematic correspondence beginning with the second and first centuries BCE, Chinese physicians had observed epidemics affecting many people at the same time, and they had become aware of identical illnesses in large numbers of individuals displaying identical symptoms over time. Thus, a concept of disease emerged, including ontological concepts of pathogenic agents – such as demons and "bugs" – entering the human body and causing more or less well-defined destruction there. Notions of an inheritance of a disease, as well as concepts of infection constitute integrated facets of this concept of disease. The pathogenic factor documented in Chinese medical history longer and with more emphasis than any other was the "wind". Originally perceived as a spirit, it changed into a natural phenomenon activated by a spirit, and, finally, into a natural phenomenon in its own right. Wind, either alone or in conjunction with further natural factors such as cold or dampness, was thought to cause a variety of illnesses and diseases, including *bi* 痺, "blockage", an example of a pathological concept that has no counterpart in modern medicine, and leprosy, an example of a transculturally valid nosological fact. The medicine of systematic correspondence excluded demons and bugs from its etiology, identifying only climatic factors as external and affects as internal causes of ailments. The notion of diseases caused by demons and bugs was continued in the pharmaceutical tradition of the social elite, as well as in folk medicine. The medicine of systematic correspondence suggested an individualistic understanding of illness. That is, any human being falling ill has his or her own reasons for succumbing, and his or her illness takes a specific course in the organism that is paralleled by the illness of another organism only by chance.

Key Terms Introduced in Lesson Four

痺	bì	the disease "blockage"
疼	téng	pain

痛	tòng	pain
屈	qū	to crouch; to bend down
小便	xiǎo biàn	urine
嗌	yì	the throat
噫	yì	to belch
咳	ké	to cough
嘔	ǒu	to vomit
脹	zhàng	to swell up
正方	zhèng fāng	prescription for a [manual] correction [treatment]
涎	xián	saliva
瘀血	yū xuě	stagnating blood
臌	gǔ	bloating
膈	gé	blockage
中	zhōng	the center (of the body)
脝	hēng	fat; bloated
滿	mǎn	swollen
下	xià	to purge
補	bǔ	to supplement
尅化	kè huà	to digest
矢	shǐ	ordure; droppings
臂	bì	an arm
凸	tū	protruding
手心	shǒu xīn	the center of the hand; palm
反胃	fǎn wèi	a stomach that turns back (the food it receives)
腫	zhǒng	to swell; a swelling
分肉	fēn ròu	the partings of the flesh
利	lì	free passage
膹 XXX	fèn chēn	swollen
瘀	yū	to stagnate
縮	suō	to shrink
膿	nóng	pus
眉	méi	the eyebrows
痹	bì	lame; paralyzed; limpness

趾	zhǐ	the toes
癢	yǎng	to itch
瘸	qué	lame; deformation
癟	biě	shrivelled
痠	suān	aching of the limbs
疙瘩	gē da	knots
傳染	chuán rǎn	to be affected [by a disease] through transmission [from someone else]
毒	dú	poison
蠱	gǔ	the *gu*(-spirit)
感冒	gǎn mào	to be affected by adverse (climatic qi)
積鬱	jī yù	accumulation
瘧	nüè	malaria
頷	hán	the jaws
腰	yāo	the lower back
陽明	yáng míng	the yang-brilliance (conduit)
巨陽	jù yáng	the great-yang (conduit)
項	xiàng	the neck
風府	fēng fǔ	the wind palace
膂	lǚ	the spinal column
骶骨	dǐ gǔ	the sacrum
缺盆	quē pén	the broken basic
募原	mù yuán	the membrane plain (alternative writing: 膜原)
傷寒	shāng hán	harm caused by cold
觸冒	chù mào	to get into touch with, as with something potentially dangerous; to be affected
時行氣	shí xíng qì	seasonally prevalent (harmful) qi
[心] 胞絡	[xīn]bāo luò	the [heart] enclosing network
乘	chéng	to seize; to avail oneself of
煩	fán	to feel distressed
脉（=脈）	mài	the [movement in the] vessels
洪	hóng	vast
瀉	xiè	to drain
虛	xū	to deplete
實	shí	to replenish

4.a *Zhū bìng yuán hòu lùn* 1
諸病源候論
Fēng bì hòu 風痺候
Symptoms of Blockage [Caused by] Wind

痺者。風寒濕三氣雜至。合而成痺。其狀。肌肉頑厚。或疼痛。由人體虛。腠理開。故受風邪也。病在陽曰風。在陰曰痺。陰陽俱病。曰風痺。其以春遇痺爲筋痺。則筋屈。筋痺不已。又遇邪者。則移入肝。其狀。夜臥則驚。飲多。小便數。夏遇痺者爲脈痺。則血凝不流。令人萎黃。脈痺不已。又遇邪者。則移入心。其狀。心下鼓。氣暴上逆。喘不通。嗌乾喜噫。長夏遇痺者爲肌痺。在肉則不仁。肌痺不已。復遇邪者。則移入脾。其狀。四肢懈惰。發咳嘔汁。秋遇痹者爲皮痹。則皮膚無所知。皮痺不已。又遇邪者。則移入於肺。其狀氣奔痛。冬遇痹者爲骨痹。則骨重不可舉。不隨而痛。骨痺不已。又遇邪者。則移入於腎。其狀喜脹。診其脈大而澀者。爲痺。脈來急者。爲痺。其湯熨鍼石。別有正方。

痺	bì	the disease "blockage"
雜	zá	mixed; confused
頑	wán	heavy; clumsy
或	huò	occasionally; in some cases
疼	téng	pain
痛	tòng	pain
屈	qū	to crouch; to bend down
已	yǐ	to come to an end; to heal
移	yí	to change residence; to move
小便	xiǎo biàn	urine
萎	wěi	to wither; to dry out
鼓	gǔ	drum
嗌	yì	the throat
乾	gān	dry
噫	yì	to belch
長夏	cháng xià	late summer
不仁	bù rén	numb; insensitivity
懈惰	xiè duò	idle; lame
咳	ké	to cough
嘔	ǒu	to vomit
奔	bēn	to run; to be in a hurry
脹	zhàng	to swell up
澀	sè	rough
正方	zhèng fāng	prescription for a [manual] correction [treatment]

Bì zhě. fēng hán shī sān qì zá zhì. hé ér chéng bì. qí zhuàng. jī ròu wán hòu. huò téng tòng. yóu rén tǐ xū. còu lǐ kāi. gù shòu fēng xié yě. bìng zài yáng yuē fēng. zài yīn yuē bì. yīn yáng jù bìng. yuē fēng bì. qí yǐ chūn yù bì wéi jīn bì. zé jīn qū. jīn bì bù yǐ. yòu yù xié zhě. zé yí rù gān. qí zhuàng. yè wò zé jìng. yǐn duō. xiǎo biàn shuò. xià yù bì zhě wéi mài bì. zé xuě níng bù liú. lìng rén wěi huáng. mài bì bù yǐ. yòu yù xié zhě. zé yí rù xīn. qí zhuàng. xīn xià gǔ. qì bào shàng nì. chuǎn bù tōng. yì gān xǐ yì. cháng xià yù bì zhě wéi jī bì. zài ròu zé bù rén. jī bì bù yǐ. fù yù xié zhě. zé yí rù pí. qí zhuàng. sì zhī xiè duò. fā ké ǒu zhī. qiū yù bì zhě wéi pí bì. zé pí fū wú suǒ zhī. pí bì bù yǐ. yòu yù xié zhě. zé yí rù yú fèi. qí zhuàng qì bēn tòng. dōng yù bì zhě wéi gǔ bì. zé gǔ zhòng bù kě jǔ. bù suí ér tòng. gǔ bì bù yǐ. yòu yù xié zhě. zé yí rù yú shèn. qí zhuàng xǐ zhàng. zhěn qí mài dà ér sè zhě. wéi bì. mài lái jí zhě. wéi bì. qí tāng yùn zhēn shí. bié yǒu zhèng fāng.

In case of a *blockage*, the three qi wind, cold, and dampness arrive together [in the body where they] unite and constitute blockage. Its appearance is such that the muscles and the flesh turn clumsy and thick. Occasionally, one may feel pain. The human body may receive wind-evil if the skin structures have opened because [the body is marked by] depletion. When the disease affects the yang [regions of the organism], it is called "wind"; if it affects the yin [regions], it is called "blockage". If both the yin and the yang [regions are affected by such an] illness, one speaks of a "wind-blockage". If one encounters a blockage during spring, it will be a sinews-blockage. In this case then, the sinews are bent. If one encounters additional evil before the sinews-blockage has ended, [the disease] will move into the liver. Its appearance then is such that one is scared in bed at night. One drinks a lot and urinates frequently. If one encounters a blockage during summer, it will be a vessel-blockage. In this case then, the blood will be blocked and cannot flow, which causes the person [afflicted] to dry out and turn yellow. If one encounters additional evil before the vessel-blockage has ended, [the disease] will move into the heart. Its appearance then is such that drumming qi from below the heart violently move upwards. They move contrary to their proper direction, one pants, and [the qi ascending] cannot pass through freely. The throat dries out and one is likely to belch. If one encounters a blockage in late summer, it will be a muscle-blockage. The flesh turns numb. If one encounters evil again, before the muscle-blockage has ended, [the disease] will move into the spleen. Its appearance then is such that the four limbs become lame. One develops cough and vomits juice[-like liquid]. If one encounters a blockage during autumn, it will be a skin-blockage. In this case then, the skin will be numb. If one encounters additional [wind] evil before the skin-blockage has ended, [the disease] will move into the lung. Its appearance then is such that one's [breathing] qi run wildly and cause pain. If one encounters a blockage during winter, it will be a bone-blockage. In this case then, the bones will be heavy and cannot be raised. They do not follow [one's orders] and are in pain. If one encounters additional evil before the bone-blockage has ended, [the disease] will move into the kidneys. Its appearance then is such that one is likely to swell up. If an examination of the [movement in the] vessels of such [a patient reveals a] strong and rough [movement] it is a blockage. If [the movement in] the vessels arrives tense, [this, too, indicates a] blockage. In addition to its [therapy by means of] hot baths, hot pressure, needles, and stones, there is also a prescription for a [manual] correction [treatment].

4.b *Xú líng tāi xiān sheng yī shū quán jí, juan* 1.2 徐靈胎先生醫書全集 (*Yī xué yuán liú lùn* 醫學源流論) Gǔ gé lùn 臌膈論 On Bloating and Blockage

臌膈同爲極大之病。然臌可治。而膈不可治。蓋臌者。有物積中。其症屬實。膈者。不能納物。其症屬虛。實者可治。虛者不可治。此其常也。臌之爲病。因腸胃衰弱。不能運化。或痰或血。或氣或食。凝結於中。以致臌脝脹滿。治之當先下其結聚。然後補養其中氣。則腸胃漸能尅化矣。內經有雞矢醴方。即治法也。後世治臌之方。亦多見效。惟臟氣已絕。臂細臍凸。手心及背平滿。青筋繞腹。種種惡症齊現。則不治。若膈症。乃肝火犯胃。木來侮土。謂之賊邪。胃脘枯槁。不復用事。惟留一綫細竅。又爲痰涎瘀血閉塞。飲食不能下達。即勉强納食。仍復吐出。蓋人生全在飲食。經云。穀入於胃。以傳于肺。五臟六腑。皆以受氣。今食既不入。則五臟六腑皆竭矣。所以得此症者。能少納穀。則不出一年而死。全不納穀。則不出半年而死。凡春得病者。死于秋。秋得病者。死于春。蓋金木相尅之時也。又有卒然嘔吐。或嘔吐而時止時發。又或年當少壯。是名反胃。非膈也。此亦可治。至于類臌之症。如浮腫水腫之類。或宜針灸。或宜洩瀉。病象各殊。治亦萬變。醫者亦宜廣求諸法。而隨宜施用也。

臌	gǔ	bloating
膈	gé	blockage
大	dà	strong; serious
症	zhèng	a pathological condition; patho-condition
中	zhōng	the center (of the body)
納	nà	to receive; to ingest; to consume (food)
運	yùn	to move
脝	hēng	fat; bloated
滿	măn	swollen
下	xià	to purge
補	bǔ	to supplement
尅	kè	to destroy
尅化	kè huà	to digest
矢	shǐ	ordure; droppings
法	fă	method
效	xiào	effect
絕	jué	to cut off
臂	bì	an arm
細	xì	fine; emaciated
凸	tū	protruding
手心	shǒu xīn	the center of the hand; palm
平	píng	equally; both
青	qīng	blue
繞	rào	to wind around
種	zhǒng	species; kind
種種	zhǒng zhǒng	all kinds; all types

齊	qí	all alike
土	tǔ	soil
枯槁	kū gǎo	to wither; to dry out
用事	yòng shì	to perform functions
綫	xiàn	a thread
涎	xián	saliva
瘀血	yū xuě	stagnating blood
達	dá	to reach to; to pass through
勉强	miǎn qiáng	to force; to compel
仍	réng	yet; still
吐	tù	to vomit
全	quán	entirely; completely
在	zài	to depend on
于	yú	in; at; with
既	jì	already
竭	jiē	to exhaust; exhausted
所以	suǒ yǐ	therefore
出	chū	to elapse; to pass
半	bàn	half
卒然	cù rán	suddenly
止	zhǐ	to halt; to stop
反胃	fǎn wèi	a stomach that turns back (the food it receives)
類	lèi	similar
浮	fú	to float; surface
腫	zhǒng	to swell; a swelling
洩瀉	xiè xiè	to drain off; to purge
象	xiàng	image; reflection
殊	shū	different
宜	yí	ought; should
施用	shī yòng	to put into use; to make use of

Gǔ gé tóng wéi jí dà zhī bìng. rán gǔ kě zhì. ér gé bù kě zhì. gài gǔ zhě. yǒu wù jī zhōng. qí zhèng shǔ shí. gé zhě. bù néng nà wù. qí zhèng shǔ xū. shí zhě kě zhì. xū zhě bù kě zhì. cǐ qí cháng yě. gǔ zhī wéi bìng. yīn cháng wèi shuāi ruò.

bù néng yùn huà. huò tán huò xuě. huò qì huò shí. níng jié yú zhōng. yǐ zhì gǔ hēng zhàng mǎn. zhì zhī dāng xiān xià qí jié jù. rán hòu bǔ yǎng qí zhōng qì. zé cháng wèi jiàn néng kè huà yǐ. nèi-jīng yǒu jī shǐ lǐ fāng. jí zhì fǎ yě. hòu shì zhì gǔ zhī fāng. yì duō jiàn xiào. wéi zàng qì yǐ jué. bì xì qí tū. shǒu xīn jí bèi píng mǎn. qīng jīn rào fù. zhǒng zhǒng è zhèng qí xiàn. zé bù zhì. ruò gé zhèng. nǎi gān huǒ fàn wèi. mù lái wǔ tǔ. wèi zhī zèi xié. wèi wǎn kū gǎo. bù fù yòng shì. wéi liú yí xiàn xì qiào. yòu wéi tán xián yū xuě bì sāi. yǐn shí bù néng xià dá. jí miǎn qiáng nà shí. réng fù tù chū. gài rén shēng quán zài yǐn shí. jīng yún. gǔ rù yú wèi. yǐ chuán yú fèi. wǔ zàng liù fǔ. jiē yǐ shòu qì. jīn shí jì bù rù. zé wǔ zàng liù fǔ jiē jiē yǐ. suǒ yǐ dé cǐ zhèng zhě. néng shǎo nà gǔ. zé bù chū yì nián ér sǐ. quán bù nà gǔ. zé bù chū bàn nián ér sǐ. fán chūn dé bìng zhě. sǐ yú qiū. qiū dé bìng zhě. sǐ yú chūn. gài jīn mù xiāng kè zhī shí yě. yòu yǒu cù rán ǒu tù. huò ǒu tù ér shí zhǐ shí fā. yòu huò nián dāng shào zhuàng. shī míng fǎn wèi. fēi gé yě. cǐ yì kě zhì. zhì yú lèi gǔ zhī zhèng. rú fú zhǒng shuǐ zhǒng zhī lèi. huò yí zhēn jiǔ. huò yí xiè xiè. bìng xiàng gè shū. zhì yì wàn biàn. yī zhě yì yí guǎng qiú zhū fǎ. ér suí yí shī yòng yě.

Bloating and blockage are both very serious diseases. And yet, bloating can be cured while blockage cannot be cured. In case of bloating, substances accumulate in [one's] center; its patho-conditions[1] belong to [the class of] repletions. In case of blockage, one is unable to ingest any substances; its patho-conditions belong to [the class of] depletions. Repletions can be cured; depletions cannot be cured. That is the rule. The disease of bloating results from a weakness of the intestines and of the stomach which [therefore] are unable to pass on and transform [any substances they may receive]. It may be phlegm or blood, or qi or food that agglomerate in the center [of the body], causing bloating and swelling. To treat this [disease], one must first purge these accumulations, and after that supplement and nourish the central qi. As a result, the intestines and the stomach will slowly recover their ability to digest. The *Neijing* has a wine made from chicken droppings as a prescription; that is an [appropriate] method for curing [this disease]. The prescriptions used in later generations to treat bloating have often shown [positive] effects too. Only when the viscera are already cut off from qi, when the arms are emaciated and the navel protrudes, when the palms and the back of one's hands are both swollen, and when blue sinews wind around the abdomen, if all these bad symptoms appear alike, in that case no cure [is possible]. As for the patho-conditions of a blockage, here the fire of the liver has offended the stomach; the wood has come to insult the soil. That is called a robber evil. The stomach duct dries out and can no longer perform its functions. Only a hole as fine as a thread remains, and that is blocked by phlegm, saliva, or stagnating blood. Neither food nor drinks can pass downwards. One forces oneself to consume food, but it is thrown up again. Man's life depends on food and beverages entirely. The classic states: The grains enter into the stomach whence they are to be transmitted to the lung. [From the lung] all the five depots and six palaces receive their qi. Here now the food no longer enters [into the stomach]. As a result, the five depots and six palaces are all exhausted. Hence, if [a patient] gets this patho-condition, and if he [is still able to] consume a small amount of grains [per day, he] will die before one year has passed. If he does not consume any grains, he will die before half a year has passed. Whenever one is affected by this disease in spring, death will occur in autumn; if one gets this disease during autumn, death will occur in spring. The reason is that these seasons are related to the mutual destruction of [the agents] metal and wood. Then there are cases where suddenly one vomits, or the vomiting stops at times, and erupts at times, and it may be that one is young of age and strong. That is called "a stomach that turns back [the food it receives]"; it is not a blockage. Such [a disease] can also be cured. As for complaints similar to bloating, such as surface swellings or water swellings, in some cases one should needle or cauterize, in others one should drain. The images of the diseases are all different, and their treatments [follow] ten thousand variations. A physician must extensively search after all possible methods and apply them in accordance with what is suitable.

Note

[1] The character 症 *zhèng* is not attested before the Song dynasty. It was introduced as a variant of the homophone 證, "evidence", "sign", to indicate a conceptual division between an underlying disease, *bing* 病, and the pathological conditions generated by this disease and to be noticed by a patient himself or an expert healer. As there is no one-to-one relationship between disease and patho-condition, the concept of "symptom", as used in Western medicine, is to be avoided. In Chinese traditional medicine, one identical disease may present itself in different pathological conditions in different patients. Conversely, patients with identical pathological signs may suffer from different underlying diseases. For a detailed discourse, see 5.d.

4.c *Jiě wéi yuán sǒu* 1 解圍元藪 Fēng lài lùn風 癩論 On the Disease [Leading to] Repudiation [That is Caused] by Wind

四時酷烈。暴悍賊邪。風也。爲病最甚。殘害最劇。古人稱癘。爲惡疾之首。患之變敗。形質頑固。不知所之。充塞脉絡之內。輸散分肉之間。榮衛不利。肌腋臏䐜。氣聚不通。使血瘀不流。筋骨弛縮。膚體腐爛。膿穢淋漓。眉髮毨落。手足痿痹。趾指墮折。寒熱痳癢。癥瘍腫瘓。荼毒疙瘩。百惡駢集。得之所由有五。一曰風水陰陽所損。地脉方向吉凶之理曰風水。星曆孤虛曰陰陽。二曰源流傳染所襲。人稟父母精血而成形。受天地造化而爲用。故觸天地不和之氣則病焉。若父母素患惡疾。必精血有毒。交感於胚胎。傳之於兒女。三曰氣穢蠱疰所犯。他人之毒。傳之閒人。曰疰。若人血氣虛。脾胃弱。偶遇惡疾之人。聞其污氣。或對語言。而病人口內之毒氣。衝於無病之人之口鼻。直入五內則發爲病。又如惡疾人登厠之後。而虛弱人或空腹人隨相繼而圊。則病人泄下穢毒之氣。未散衝上。從無病人口鼻直入於臟腑。四曰保養失度所發。五曰感冒積鬱所生。

酷烈	kù liè	fierce
悍	hàn	fierce; violent

殘害	cán hài	to destroy; to injure
劇	jù	troublesome; distressing
稱	chēng	to call; to name
敗	bài	to destroy
質	zhì	substance; matter. Here: disposition
頑固	wán gù	obstinate
之	zhī	to arrive at; to go to
輸	shū	to transport
散	sàn	to disperse; to distribute
分肉	fēn ròu	the partings of the flesh
利	lì	free passage
膹䐜	fèn chēn	swollen
瘀	yū	to stagnate
弛	chí	to relax
縮	suō	to shrink
爛	làn	to decay; rotten
膿	nóng	pus
淋漓	lín lí	to drip
眉	méi	the eyebrows
毷落	mào luò	used here for *tuò luò* 毤落, to shed feathers or fur
落	luò	to fall; to lose
痹	bì	lame; paralyzed; limpness
趾	zhǐ	the toes
墮	duò	to fall
癢	yǎng	to itch
瘸	qué	lame; deformation
癟	biě	shrivelled
痠	suān	aching of the limbs
荼毒	tú dú	poison
疙瘩	gē da	knots
惡	è	vice
駢	pián	joined together
方向	fāng xiàng	direction
吉	jí	auspicious

凶	xiōng	inauspicious
星曆	xīng lì	the sidereal calendar
孤虛	gū xū	lucky and unlucky (days of the calendar)
傳染	chuán rǎn	to be affected [by a disease] through transmission [from someone else]
襲	xí	to inherit; heritage
造化	zào huà	to create
觸	chù	to have contact with
素	sù	originally
兒	ér	son; boy
蠱	gǔ	the *gu*(-spirit)
他	tā	other; another
閒人	xián rén	unaffected people
偶	ǒu	accidental
聞	wén	to smell
對語	duì yǔ	conversation; dialogue
衝	chōng	to pass through
直	zhí	directly
登厠	dēng cè	to mount a privy
繼	jì	to follow
圊	qīng	to visit a privy
失度	shī dù	out of proportion
感冒	gǎn mào	to be affected by adverse (climatic qi)
積鬱	jī yù	accumulation

Sì shí kù liè. bào hàn zèi xié. fēng yě. wéi bìng zuì shèn. cán hài zuì jù. gǔ rén chēng lì. wéi è jí zhī shǒu. huàn zhī biàn bài. xíng zhì wán gù. bù zhī suǒ zhī. chōng sāi mài luò zhī nèi. shū sàn fēn ròu zhī jiān. róng wèi bù lì. jī yè fèn chēn. qì jù bù tōng. shì xuě yū bù liú. jīn gǔ chí suō. fū tǐ fǔ làn. nóng huì lín lí. méi fà mào luò. shǒu zú wěi bì. zhǐ zhǐ duò zhé. hán rè má yǎng. Qué biě zhǒng suān. tú dú gē da. bǎi è pián jí. dé zhī suǒ yóu yǒu wǔ. yī yuē fēng shuǐ yīn yáng suǒ sǔn. dì mài fāng xiàng jí xiōng zhī lǐ yuē fēng shuǐ. xīng lì gū xū yuē yīn yáng. èr yuē yuán liú chuán rǎn suǒ xí. rén bǐng fù mǔ jīng xuě ér chéng xíng. shòu tiān dì zào huà ér wéi yòng. gù chù tiān dì bù hé zhī qì zé bìng yān. ruò fù mǔ sù huàn è jí. bì jīng xuě yǒu dú. jiāo gǎn yú pēi tāi. chuán zhī yú ér nǚ. sān yuē qì huì gǔ zhù suǒ fàn. tā rén zhī dú. chuán zhī xián rén. yuē zhù. ruò rén xuě qì xū. pí wèi ruò. ǒu yù è jí zhī rén. wén qí wū qì. huò duì yǔ yán. ér bìng rén kǒu nèi zhī dú qì. chōng yú wú bìng zhī rén zhī kǒu bí. zhí rù wǔ nèi zé fā wéi bìng. yòu rú è jí rén dēng cè zhī hòu. ér xū ruò rén huò kōng fù rén suí xiāng jì ér qīng. zé bìng rén xiè xià huì dú zhī qì. wèi sàn chōng shàng. cóng wú bìng rén kǒu bí zhí rù yú zàng fǔ. sì yuē bǎo yǎng shī dù suǒ fā. wǔ yuē gǎn mào jī yù suǒ shēng.

A robber evil that is fierce and violent during all four annuals seasons, that is the wind. It causes a disease that is most harmful and extremely distressing. In ancient times the people called it *li*,[1] and they considered it as the worst of all vicious illnesses. To suffer from this [illness means that one's] physical appearance and disposition undergo destruction and change. It is an obstinate [illness], and one does not know where it will turn. It fills and blocks the interior of the [conduit] vessels and network [vessels], and it spreads into the partings of the flesh. The camp and guardian qi can no [longer] pass freely. The flesh and the armpits swell; the qi accumulate and do not pass through [the body any longer]. That causes the blood [stream] to stagnate, and stop flowing. The sinews and the bones relax and shrink, the skin and the body rot. Pus and foul [liquids] drip out [of these lesions]. The eyebrows and the hair fall out; the hands and the feet are paralyzed. The toes and the fingers break and fall off; one feels spells of cold and heat, numbness and itching. Deformations through shrivelling occur as well as swellings; one's limbs ache; poison [seems to penetrate the body; externally it is covered with] knots. All possible vices come together. One may get this [illness] from five sources. The first is called "injury because of wind and water[2] or yin and yang." The principles of the auspicious or inauspicious directions of the vessels penetrating the earth are called "wind and water". The lucky and unlucky [days of the] calendar are called "yin and yang". [3] The second is called "inheritance because of a transmission that flows from one's source." Human physical appearance is generated because a father contributes his semen, and a mother contributes her blood; it may function because it receives the creative [qi] of heaven and earth. If, therefore, one has contact with qi that are not in accord with heaven and earth, illnesses will follow. If a father or a mother had suffered originally from a vicious illness, their semen or blood must carry the poison. It affects the fetus and will be transmitted to the son or daughter. The third is called "attack from qi filth or *gu*-possession."[4] If another person's poison is transmitted to a [hitherto] unaffected person, that is called "possession". If someone whose blood and qi are depleted, and whose spleen and stomach are weak, accidentally meets a person suffering from a vicious illness, he may smell this [person's] unclean qi or in the course of a conversation the poisonous qi from the mouth of the sick person may pass through the mouth or nose of the healthy person directly into his five interior [depots], and emerge there as illness. Or it may be that a person suffering from a vicious illness has been to a privy and a depleted and weak person, or someone with an empty abdomen follows him to go to that latrine. Then the qi filth passed down by the sick person has not yet dispersed and passes upwards through the healthy person's mouth or nose and enters directly into [this person's] depots and palaces. The fourth is called "emergence from a nourishment that is out of proportion". The fifth is called "generation through an affection by adverse [climatic qi] and their accumulations [in the body]."

Notes

[1] This disease corresponds to the European concept of leprosy prior to the discovery of the myco-bacterium leprae and the exact identification of "Hansen's disease". Confucian ethics permitted repudiation of a marriage contract when a wife was found to suffer from 風癩 *feng lai*, leprosy. The term "repudiation" may also refer to an exclusion of such patients from society altogether, a practice that was documented in early Han-sources and was advocated by the Tang physician Sun Simiao. The term 癩, based on 賴 *lai*, "repudiation", closely parallels the German designation of *Aussatz* for leprosy.

[2] Generally translated as "the geomantic system".

[3] Commentary by the author himself, Shěn Zhīwèn 沈之問.

[4] For the *gu*-spirit, see Paul U. Unschuld, *Medicine in China. A History of Ideas*. Univ. of California Press. Berkeley, Los Angeles, London. 1985, 46-50.

4.d *Huáng dì nèi jīng, Sù wèn* 35
黃帝內經·素問
Nüè lùn瘧論
On Malaria

黃帝問曰。夫痎瘧皆生於風。其蓄作有時者。何也。岐伯對曰。瘧之始發也。先起於毫毛。伸欠乃作。寒慄鼓頷。腰脊俱痛。寒去則內外皆熱。頭痛如破。渴欲冷飲。帝曰。何氣使然。願聞其道。岐伯曰。陰陽上下交爭。虛實更作。陰陽相移也。陽幷於陰。則陰實而陽虛。陽明虛則寒慄鼓頷也。巨陽虛則腰背頭項痛。三陽俱虛則陰氣勝。陰氣勝則骨寒而痛。寒生於內。故中外皆寒。陽盛則外熱。陰虛則內熱。外內皆熱則喘而渴。故欲冷飲也。此皆得之夏傷於暑。熱氣盛。藏於皮膚之內。腸胃之外。此榮氣之所舍也。此令人汗空疏。腠理開。因得秋氣。汗出遇風。及得之以浴。水氣舍於皮膚之內。與衛氣幷居。衛氣者。晝日行於陽。夜行於陰。此氣得陽而外出。得陰而內薄。內外相薄。是以日作。帝曰。其間日而作者何也。岐伯曰。其氣之舍深。內薄於陰。陽氣獨發。陰邪內著。陰與陽爭不得出。是以間日而作也。帝曰。善。其作日晏與其日早

者。何氣使然。歧伯曰。邪氣客於風府。循膂而下。衛氣一日一夜。大會於風府。其明日日下一節。故其作也晏。此先客於脊背也。每至於風府則腠理開。腠理開則邪氣入。邪氣入則病作。以此日作稍益晏也。其出於風府。日下一節。二十五日下至骶骨。二十六日入於脊內。注於伏膂之脉。其氣上行。九日出于缺盆之中。其氣日高。故作日益早也。其間日發者。由邪氣內薄於五藏。橫連募原也。其道遠。其氣深。其行遲。不能與衛氣俱行。不得皆出。故間日乃作也。

蓄	xù	to collect
作	zuò	to be active
歧伯	qí bó	Qi Bo, legendary informant of Huang Di on medicine
伸	shēn	to stretch
欠	qiàn	to yawn
慄	lì	to tremble; to shiver
鼓	gŭ	to chatter, as jaws or teeth
頷	hán	the jaws
腰	yāo	the lower back
爭	zhēng	struggle
更	gèng	to change; alternately
陽明	yáng míng	the yang-brilliance (conduit)
巨陽	jù yáng	the great-yang (conduit)
項	xiàng	the neck
汗空	hàn kōng	a sweat opening
疏	shū	lax; separated; open
浴	yù	to wash; to bathe
舍	shě	to reside; to settle; to lodge

薄	bó	to strike
間日	jiàn rì	to skip a day
著	zhuó	to be attached to
晏	yàn	late
風府	fēng fǔ	the wind palace
膂	lǚ	the spinal column
也	yě	also
每	měi	each
益	yì	more; to increase
骶骨	dǐ gǔ	the sacrum
缺盆	quē pén	the broken basin (i.e. the supraclavicular fossa)
橫連	héng lián	to attach horizontally
募原	mù yuán	the membrane plain (alternative writing: 膜原)
遲	chí	to be slow

Huáng dì wèn yuē. fū jiē nüè jiē shēng yú fēng. qí xù zuò yǒu shí zhě. hé yě. qí bó duì yuē. nüè zhī shǐ fā yě. xiān qǐ yú háo máo. shēn qiàn nǎi zuò. hán lì gǔ hán. yāo jí jù tòng. hán qù zé nèi wài jiē rè. tóu tòng rú pò. kě yù lěng yǐn. dì yuē. hé qì shǐ rán. yuàn wén qí dào. qí bó yuē. yīn yáng shàng xià jiāo zhēng. xū shí gèng zuò. yīn yáng xiāng yí yě. yáng bìng yú yīn. zé yīn shí ér yáng xū. yáng míng xū zé hán lì gǔ hán yě. jù yáng xū zé yāo bèi tóu xiàng tòng. sān yáng jù xū zé yīn qì shèng. yīn qì shèng zé gǔ hán ér tòng. hán shēng yú nèi. gù zhōng wài jiē hán. yáng shèng zé wài rè. yīn xū zé nèi rè. wài nèi jiē rè zé chuǎn ér kě. gù yù lěng yǐn yě. cǐ jiē dé zhī xià shāng yú shǔ. rè qì shèng. cáng yú pí fū zhī nèi. cháng wèi zhī wài. cǐ róng qì zhī suǒ shě yě. cǐ lìng rén hàn kōng shū. còu lǐ kāi. yīn dé qiū qì. hàn chū yù fēng. jí dé zhī yǐ yù. shuǐ qì shě yú pí fū zhī nèi. yǔ wèi qì bìng jū. wèi qì zhě. zhòu rì xíng yú yáng. yè xíng yú yīn. cǐ qì dé yáng ér wài chū. dé yīn ér nèi bó. nèi wài xiāng bó. shī yǐ rì zuò. dì yuē. qí jiàn rì ér zuò zhě hé yě. qí bó yuē. qí qì zhī shě shēn. nèi bó yú yīn. yáng qì dú fā. yīn xié nèi zhù. yīn yǔ yáng zhēng bù dé chū. shī yǐ jiàn rì ér zuò yě. dì yuē. shàn. qí zuò rì yàn yǔ qí rì zǎo zhě. hé qì shǐ rán. qí bó yuē. xié qì kè yú fēng fǔ. xūn lǚ ér xià. wèi qì yí rì yí yè. dà huì yú fēng fǔ. qí míng rì rì xià yì jié. gù qí zuò yě yàn. cǐ xiān kè yú jí bèi yě. měi zhì yú fēng fǔ zé còu lǐ kāi. còu lǐ kāi zé xié qì rù. xié qì rù zé bìng zuò. yǐ cǐ rì zuò shāo yì yàn yě. qí chū yú fēng fǔ. rì xià yì jié. èr shí wǔ rì xià zhì dǐ gǔ. èr shí liù rì rù yú jí nèi. zhù yú fú lǚ zhī mài. qí qì shàng xíng. jiǔ rì chū yú quē pén zhī zhōng. qí qì rì gāo. gù zuò rì yì zǎo yě. qí jiàn rì fā zhě. yóu xié qì nèi bó yú wǔ zàng. héng lián mù yuán yě. qí dào yuǎn. qí qì shēn. qí xíng chí. bù néng yǔ wèi qì jù xíng. bù dé jiē chū. gù jiàn rì nǎi zuò yě.

Huang Di asked: Now, all [cases of] *jie* and malaria are generated by wind. Their collecting and being active occurs at [specific] times. Why?
Qi Bo: When *malaria* begins to break out, it first emerges from the finest body hair. [The patient] stretches and yawns and then [the disease] is active. [The patient] shivers from cold and his jaws chatter. Both the lower back and the spine experience pain. When the cold leaves, then [the patient feels] hot everywhere in the inner and outer [regions of his body]. His head aches as if it [were about to] burst. He is thirsty and longs for cold beverages.
Huang Di: Which qi causes this to be so; I should like to hear its Way.
Qi Bo: Yin and yang [qi] rise and descend, interacting in struggle. Depletion and repletion occur alternately. The yin [qi] and the yang [qi] move into each other's [section]. When the yang [qi] collects in the yin [section], then the yin [section] has a repletion, while the yang [section] is depleted. When the yang brilliance is depleted, then one shivers from cold and the jaws chatter. When the great yang is depleted, then the lower back and the backbone, as well as the head and the neck have pain. When all three yang are depleted, then the yin qi dominates. When the yin qi dominates, then the bones are cold and ache. The cold is generated inside. Hence, the center and the outside are all cold. When the yang abounds, then the outside is hot. When the yin is depleted, then the inside is hot. When outside and inside are both hot, then [the patient] pants and is thirsty. Hence, he longs for something cold to drink. All these [states] are acquired from harm by summerheat during summer. The heat qi abounds; it is stored inside the skin and outside of the intestines and the stomach. This is where the camp qi lodges.[1] This lets the person's sweat openings widen. The skin structures open. If subsequently [that person] is affected by autumn qi, sweat leaves [the body] and encounters wind. One may also be affected by it through bathing. [In this case] the water qi lodges inside the skin and resides [there] together with the guardian qi. The guardian qi moves through the yang [sections] during daytime and it moves through the yin [sections] during the night. When this qi meets the yang, it leaves to the outside; when it meets the yin, it strikes at the inside. The inside [qi] and the outside [qi] strike at each other. Hence, [the disease] is active each day.
Huang Di: When it skips a day [before it] is active [again], why is that?
Qi Bo: When this qi lodges in the depth, it strikes at the yin [qi] internally. The yang qi breaks out alone, the yin evil remains attached inside. The yin [qi] struggles with the yang [qi] and cannot leave. Hence, [the disease] skips a day

[before it] is active [again].

Huang Di: Good! When it is active [progressively] later each day, and [afterwards progressively] earlier each day, which qi causes it to be like this?

Qi Bo: The evil qi settles in the wind palace [first, whence] it descends along the spinal column. Each day and each night, the guardian qi has a big meeting at the wind palace. The next day, [the evil qi] descends one [vertebral] joint each day. Hence, it is active [progressively] later [each day]. This [qi] at first settles in the backbone. Everytime when it reaches the wind palace, then the skin structures open. When the skin structures open, then [further] evil qi enters. When [further] evil qi enters, then the disease is active. This way [the disease] is active a little later each day.[2] When the [evil qi] has left the wind palace, it descends one [vertebral] joint each day. After descending for 25 days, it reaches the sacrum. On the 26th day, it enters into the spine and pours into the vessel hidden in the spinal column. The qi rises and on the ninth day it leaves through the broken basin. The qi [ascends] higher each day. Hence, it is active a little earlier each day. As for "it skips a day [before it] is active [again]," that is because the evil strikes at the five depots internally and attaches itself horizontally to the membrane plain. Its path is far, the qi is in the depth, and its movement is slow. It cannot move alongside the guardian qi. It cannot leave together [with the guardian qi]. Hence, it skips a day [before it] is active [again].[3]

Notes

[1, 2, 3] Presumably an ancient anonymous commentary to an older layer of the text that was integrated into the main text in later copies.

4.e *Zhù jiě shāng hán lùn* 2
註解傷寒論
Shāng hán lì 傷寒例
The Principles of Harm Caused by Cold

陰陽大論云。春氣溫和。夏氣暑熱。秋氣清涼。冬氣冷冽。此則四時正氣之序也。冬時嚴寒。萬類深藏。君子固密。則不傷於寒。觸冒之者。乃名傷寒耳。其傷於四時之氣。皆能爲病。以傷寒爲毒者。以其最成殺厲之氣也。中而即病者。名曰傷寒。不即病者。寒毒藏於肌膚。至春變爲溫病。至夏變爲暑病。暑病者。熱極重於溫也。是以辛苦之人。春夏多溫熱病。皆由冬時觸寒所致。非時行之氣也。凡時行者。春時應暖。而復大寒。夏時應大熱。而反大涼。秋時應涼。而反大熱。冬時應寒。而反大溫。此非其時而有其氣。是以一歲之中。長幼之病多相似者。此則時行之氣也。...。從霜降以後。至春分以前。凡有觸冒霜露。體中寒即病者。謂之傷寒也。九月十月。寒氣尚微。爲病則輕。十一月十二月。寒冽已嚴。爲病則重。正月二月。寒漸將解。爲病亦輕。此以冬時不調適。有傷寒之人。即爲病也。其冬有非節之暖者。名曰冬溫。冬溫之毒。與傷寒大異。...。凡傷於寒。則爲病熱。熱雖甚。不死。若兩感於寒而病者。必死。

陰陽大論	yīn yáng dà lùn	Yin yang da lun, Comprehensive Treatise on Yin and Yang; a larger treatise no longer extant, with some passages surviving as quotes in the present text and in the *Huang Di nei jing su wen*
和	hé	pleasant
涼	liáng	cool; fresh
冽	liè	biting cold
序	xù	series; order
嚴	yán	strict; severe
君子	jūn zǐ	the noble man; the gentleman
密	mì	close; sealed
傷寒	shāng hán	harm caused by cold
觸冒	chù mào	to get into touch with, as with something potentially dangerous; to be affected
厲	lì	to grind; to destroy
即	jí	instantly; immediately
辛苦	xīn kǔ	tired; suffering
觸	chù	to be affected by
暖	nuǎn	warm; mild
時行氣	shí xíng qì	seasonally prevalent (harmful) qi
長幼	zhǎng yòu	old and young
霜降	shuāng jiàng	"frost's descent", a solar term denoting the middle of the ninth month
至	zhì	until
春分	chūn fēn	spring equinox, in the middle of the second month
已	yǐ	extremely; intensive particle
正月	zhēng yuè	first month of the year
解	jiě	to loosen
調	tiáo	to adjust

非節	fēi jié	unseasonable; out of season
節	jié	season

Yīn yáng dà lùn yún. chūn qì wēn hé. xià qì shǔ rè. qiū qì qīng liáng. dōng qì lěng liè. cǐ zé sì shí zhèng qì zhī xù yě. dōng shí yán hán. wàn lèi shēn cáng. jūn zǐ gù mì. zé bù shāng yú hán. chù mào zhī zhě. nǎi míng shāng hán ěr. qí shāng yú sì shí zhī qì. jiē néng wéi bìng. yǐ shāng hán wéi dú zhě. yǐ qí zuì chéng shā lì zhī qì yě. zhōng ér jí bìng zhě. míng yuē shāng hán. bù jí bìng zhě. hán dú cáng yú jī fū. zhì chūn biàn wéi wēn bìng. zhì xià biàn wéi shǔ bìng. shǔ bìng zhě. rè jí zhòng yú wēn yě. shī yǐ xīn kǔ zhī rén. chūn xià duō wēn rè bìng. jiē yóu dōng shí chù hán suǒ zhì. fēi shí xíng zhī qì yě. fán shí xíng zhě. chūn shí yīng nuǎn. ér fù dà hán. xià shí yīng dà rè. ér fǎn dà liáng. qiū shí yīng liáng. ér fǎn dà rè. dōng shí yīng hán. ér fǎn dà wēn. cǐ fēi qí shí ér yǒu qí qì. shī yǐ yí suì zhī zhōng. zhǎng yòu zhī bìng duō xiāng sì zhě. cǐ zé shí xíng zhī qì yě. ... cóng shuāng jiàng yǐ hòu. zhì chūn fēn yǐ qián. fán yǒu chù mào shuāng lù. tǐ zhōng hán jí bìng zhě. wèi zhī shāng hán yě. jiǔ yuè shí yuè. hán qì shàng wēi. wéi bìng zé qīng. shí yí yuè shí èr yuè. hán liè yǐ yán. wéi bìng zé zhòng. zhēng yuè èr yuè. hán jiàn jiāng jiě. wéi bìng yì qīng. cǐ yǐ dōng shí bù tiáo shì. yǒu shāng hán zhī rén. jí wéi bìng yě. qí dōng yǒu fēi jié zhī nuǎn zhě. míng yuē dōng wēn. dōng wēn zhī dú. yǔ shāng hán dà yì. ... . fán shāng yú hán. zé wéi bìng rè. rè suī shèn. bù sǐ. ruò liǎng gǎn yú hán ér bìng zhě. bì sǐ.

The "Comprehensive Discourse on Yin and Yang" states: The qi of spring are warm and pleasant; the qi of summer are hot and fiery; the qi of autumn are clear and cool; the qi of winter are bitingly cold. This, then, is the order of the regular qi associated with the four seasons. In winter, when it is severely cold, all species [of living beings] hide themselves in the depth. [Similarly,] the noble man covers himself tightly, and, consequently, he will not be harmed by the cold. If one is affected [by the qi of winter], that is called harm caused by cold. All harm received from any of the qi of the four seasons may result in a disease, but the harm caused by cold is considered to be [the greatest] poison because qi are involved here that cause more deaths and destruction than [all the others]. If one is struck and falls ill immediately, this is called harm caused by cold. If one does not fall ill immediately, the cold-poison may stay in the flesh or in the skin. In spring then, it may turn into a warmth illness; in summer it may turn into a heat illness. Heat illnesses go along with extreme heat and are more severe than warmth [illnesses]. If, therefore, people whose life is tiring suffer from warmth or heat illnesses during spring and summer, this is always because they were affected by cold during winter. Seasonally prevalent [harmful] qi are not involved. As for the seasonally prevalent [harmful qi, that is to say:] during spring, when it should be warm, it is, again, very cold; or in summer, when it should be very hot, it is, on the contrary, very cool; or during autumn, when it should be cool, it is, on the contrary, very hot; or during winter, when it should be cold, it is, on the contrary, very warm. In these cases there are qi present that are out of season. Hence, if in the course of one year, old and young suffer from very similar illnesses, that is due to seasonally prevalent [harmful] qi. ... Whenever someone is affected by frost or dew [in the period stretching] from after "frost descends" to before spring equinox, and if that [person] falls ill because his body was hit by cold, that is called harm caused by cold. During the ninth and the tenth month, the cold qi is still weak; if it causes a disease, it will be minor. During the eleventh and twelfth month, the cold has become extremely severe; if it causes a disease [during that time], it will be serious. During the first and the second month [of the new year], the cold loosens its grip gradually; if it causes a disease [now], it will be minor again. The situation is [always] such that because they cannot adapt to the season of winter, people are harmed by cold, and this results in a disease.[1] If during winter an unseasonal warmth occurs, that is called winter warmth. The poison of winter warmth is very different from harm caused by cold. ... Whenever one has been harmed by cold, he will be ill with heat. That heat may be extreme but one does not die. If, however, both [one's internal and external regions in the body] are affected by the cold and fall ill, death is inevitable.

Note

1 Main text by the later Han dynasty author Zhang Ji 張機 (ca. 200 CE). The commentary was added by Cheng Wuji 成無己 during the Song dynasty.

4.f *Pí wèi lùn 2* 脾胃論 Yǐn shí láo juàn suǒ shāng shǐ wéi rè zhōng lùn 飲食勞倦所傷始爲熱中論On [the Fact that] Harm Caused by Drinking and Eating, Taxation and Fatigue Begins with Heat in One's Center

---

古之至人。窮於陰陽之化。究乎生死之際。所著內外經。悉言人以胃氣爲本。蓋人受水穀之氣以生。所謂清氣。營氣。運氣。衛氣。春升之氣。皆胃氣之別稱也。夫胃爲水穀之海。飲食入胃。遊溢精氣。上輸於脾。脾氣散精。上歸於肺。通調水道。下輸膀胱。水精四布。五經幷行。合於四時五臟陰陽。揆度以爲常也。若飲食失節。寒溫不適。則脾胃乃傷。喜怒憂恐。損耗元氣。既脾胃氣衰。元氣不足。而心火獨盛。心火者。陰火也。起於下焦。其系繫于心。心不主令。相火代之。相火。下焦胞絡之火。元氣之賊也。火與元氣不兩立。一勝則一負。脾胃氣虛。則下流於腎。陰火得以乘其土位。故脾證始得。則氣高而喘。身熱而煩。其脉洪大而頭痛。或渴不止。其皮膚不任風寒。而生寒熱。蓋陰火上衝。則氣

高喘而煩熱。爲頭痛。爲渴。而脉洪。脾胃之氣下流。使穀氣不得升浮。是春生之令不行。則無陽以護其營衛。則不任風寒。乃生寒熱。此皆脾胃之氣不足所致也。然而與外感風寒所得之證。頗同而實異。內傷脾胃。乃傷其氣。外感風寒。乃傷其形。傷其外爲有餘。有餘者瀉之。傷其內爲不足。不足者補之。內傷不足之病。苟誤認作外感有餘之病。而反瀉之。則虛其虛也。實實虛虛。如此死者。醫殺之耳！

至人	zhì rén	someone who has reached highest perfection; a sage
著	zhù	to write, as a book
內外經	nèi wài jīng	short for *Nei jing* ("Inner Classic") and *Wai jing* ("Outer Classic"), referring to ancient writings listed in the bibliographical section of the History of the Han dynasty
悉	xī	all
運氣	yùn qì	moving qi
升	shēng	to ascend
溢	yì	to flow out
歸	guī	to return; to turn to; to end up somewhere
調	diào	to move; to transfer
布	bù	to spread
五經	wǔ jīng	the five conduits
幷	bìng	together
揆度	kuí duó	to consider; to estimate
失節	shī jié	to lose rhythm; irregular
適	shì	to adapt oneself to
耗	hào	to destroy; to diminish

元氣	yuán qì	to original qi
獨	dú	alone; isolated
下焦	xià jiāo	the lower [section of the triple] burner
主	zhǔ	to rule; to govern
令	lìng	an order
相	xiàng	a minister
相火	xiàng huǒ	the minister fire
代	dài	to substitute; to act on behalf of
[心]胞絡	[xīn]bāo luò	the [heart] enclosing network
立	lì	to stand; to exist
勝	shèng	to dominate
負	fù	to succumb
乘	chéng	to seize; to avail oneself of
位	wèi	position
煩	fán	vexed
脉（=脈）	mài	the [movement in the] vessels
洪	hóng	vast
任	rèn	to tolerate; to stand
行	xíng	to pass on; to carry out
頗	pō	very
實	shí	substance; substantial
餘	yú	superabundance
瀉	xiè	to drain
苟	gǒu	if
認作	rèn zuò	to identify as
反	fǎn	in contrast
虛	xū	to deplete
實	shí	to replenish

Gǔ zhī zhì rén. qióng yú yīn yáng zhī huà. jiū hū shēng sǐ zhī jì. suǒ zhù nèi wài jīng. xī yán rén yǐ wèi qì wéi běn. gài rén shòu shuǐ gǔ zhī qì yǐ shēng. suǒ wèi qīng qì. yíng qì. yùn qì. wèi qì. chūn shēng zhī qì. jiē wèi qì zhī bié chēng yě. fū wèi wéi shuǐ gǔ zhī hǎi. yǐn shí rù wèi. yóu yì jīng qì. shàng shū yú pí. pí qì sàn jīng. shàng guī yú fèi. tōng tiáo shuǐ dào. xià shū páng guāng. shuǐ jīng sì bù. wǔ jīng bìng xíng. hé yú sì shí wǔ zàng yīn yáng. Kuí duó yǐ wéi cháng yě. ruò yīn shí shī jié. hán wēn bù shì. zé pí wèi nǎi shāng. xǐ nù yōu kǒng. sǔn hào yuán qì. jì pí wèi qì shuāi. yuán qì bù zú. ér xīn huǒ dú shèng. xīn huǒ zhě. yīn huǒ yě. qǐ yú xià jiāo. qí xì jì yú xīn. xīn bù zhǔ lìng. xiàng huǒ dài zhī. xiàng huǒ. xià jiāo bāo luò zhī huǒ. yuán qì zhī zèi yě. huǒ yǔ yuán qì bù liǎng lì. yī shèng zé yī fù. pí wèi qì xū. zé xià liú yú shèn. yīn huǒ dé yǐ chéng qí tǔ wèi. gù pí zhèng shǐ dé. zé qì gāo ér chuǎn. shēn rè ér fán. qí mài hóng dà ér tóu tòng. huò kě bù zhǐ. qí pí fū bù rèn fēng hán. ér shēng hán rè. gài yīn huǒ shàng chōng. zé qì gāo chuǎn ér fán rè. wéi tóu tòng. wéi kě. ér mài hóng. pí wèi zhī qì xià liú. shǐ gǔ qì bù dé shēng fú. shī chūn shēng zhī lìng bù xíng. zé wú yáng yǐ hù qí yíng wèi. zé bù rèn fēng hán. nǎi shēng hán rè. cǐ jiē pí wèi zhī qì bù zú suǒ zhì yě. rán ér yǔ wài gǎn fēng hán suǒ dé zhī zhèng. pō tóng ér shí yì. nèi shāng pí wèi. nǎi shāng qí qì. wài gǎn fēng hán. nǎi shāng qí xíng. shāng qí wài wéi yǒu yú. yǒu yú zhě xiè zhī. shāng qí nèi wéi bù zú. bù zú zhě bǔ zhī. nèi shāng bù zú zhī bìng. gǒu wù rèn zuò wài gǎn yǒu yú zhī bìng. ér fǎn xiè zhī. zé xū qí xū yě. shí shí xū xū. rú cǐ sǐ zhě. yī shā zhī ěr！

In ancient times, the sages thoroughly investigated the transformations of yin and yang, and they examined into the borderline of life and death. In all their writings, [be they called] "Inner [Classic]" or "Outer Classic", they stated: Man needs the qi of the stomach as his basis. That is to say, man absorbs the qi of water and of the grains in order to live; the clear qi, the camp qi, the moving qi, the guardian qi, and the qi ascending in spring, these are all additional designations of the qi of the stomach. The stomach is the sea of water and of the grains. Food and beverages enter the stomach whence they flow out as essence qi. They are transported upwards into the spleen, and their essence is distributed [further on] by the qi of the spleen so as to end up in the lung. [From here] they move into the [body's] water ways and are transported downward into the urinary bladder. The water spreads the essence [qi] through [all] the four [sections of the body]; it passes through [all] the five conduits alike. The agreement [of these processes] with the yin and yang [qi] of the five depots and the [course of the] four seasons, that is considered to be normal. If however one drinks and eats without restraints, and if [one's consumption of beverages and food] fails to correspond to the cold or warmth [of the four seasons], this will cause harm to both spleen and stomach. [Also, excessive] joy and anger, as well as [excessive] mourning and fear injure one's original qi. If the qi of the spleen and of the stomach are weakened, and if not enough original qi is present, an isolated fire will flare up in the heart. This fire in the heart is a yin fire; it rises from the lower burner, and ties itself[1] to the heart. [The reason is that when] the heart fails to be in control [of the organism] and to give orders, the minister fire will assume its position. The minister fire, though, is a fire [that arises from the] lower [section of the triple] burner [and ties up with the heart] enclosing network. It causes destruction to the original qi. [This minister] fire and the original qi cannot exist both side by side. [In their struggle] one will dominate and one will succumb. In case the qi of spleen and stomach are depleted, [the essence digested from beverages and food will not move up into the lung but] will flow down into the kidneys. That, [in turn,] enables the yin fire to seize the position [that should be occupied by qi associated with the] soil.[2] Consequently, the first symptoms of [a disease in] spleen [and stomach are as follows]. One's qi will rise high which results in panting. The body will be hot, and feels vexed. The [movement in the patient's] vessels is vast and strong, and he suffers from headache or from an unquenchable thirst. His skin cannot stand wind and cold, and fits of cold and heat emerge. [The reason for these symptoms is that if] a yin fire moves upwards, the qi will rise high and one pants. One feels distressed and hot; one has headaches, one is thirsty, and the [movement in the] vessels is vast. When the qi of spleen and stomach flow downwards, and do not let the qi of the grains [that one has consumed] rise and ascend to the surface, [that means that] the orders of spring to generate life cannot be carried out. Hence, no yang [qi] will be present to preserve the camp and guardian [qi], and [the body] cannot stand wind and cold, and develops [fits of] cold and heat. All of these [signs] result from an insufficiency of the qi of spleen and stomach. These [signs] are quite similar to the signs resulting from an external affection by wind and cold, but they are substantially different. If spleen and stomach are harmed from within [the body], one's qi will be harmed. If wind and cold have affected one from outside [the body], one's physical appearance will be harmed. Harm caused externally results in superabundance, and in case of superabundance one has to drain it. Harm caused internally results in an insufficiency, and in case of an insufficiency one has to supplement it. If, however, a disease consisting of an insufficiency resulting from harm caused internally is misidentified as a disease consisting of superabundance resulting from harm caused externally, and if the [patient] is drained in contrast [to what his disease requires], then his depletion is further depleted. If someone dies because his repletion was further replenished, or because his depletion was further depleted, he was killed by the physician.

Notes

[1] "Yin fire" refers to the minister fire originating from a yin position in or between the kidneys. It may move upward through the foot-minor-yin conduit of the kidneys, and enter the hand-ceasing-yin conduit of the heart-enclosing-network in the chest.

[2] In the system of correspondences based on the five agents, spleen and stomach are associated with the agent soil.

Lesson Five

Diagnostics: General Principles

Because all the organism's functional units were associated, in the medicine of systematic correspondence, with secondary functions, as, for instance, voice, vision, hearing, odor, one's desires for a specific flavor, or the production of liquids such as tears and saliva, any disease affecting one or more of the functional units constituting the organism could be recognized, it was assumed, from changes in these secondary functions. Hence a practitioner was supposed to observe a patient's complexion, to listen to his voice and smell his odors, and to ask him questions to find out about any changes the patient was aware of himself. In addition, physiological signs were identified as indicating sub-manifest or latent stages of a disease, possibly unknown to the patients themselves. In this regard the feeling of the pulse played a major role (see Lesson Six). A physician practicing on the basis of the theories of systematic correspondence had, ideally, to take a wide range of factors into account, first to determine origin, seat, and future course of a disease, and second to conduct an appropriate therapy. Social factors as well as habits of lifestyle and individual conditions were emphasized by authors as parameters in a physician's decision-making. The most important starting point for therapeutic intervention, though, was thought to be an exact identification of the history of the disease to be treated inside the organism. To employ a successful therapeutic strategy, a healer had to know whether a disease was still located in the first functional unit it had affected, and whether it had already spread to one or more additional functional units. These secondary affections had to be differentiated again, on the basis of the five-agents doctrine, in accordance with their different relations with the unit from which the disease had originated. Prognosis and treatment of a disease transmitted, for instance, from the kidneys to the heart were different from those of a disease transmitted from the kidneys to the liver.

Key Terms Introduced in Lesson Five

主	zhǔ	to be responsible, as a conduit or depot for the condition of an external organ or section of the body
針灸	zhēn jiǔ	acupuncture and moxibustion
少腹	shào fù	the lower abdomen
眥	zì	the corner of an eye; canthus
大眥	dà zì	the inner canthus
小眥	xiǎo zì	the outer canthus
黑珠	hēi zhū	the dark (section of the) eyeball
白珠	bái zhū	the white (section of the) eyeball
胞	bāo	an eyelid
上胞	shàng bāo	the upper eyelid
下胞	xià bāo	the lower eyelid
真氣	zhēn qì	true qi; i.e. man's congenital qì
太陽經	tài yáng jīng	the major-yang conduit
引	yǐn	to pull/conduct (qi into a specific conduit)
引經藥	yǐn jīng yào	drugs conducting/pulling (qi) into specific conduits
望聞問切	wàng wén wèn qiè	the four diagnostic approaches: to look (at a patient's complexion), to smell (his breath) and listen (to the pitch of his voice), to ask (him about his condition), and to press (his vessels to feel the movement within them)
切脈	qiè mài	to press the vessels
寸口	cùn kǒu	the inch-opening; a location at the wrists where the movement in the vessels can be felt
患人	huàn rén	a patient
便	biàn	urine and stools
悶	mèn	pressing (sensation in one's chest)
素	sù	congenital; all along
聾	lōng	deaf; hard of hearing
月水	yuè shuǐ	the monthly water; menstrual blood
尺	chǐ	the foot-section, at the wrists

滑	huá	smooth
膊	bó	the upper arm; the shoulder
症	zhèng	a pathological condition; patho-condition
自汗	zì hàn	to sweat without apparent external reason, such as hot weather, thick clothing, etc.
本症	běn zhèng	the typical patho-conditions accompanying an illness
泄瀉	xiè xiè	diarrhea
痞	pǐ	obstruction; blocked (qi in the chest)
兼症	jiān zhèng	adjunct patho-conditions accompanying an illness
往來寒熱	wǎng lái hán rè	alternating fits of cold and heat
痢	lì	dysentery
兼病	jiān bìng	additional disease
法	fǎ	pattern
按	àn	to feel (the vessels in order to examine the movement within them)
弦	xián	string(-like movement in the vessels)
鉤	gōu	hook(-like movement in the vessels)
代	dài	intermittent (movement in the vessels)
毛	máo	hair(-like movement in the vessels)
石	shí	stone(-like movement in the vessels)
相勝	xiāng shèng	the mutual destruction (among the five agents)
相生	xiāng shēng	the mutual generation (among the five agents)
正經	zhèng jīng	the regular conduits
自病	zì bìng	to fall ill by itself (as of a regular conduit, in contrast to an illness transmitted from another depot or conduit)
五邪	wǔ xié	the five evils
傷暑	shāng shǔ	to be harmed by summer-heat
中濕	zhòng shī	to be struck by dampness
中風	zhòng fēng	to be struck by wind
焦	jiāo	burnt (breath odor)
臭	xiù	odor

香	xiāng	aromatic
臊	sāo	fetid
腐	fŭ	foul
腥	xīng	fishy
散	sàn	dispersed (movement in the vessels)
收	shōu	to contract (as one's limbs)
呻	shēn	to groan
洒洒	xiăn xiăn	to shiver
咳	ké	to cough
泣	qì	tears
涎	xián	saliva
涕	tī	snivel
唾	tuò	spittle
小腹	xiăo fù	the lower abdomen
脛	jìng	the shinbone
沉	chén	in the depth (as a movement in the vessels)
濡	rú	soft (movement in the vessels)

5.a *Yī xué liù yào* 醫學六要 (Gǔ jīn tú shū jí chéng yī bù quán lù 古今圖書集成醫部全錄, Yī bù huì kǎo 醫部彙考110) Míng bù dìng jīng 明部定經 Understand the Section [Where a Disease is Located] and Determine the Conduit [Where the Treatment is to be Applied]

夫臟腑陰陽。各有其經。四肢筋骨。各有所主。明其部以定經。循其流以尋源。捨此而欲知病之所在。猶適燕而南行。豈不愈勞而愈遠哉。方書云。不讀十二經絡。開口動手便錯。誠確論也。世人以經絡爲針灸家書。皆懵然罔究。妄舉妄譚。即如頭痛一證。左右分經。前後異位。同一腹痛也。而有中脘當臍少腹之分。同一害眼也。而有大眥小眥。黑珠白珠。上胞下胞之異。在肺而用心藥。則肺病不去。而復損心經。在血而用氣藥。則真氣反傷。而血病益滋。東垣曰。傷寒邪在太陽經。誤用葛根湯。則引邪入陽明。是葛根乃陽明引經藥。非太陽經藥也。即此而推之。則夭於藥者。不知其凡幾矣。仁人君子。慎勿輕議。當留心于明部定經焉。

主	zhǔ	to be responsible, as a conduit or depot, for the condition of an external organ or section of the body
定	dìng	to identify; to determine
捨	shě	to reject; to determine
所在	suǒ zài	location
適	shì	to follow; to go to
燕	yàn	(the state of) Yan (in the far North)
南	nán	the South
愈	yù	very (愈 ... 愈…: the more … the more)
勞	láo	exhausting
遠	yuǎn	long; distant
方書	fāng shū	title of a book; possibly referring to a text compiled by Xú Dùzhēn 徐杜真 of the Yuan era
便	biàn	particle indicating an immediate temporal sequence
錯	cuò	mistake
誠	chéng	truly
確	què	correct
論	lùn	statement
世人	shì rén	mankind; all the people
針灸	zhēn jiǔ	acupuncture and moxibustion
家	jiā	a specialist
懵	mēng	ignorant
妄	wàng	absurd; foolish; false
舉	jǔ	an activity; something one "takes up"
譚	tán	to boast; claim
少腹	shào fù	the lower abdomen
眥	zì	the corner of an eye; canthus
大眥	dà zì	the inner canthus
小眥	xiǎo zì	the outer canthus
黑珠	hēi zhū	the dark (section of the) eyeball
白珠	bái zhū	the white (section of the) eyeball
胞	bāo	an eyelid

上胞	shàng bāo	the upper eyelid
下胞	xià bāo	the lower eyelid
復	fù	additional
真氣	zhēn qì	true qi; i.e. man's congenital qì
東垣	dōng yuán	Dongyuan, style-name of Lǐ Gǎo 李杲 (1180-1251); author of medical texts
太陽經	tài yáng jīng	the major-yang conduit
葛根湯	gé gēn tāng	"decoction with *gegen* (i.e. the roots of Pueraria lobata (Willd.) Ohwi)"
引	yǐn	to pull/conduct (qi into a specific conduit)
引經藥	yǐn jīng yào	drugs conducting/pulling (qi) into specific conduits
推	tuī	to draw conclusions; to continue a line of thought
幾	jǐ	how many?
仁	rén	the attitude of humaneness
輕	qīng	light-minded
議	yì	to deliberate; to propose
留心	liú xīn	to focus attention

Fū zàng fǔ yīn yáng. gè yǒu qí jīng. sì zhī jīn gǔ. gè yǒu suǒ zhǔ. míng qí bù yī dìng jīng. xūn qí liú yǐ xún yuán. shě cǐ ér yù zhī bìng zhī suǒ zài. yóu shì yàn ér nán xíng. qǐ bù yù láo ér yù yuǎn zāi. fāng shū yún. bù dú shí èr jīng luò. kāi kǒu dòng shǒu biàn cuò. chéng què lùn yě. shì rén yǐ jīng luò wéi zhēn jiǔ jiā shū. jiē mēng rán wǎng jiū. wàng jǔ wàng tán. jí rú tóu tòng yí zhèng. zuǒ yòu fēn jīng. qián hòu yì wèi. tóng yī fù tòng yě. ér yǒu zhōng wǎn dāng qí shào fù zhī fēn. tóng yī hài yǎn yě. ér yǒu dà zì xiǎo zì. hēi zhū bái zhū. shàng bāo xià bāo zhī yì. zài fèi ér yòng xīn yào. zé fèi bìng bù qù. ér fù sǔn xīn jīng. zài xuě ér yòng qì yào. zé zhēn qì fǎn shāng. ér xuě bìng yì zī. dōng yuán yuē. shāng hán xié zài tài yáng jīng. wù yòng gé gēn tāng. zé yǐn xié rù yáng míng. shī gé gēn nǎi yáng míng yǐn jīng yào. fēi tài yáng jīng yào yě. jí cǐ ér tuī zhī. zé yāo yú yào zhě. bù zhī qí fán jǐ yǐ. rén rén jūn zǐ. shèn wù qīng yì. dāng liú xīn yú míng bù dìng jīng yān.

All the [body's] depots and palaces with their yin and yang [qi] have their specific conduits; all the four limbs, the sinews, and the bones have a [conduit] responsible for [their condition]. One [should] understand the section [of the body where the symptoms appear], in order to identify the conduit [that must be treated, in the same way as] one follows a stream [backward] in order to trace its source. If one disregarded these [principles] and still wished to know where a disease was located, that would be the same as if one wished to go to [the northern state of] Yan but went South. The more one toiled, the farther away [from Yan one would move]! The *Fangshu* says: "If one does not study the *Twelve Counduits and Network [Vessels]*[1], one will already make a mistake if one only opens the mouth or moves one's hand!" That is truly a correct statement! All the people nowadays regard the *[Twelve] Conduits and Network [Vessels]* as a book [written] for acupuncture and moxibustion specialists [only but not for those who intend to apply pharmaceutical drugs]. Hence, in their ignorance, they fail to carry out thorough investigations, and their activities are as absurd as are their claims. If, for example, [one considers] only the one symptom of headache, one must distinguish whether a conduit on the right or on the left [side of the head is affected], and it makes a difference whether [the pain] is located in the front or in the back [of the head]. As for identical [symptoms of] abdominal pain, one must distinguish between [pain in] the central duct [of the stomach, pain located] exactly at the navel, [and pain located] in the lower abdomen. Or, in case of identical injuries of the eyes, one must distinguish between the inner canthus, the outer canthus, the dark [section of the] eyeballs, and the white [section of the] eyeballs, the upper eyelids, and the lower eyelids. If an [illness] is located in the lung, and one uses a heart drug [to treat it], the disease in the lung will not be eliminated, but additional harm will result in the conduit associated with the heart. Or, if [a disease] is located in the blood, and one uses drugs [suitable for treating diseases affecting the] qi, then, contrary [to one's intentions], the true qi will be harmed and the disease in the blood will be further increased. [Li] Dongyuan has stated: "If evil [qi resulting from] harm caused by cold are located in the major-yang conduit, and one mistakenly uses the decoction with *gegen*, one will draw the evil [qi] into the yang-brilliance [conduit]." *Gegen* is a drug that draws [qi] into the yang-brilliancee conduit, it is not a drug [associated with] the major-yang conduit. If one continues this line a little further, it is hard to know how many [people] had to die young because of the drugs [prescribed to them]! Humane gentlemen will be careful not to make any light-minded proposals; they should focus their attention on an understanding of the [body's] sections [where the symptoms appear] and on an identification of the conduits [where the disease is located].

Note

[1] It is not entirely clear whether the author refers here to a specific text (a book entitled *Shi er jing luo* was compiled by the Yuan author Ge Qiansun 葛乾孫), or to the knowledge on the conduits in general.

5.b *Gŭ jīn yī tǒng dà quán* 3
古今醫統大全
(Yì yī tōng kǎo翼醫通考)
Wàng wén wèn qiè dìng 望聞問切訂
Specification of [the Four Diagnostic Methods, including] Looking, Smelling/Listening, Asking, and [Vessel] Pressing

---

按望聞問切四字。誠爲醫之綱領。若得四字之旨。則於醫學。可謂至矣。今人惟問一端而已。其於望聞亦淺淺耳。至於切脈。則又謂居三者之末。而猶復輕視之。故所以卒鮮有精于脉者。間有言者。亦不過左心小腸肝膽腎之說耳。經位不別。其何以察虛實生死之幾耶。殊不知四者之要。則又在切之之功也。其望聞問之三者。先以得其病情之端。而後總切脈於寸口。確乎知始病之源。而方今延流於何臟何經。若虛若實。或死或生。準候酌方。必有賴於切脈。而後可以爲圖治之效矣。斯其次第之序。初近患人。先望而聞。次問而切。固理之不容易也。然則切脈果可輕與。

按	àn	as for
望聞問切	wàng wén wèn qiè	the four diagnostic approaches: to look (at a patients complexion), to smell (his breath) and listen (to the pitch of his voice), to ask (him about his condition), and to press (his vessels to feel the movement within them)
字	zì	a word
綱領	gāng lǐng	a pervasive principle
旨	zhǐ	meaning
醫學	yī xué	the medical teachings
至	zhì	accomplished
端	duān	one aspect; one end
切脈	qiè mài	to press the vessels
末	mò	an end
猶	yóu	especially
輕視	qīng shì	to consider as unimportant; to hold in disdain
鮮	xiǎn	rare; few; seldom
精	jīng	to be versed in; to be an expert
間有	jiàn yǒu	if occasionally
不過	bù guò	only; but
何以	hé yǐ	by what means; how
察	chá	to investigate; to find out
幾	jǐ	minute
殊不	shū bù	definitely not; not at all
要	yào	important; essential point
寸口	cùn kǒu	the inch-opening; a location at the wrists where the movement in the vessels can be felt
延	yán	to extend
準	zhǔn	to weigh; to compare
候	hòu	sign of a disease
酌	zhuó	to deliberate; to think about
圖	tú	to plan; to seek; to envisage
效	xiào	success
次第之序	cì dì zhī xù	a sequential order

近	jìn	to approach
患人	huàn rén	a patient
理	lǐ	to manage; to order
容易	róng yì	easy
果	guǒ	really
與	yǔ	final interrogative particle

Àn wàng wén wèn qiè sì zì. chéng wéi yī zhī gāng lǐng. ruò dé sì zì zhī zhǐ. zé yú yī xué. kě wèi zhì yǐ. jīn rén wéi wèn yì duān ér yǐ. qí yú wàng wén yì qiǎn qiǎn ěr. zhì yú qiè mài. zé yòu wèi jū sān zhě zhī mò. ér yóu fù qīng shì zhī. gù suǒ yǐ zú xiǎn yǒu jīng yú mài zhě. jiàn yǒu yán zhě. yì bù guò zuǒ xīn xiǎo cháng gān dǎn shèn zhī shuō ěr. jīng wèi bù bié. qí hé yǐ chá xū shí shēng sǐ zhī jī yé. shū bù zhī sì zhě zhī yào. zé yòu zài qiè zhī zhī gōng yě. qí wàng wén wèn zhī sān zhě. xiān yǐ dé qí bìng qíng zhī duān. ér hòu zǒng qiè mài yú cùn kǒu. què hū zhī shǐ bìng zhī yuán. ér fāng jīn yán liú yú hé zàng hé jīng. ruò xū ruò shí. huò sǐ huò shēng. zhǔn hòu zhuó fāng. bì yǒu lài yú qiè mài. ér hòu kě yǐ wéi tú zhì zhī xiào yǐ. sī qí cì dì zhī xù. chū jìn huàn rén. xiān wàng ér wén. cì wèn ér qiè. gù lǐ zhī bù róng yì yě. rán zé qiè mài guǒ kě qīng yǔ.

The four words "to look", "to smell and to listen", "to ask", and "to press" are the basic theme running through medicine. If one has grasped the meaning of these four words, he may be called accomplished in the medical teachings. Today, the people [resort] only to one part [of these four diagnostic techniques, that is, to] asking, and to nothing else. Their [knowledge of the techniques of] looking [at a patient's complexion, and of] smelling and listening [to recognize his odor and the pitch of his voice] is quite shallow, and when it comes to [the technique of] pressing the [patient's] vessels [in order to feel the movement within these vessels], then they say that it is placed at the end of the three [techniques mentioned already], and hold it in particular disdain. Hence there are, as a result, only very few [who may be considered as] experts in vessel [diagnosis]. If occasionally someone speaks [on this topic], he will make but [very general] statements such as that [movements associated with] the heart, the small intestine, the liver, the gallbladder, and the kidneys are [to be felt] on the left. If, [however,] one fails to distinguish among the locations of the conduits, how is one going to find out the minute [signs of] depletion and repletion, of survival or [impending] death? [These people] are definitely unaware of [the fact that] the importance of the four [diagnostic techniques] culminates in the results achieved through pressing the [vessels of a patient]. The three [techniques of] looking, smelling/listening, and asking are [applied] first in order to understand the primordial cause underlying the illness condition [at hand]. Only then, summing up [the information gained through these three techniques], one presses the vessels at the inch-opening to correctly know the source whence the illness emerged, [to find out] into which of the depots and into which conduit [the evil qi] have flowed, [to determine] whether it is a case of depletion or repletion, and whether [the patient] will die or survive, and, [finally, in order] to weigh the signs and to think about a [suitable] prescription – [all these steps] must rely on the pressing of the vessels, and only after [these measures have been taken] will it be possible to envisage the success of one's treatment. This is the sequential order [of the four diagnostic techniques]: Upon approaching a patient, one should first look [at his complexion] and smell [his odor], and listen [to the pitch of his voice]. Then one asks [him about his complaints, preference for a specific flavor, etc.], and presses [his vessels]. To structure [this data] is certainly not easy! How could anybody consider the pressing of the vessels [for diagnostic purposes] as unimportant?

5.c *Yī xué liù yào* 醫學六要 (Gǔ jīn tú shū jí chéng yī bù quán lù 古今圖書集成醫部全錄· Yī bù huì kǎo 醫部彙考 92) Wèn bìng bì xiáng 問病必詳 Questions Addressed to a Patient Must be Detailed

---

凡診病必先問所看何人。或男或女。或老或幼。或婢妾。或僮僕。次問得病之日。受病之原。及飲食胃氣如何。便利如何。曾服何藥。日間何如。夜寐何如。膈間有無脹悶痛處。問病不答必耳聾。即當詢之是素聾否。不則病久。或汗下過傷虛聾。問而懶言點頭。是中氣虛。昏憒不知人。是暴厥耶。抑久病耶。婦人當問月水如何。寡婦氣血凝滯。兩尺多滑。不可誤斷爲胎。室女同。心腹脹痛。問是舊病舉耶。或新起耶。診病必問所欲何味。所嗜何物。或縱酒。或齋素。喜酸則知肝虛。喜甘則知脾弱。頭身臂膊作痛。必問曾病惡瘡否。

看	kàn	to examine; to look at
或	huò	whether
婢	bì	a female servant
妾	qiè	a female servant; a concubine
僮	tóng	a boy; a servant

僕	pú	a servant
原	yuán	a source; an origin
便	biàn	urine and stools
寐	mèi	to sleep
悶	mèn	pressing (sensation in one's chest)
素	sù	congenital; all along
聾	lōng	deaf; hard of hearing
詢	xún	to inquire about
否	foǔ	or not
懶	lǎn	unwilling; lazy
點	diǎn	to nod
昏憒	hūn kuì	dazed; confused
抑	yì	or; or if
婦	fù	woman
月水	yuè shuǐ	the monthly water; menstrual blood
寡婦	guǎ fù	a widow
尺	chǐ	the foot(-long section of the lower arm); i.e. a section stretching from the "gate" line near the wrist to the foot-marsh insertion hole near the elbow bend
多	duō	frequent
滑	huá	smooth
斷	duàn	to decide; to conclude
室女	shì nǚ	an unmarried girl
嗜	shì	to long for; to lust after
縱	zòng	to be indulgent; to give oneself to
齋	zhāi	to abstain; to fast
素	sù	vegetarian
膊	bó	the upper arm; the shoulder

Fán zhěn bìng bì xiān wèn suǒ kàn hé rén. huò nán huò nǚ. huò lǎo huò yòu. huò bì qiè huò tóng pú. cì wèn dé bìng zhī rì. shòu bìng zhī yuán. jí yǐn shí wèi qì rú hé. biàn lì rú hé. cēng fú hé yào. rì jiān hé rú. yè mèi hé rú. gé jiān yǒu wú zhàng mèn tòng chù. wèn bìng bù dá bì ěr lōng. jí dāng xún zhī shī sù lōng foŭ. bù zé bìng jiŭ. huò hàn xià guò shāng xū lōng. wèn ér lăn yán diăn tóu. shī zhōng qì xū. hūn kuì bù zhī rén. shī bào jué yé. yì jiŭ bìng yé. fù rén dāng wèn yuè shuĭ rú hé. guă fù qì xuĕ níng zhì. liăng chĭ duō huá. bù kĕ wù duàn wéi tāi. shì nǚ tóng. xīn fù zhàng tòng. wèn shī jiù bìng jŭ yé. huò xīn qĭ yé. zhĕn bìng bì wèn suŏ yù hé wèi. suŏ shì hé wù. huò zòng jiŭ. huò zhāi sù. xĭ suān zé zhī gān xū. xĭ gān zé zhī pí ruò. tóu shēn bì bó zuò tòng. bì wèn cēng bìng è chuāng foŭ.

In diagnosing a disease, first of all one must always ask what kind of a person one examines, whether it is a male, or a female, an old or a young [patient], a female servant, or a male servant. Next, one inquires about the day [that person] got the illness, and the source from which it was received. Furthermore, [one asks] about [the patient's] drinking and eating [habits] and about his stomach qi, about the passage of urine and stools, what pharmaceutical drugs he has taken already, how he passes his daytime, and how he sleeps at night, and whether he feels any swellings, pressing, or painful areas in the region of the diaphragm. If one asks the patient and he does not answer, his ears must be hard of hearing. In this case one should inquire whether he has been deaf all along. If not, it may be an older illness, or excessive sweating or purging have caused harm leading to deafness resulting from depletion. If one asks [the patient] and he is unwilling to speak, and simply nods his head, his central qi are depleted. If he is confused and does not recognize anybody, [one should examine] if it is a case of violently rising [yang qi], or if it is an old illness. Women should be asked about their monthly period; if widows [show signs of] congealing and stagnating qi and blood, and if [the movement in the vessels] at the foot [section] of both [wrists] is frequent and smooth, one must not mistakenly conclude the presence of a fetus in the womb. The same applies to unmarried girls. If swellings and pain occur in the [regions of] heart and abdomen, one inquires whether they are caused by an older illness, or whether they have emerged [as signs of a] new [illness]. In diagnosing a disease, one must ask [the patient] what kind of flavor he wishes [to consume], and what other things he longs for; whether he gives himself to wine, or whether he fasts or eats only vegetarian food. If [the patient] likes [to eat] sour [food], one knows that his liver is depleted; if he likes sweet [flavor], one realizes that his spleen is weak. If his head, his body, his arms, and his shoulders ache, one must ask whether he has previously suffered from any bad sores.

5.d *Xú líng tāi xiān sheng yī shū quán jí, juan* 1/2 徐靈胎先生 醫書全集 (Yī xué yuán liú lùn 醫學源流論) Bìng zhèng bù tóng lùn 病症不同論 On Discrepancies between Diseases and Patho-Conditions

---

凡病之總者。謂之病。而一病必有數症。如太陽傷風是病也。其惡風。身熱。自汗。頭痛是症也。合之而成其爲太陽病。此乃太陽病之本症也。若太陽病而又兼泄瀉。不寐。心煩。痞悶。則又爲太陽病之兼症矣。如瘧病也。往來寒熱。嘔吐。畏風。口苦是症也。合之而成爲瘧。此乃瘧之本症也。若瘧而兼頭痛。脹滿。嗽逆。便閉。則又爲瘧疾之兼症矣。若瘧而又下痢數十行。則又不得謂之兼症。謂之兼病。蓋瘧爲一病。痢又爲一病。而二病又各有本症。各有兼症。不可勝舉。以此類推。則病之與症。其分併何啻千萬。不可不求其端而分其緒也。而治之法。或當合治。或當分治。或當先治。或當後治。或當專治。或當不治。尤在視其輕重緩急。而次第奏功。一或倒行逆施。雜亂無紀。則病變百出。雖良工不能挽回矣。

惡	wù	to hate; to have an aversion
自汗	zì hàn	to sweat without apparent external reason, such as hot weather, thick clothing, etc.
本症	běn zhèng	the typical patho-conditions accompanying a disease
兼	jiān	to unite; additional; joint
泄瀉	xiè xiè	diarrhea
痞	pǐ	obstruction; blocked (qi in the chest)
兼症	jiān zhèng	adjunct patho-conditions accompanying a disease
往來寒熱	wǎng lái hán rè	alternating fits of cold and heat
畏	wèi	to fear
痢	lì	dysentery
兼病	jiān bìng	additional disease
不可勝舉	bù kě shèng jǔ	cannot all be named here one by one
類推	lèi tuī	to conclude by analogy
何啻千萬	hé chì qiān wàn	a countless multitude (lit.: how could it be only thousands of myriads?)
不可不	bù kě bù	it is impossible not to; one must
緒	xù	the end of a ball of thread
法	fǎ	pattern
專	zhuān	especially; in particular
尤在	yóu zài	the most important is ...
次第	cì dì	sequence; in order
奏功	zòu gōng	to have the intended effect
一或	yì huò	in case; if
倒行逆施	dào xíng nì shī	to move contrary (to all rules)
雜亂無紀	zá luàn wú jì	no order whatsoever
良	liáng	good
挽回	wǎn huí	to bring back (health)

Fán bìng zhī zǒng zhě. wèi zhī bìng. ér yí bìng bì yǒu shù zhèng. rú tài yáng shāng fēng shī bìng yě. qí wù fēng. shēn rè. zì hàn. tóu tòng shī zhèng yě. hé zhī ér chéng qí wéi tài yáng bìng. cǐ nǎi tài yáng bìng zhī běn zhèng yě. ruò tài yáng bìng ér yòu jiān xiè xiè. bù mèi. xīn fán. pǐ mèn. zé yòu wéi tài yáng bìng zhī jiān zhèng yǐ. rú nüè bìng yě. wǎng lái hán rè. ǒu tù. wèi fēng. kǒu kǔ shī zhèng yě. hé zhī ér chéng wéi nüè. cǐ nǎi nüè zhī běn zhèng yě. ruò nüè ér jiān tóu tòng. zhàng mǎn. sòu nì. biàn bì. zé yòu wéi nüè jí zhī jiān zhèng yǐ. ruò nüè ér yòu xià lì shù shí xíng. zé yòu bù dé wèi zhī jiān zhèng. wèi zhī jiān bìng. gài nüè wéi yí bìng. lì yòu wéi yí bìng. ér èr bìng yòu gè yǒu běn zhèng. gè yǒu jiān zhèng. bù kě shèng jǔ. yǐ cǐ lèi tuī. zé bìng zhī yǔ zhèng. qí fēn bìng hé chì qiān wàn. bù kě bù qiú qí duān ér fēn qí xù yě. ér zhì zhī fǎ. huò dāng hé zhì. huò dāng fēn zhì. huò dāng xiān zhì. huò dāng hòu zhì. huò dāng zhuān zhì. huò dāng bù zhì. yóu zài shì qí qīng zhòng huǎn jí. ér cì dì zòu gōng. yì huò dào xíng nì shī. zá luàn wú jì. zé bìng biàn bǎi chū. suī liáng gōng bù néng wàn huí yǐ.

Any disease in its entirety is called "disease", but one single disease inevitably has a number of patho-conditions. For instance, when the major-yang [conduit and depot] have been harmed by wind, that is the disease. An aversion against wind, a hot body, sweating without external reason, and headache are the patho-conditions [accompanying this disease]. Together, these [patho-conditions] constitute a major-yang disease; they are the patho-conditions typical of a major-yang disease. If [someone suffers from] a major-yang disease, and in addition [suffers from] diarrhea and inability to sleep; if he has an uneasy fealing in his heart, combined with pressure in his chest due to [qi] blocked there, these, then, are adjunct patho-conditions of a major-yang disease. Or take, as another example, the *nüe*-disease. Alternating fits of cold and heat, vomiting, a fear of wind, and a bitter taste in one's mouth, these are the patho-conditions that together constitute the *nüe*-disease. They are the patho-conditions typical of *nüe*. If a *nüe*[-disease] is accompanied by headache and swellings, together with [a feeling of] fullness, by coughing and retention of stools and urine, these, then are adjunct patho-conditions of the *nüe*-disease. If, however, a *nüe*[-disease] occurs simultaneously with a *li*-diarrhea [of such a severity] that it passes tens of times [a day], then this cannot be called an adjunct patho-condition; it must be called an additional disease. *Nüe* is one disease, and *li*-diarrhea is a disease too, and both these diseases have their respective typical patho-conditions and also their respective adjunct patho-conditions. I cannot list all [possibilities of typical and adjunct diseases and patho-conditions] here one by one. From this one can draw the conclusion that diseases and patho-conditions may appear combined in countless variations. Hence it is essential to search for their beginnings, and to sort out their different ends. And as far as the therapeutic patterns [to be applied] are concerned, in some cases [different diseases or patho-conditions] are to be treated jointly, in others they are to be treated separately. Some must be treated first, others must be treated later. Some must be the focus of a therapy, others should not be treated at all. It is most important to investigate which [disease] is minor and which is serious, which is slow and which proceeds quickly, and then [to treat them in an appropriate] sequence to achieve the intended success. If, however, one applies therapies that are contrary [to the disease's requirements], and that are confused and follow no rules, then the disease [treated] will appear in many new variations, and even a good practitioner will, in the end, not be able to restore [the patient's health].

5.e *Huáng dì nèi jīng, Tài sù* 15
黃帝內經·太素
Sè mài chǐ zhěn 色脈尺診 160
The Examination of [a Patient's] Complexion, [Movement in the] Vessels, and [Skin Condition in his Arm's] Foot [Section]

黃帝問岐伯曰。餘聞之。見其色。知其病。命曰明。按其脈。知其病。命曰神。問其病而知其處。命曰工。余願聞之。見而知之。按而得之。問而極之。爲之奈何。岐伯答曰。夫色脈與尺之相應也。如桴鼓影響之相應也。不得相失也。此亦本末根葉之出候也。故根死則葉枯矣。色脈形肉不得相失也。故知一則爲工。知二則爲神。知三則神且明矣。黃帝問曰。願卒聞之。岐伯答曰。色青者其脈弦。色赤者其脈鉤。色黃者其脈代。色白者其脈毛。色黑者其脈石。見其色而不得其脈。反得其相勝之脈。則死矣。得其相生之脈。則病已矣。黃帝問岐伯曰。五藏之所生變化之病形何如。岐伯答曰。必先定其五色五脈之應。其病乃可別也。黃帝問曰。色脈已定。別之奈何。岐伯答曰。調其脈之緩急。小大。滑澀。

而病變定矣。黃帝問曰。調之奈何。岐伯答曰。脈急者。尺之皮膚亦急。脈緩者。尺之皮膚亦緩。脈小者。尺之皮膚亦減而少氣。脈大者。尺之皮膚亦賁而起。脈滑者。尺之皮膚亦滑。脈濇者。尺之皮膚亦濇。凡此六變者。有微有甚。故善調尺者。不待於寸口。善調脈者。不待於色。能參合而行之者。可以爲上工。上工十全九。行二者爲中工。中工十全七。行一者爲下工。下工十全六。

岐伯	qí bó	alternative writing to 歧伯 Qí Bó
命	mìng	used for 名 *míng*; to name
按	àn	to feel (the vessels in order to examine the movement within them)
極	jí	thorough; (to reach a) final (conclusion)
爲	wéi	to do
桴鼓	fú gǔ	drumstick and drum [need to come together to produce a sound]
影響	yǐng xiǎng	shadow and echo
失	shī	to lose; to fail
葉	yè	a leaf
出候	chū hòu	appearance; manifestation
卒	zú	completely; in all details
弦	xián	string(-like movement in the vessels)
鈎	gōu	hook(-like movement in the vessels)
代	dài	intermittent (movement in the vessels)
毛	máo	hair(-like movement in the vessels)
石	shí	stone(-like movement in the vessels)
相勝	xiāng shèng	the mutual destruction (among the five agents)
相生	xiāng shēng	the mutual generation (among the five agents)

調	diào	to investigate
小	xiǎo	minor (movement in the vessels)
濇	sè	rough
不待於	bù dái yú	not to depend on
上	shàng	superior
下	xià	inferior
全	quán	to cure

Huáng dì wèn qí bó yuē. yú wén zhī. jiàn qí sè. zhī qí bìng. mìng yuē míng. àn qí mài. zhī qí bìng. mìng yuē shén. wèn qí bìng ér zhī qí chù. mìng yuē gōng. yú yuàn wén zhī. jiàn ér zhī zhī. àn ér dé zhī. wèn ér jí zhī. wéi zhī nài hé. qí bó dá yuē. fū sè mài yǔ chǐ zhī xiāng yìng yě. rú fú gǔ yǐng xiǎng zhī xiāng yìng yě. bù dé xiāng shī yě. cǐ yì běn mò gēn yè zhī chū hòu yě. gù gēn sǐ zé yè kū yǐ. sè mài xíng ròu bù dé xiāng shī yě. gù zhī yī zé wéi gōng. zhī èr zé wéi shén. zhī sān zé shén qiě míng yǐ. huáng-dì wèn yuē. yuàn zú wén zhī. qí bó dá yuē. sè qīng zhě qí mài xián. sè chì zhě qí mài gōu. sè huáng zhě qí mài dài. sè bái zhě qí mài máo. sè hēi zhě qí mài shí. jiàn qí sè ér bù dé qí mài. fǎn dé qí xiāng shèng zhī mài. zé sǐ yǐ. dé qí xiāng shēng zhī mài. zé bìng yǐ yǐ. Huáng dì wèn qí bó yuē. wǔ zàng zhī suǒ shēng biàn huà zhī bìng xíng hé rú. qí bó dá yuē. bì xiān dìng qí wǔ sè wǔ mài zhī yìng. qí bìng nǎi kě bié yě. Huáng dì wèn yuē. sè mài yǐ dìng. bié zhī nài hé. qí bó dá yuē. diào qí mài zhī huǎn jí. xiǎo dà. huá sè. ér bìng biàn dìng yǐ. Huáng dì wèn yuē. diào zhī nài hé. qí bó dá yuē. mài jí zhě. chǐ zhī pí fū yì jí. mài huǎn zhě. chǐ zhī pí fū yì huǎn. mài xiǎo zhě. chǐ zhī pí fū yì jiǎn ér shǎo qì. mài dà zhě. chǐ zhī pí fū yì fén ér qǐ. mài huá zhě. chǐ zhī pí fū yì huá. mài sè zhě. chǐ zhī pí fū yì sè. fán cǐ liù biàn zhě. yǒu wēi yǒu shèn. gù shàn diào chǐ zhě. bù dái yú cùn kǒu. shàn diào mài zhě. bù dái yú sè. néng cān hé ér xíng zhī zhě. kě yǐ wéi shàng gōng. shàng gōng shí quán jiǔ. xíng èr zhě wéi zhōng gōng. zhōng gōng shí quán qī. xíng yī zhě wéi xià gōng. xià gōng shí quán liù.

Huang Di asked Qi Bo: I have heard that someone who looks at the complexion [of a patient] and recognizes his disease may be called enlightened, that someone who touches the [patient's] vessels and recognizes his disease may be called a spirit, and that someone who asks the patient and then knows the location of the [disease] may be called [merely] a practitioner. I should like to hear how it can be done that one takes a look [at the complexion] and recognizes the [disease], that one touches the [vessels] and gets a [correct diagnosis], and that one asks [the patient] and reaches the final [conclusion concerning the location of the disease].

Qi Bo: The mutual correspondence among one's complexion, the [movement in one's] vessels, and the [condition of the skin at one's] foot-section [of the lower arm] is comparable to the mutual correspondence among drumstick and drum, and also to [that among an item and its] shadow [or a sound and its] echo. They cannot be separated from each other! [As a further analogy, one might point out the correspondences in] the appearances of beginning and end, of root and leaves. That is to say, when a root has died, the leaves will wither. [Similarly,] the complexion, the [movement in the] vessels, and the [condition of the] flesh of one's physical body cannot be separated from each other. Now, if someone knows one [of these three diagnostic variables], he is [merely] a practitioner; if he knows two, he is a spirit; and if he knows all three of them, he is a spirit and enlightened.

Huang Di asked: I should like to hear about this in all detail.

Qi Bo: In case a complexion is blue, the respective [movement in the] vessels is string[-like]. In case a complexion is red, the respective [movement in the] vessels is hook[-like]. In case a complexion is yellow, the respective [movement in the] vessels is intermittent; in case a complexion is white, the respective [movement in the] vessels is hair[-like]; in case a complexion is black, the respective [movement in the] vessels is stone[-like]. [1] If one sees a particular complexion, but does not get the respective [movement in the] vessels, and, on the contrary, gets a [movement in the] vessels [associated with a superior agent in the order of] mutual destruction, that means death [to the patient]. [2] If, however, one gets a [movement in the] vessels [that is associated with a mother agent in the order of] mutual generation,[3] the disease can be cured.

Huang Di asked Qi Bo: How about the changes of the physical manifestations of diseases as they are generated by the five depots?

Qi Bo answered: First of all one has to determine whether the five [types of] complexion and the five [types of movements in the] vessels correspond to each other, and then one can distinguish what diseases are present.

Huang Di asked: How can the [diseases] be distinguished, once complexion and [movement in the] vessels have been determined?

Qi Bo answered: One investigates whether the [movement in the] vessels is relaxed or tense, minor or strong, smooth or rough, and then the changes [in the physical appearance caused by a] disease can be determined.

Huang Di asked: How can this be investigated?

Qi Bo answered: If the [movement in the] vessels is tense, the skin at the foot-section should be tense too. If the [movement in the] vessels is minor, the skin at the foot-section should be reduced too, and its qi should be few.

If the [movement in the] vessels is strong, the skin at the foot-section should be vigorous too, and rise. If the [movement in the] vessels is smooth, the skin at the foot-section should be smooth too. If the [movement in the] vessels is rough, the skin at the foot-section should be rough too. All these six changes [in the physical appearance resulting from a disease] may be light or extreme. Hence, someone who knows very well how to investigate [the condition of the skin at] the foot-section, will not have to depend on [an examination of his patient's] inch-opening, and someone who knows very well how to investigate the [movement in the] vessels [at the inch-opening] will not have to depend on [an examination of the patient's] complexion. Those who are able to take all [diagnostic techniques] into consideration and apply them in practice, they are superior practitioners; a superior practitioner cures nine out of ten [cases]. Those who apply two [of these techniques in practice] are mediocre practitioners; a mediocre practitioner cures seven out of ten [cases]. Those who apply one [of these techniques in practice] are inferior practioners; an inferior practitioner cures six out of ten [cases].

Notes

[1] In the five-agents system of correspondences, a blue color and a string-like movement in the vessels are associated with the liver; the color red and a hook-like movement are associated with the heart; the color yellow and an intermittent movement in the vessels are associated with the spleen; the color white and a hair-like movement correspond to the lung; a black complexion and a stone-like movement in the vessels correspond to the kidneys.

[2] The order of mutual destruction/domination of the five agents is as follows: Metal is superior to (i.e. cuts) wood; wood is superior to (i.e. penetrates) soil; soil is superior to (i.e. restrains as a dike the flow of) water; water is superior to (i.e. extinguishes) fire; and fire is superior to (i.e. melts) metal.

[3] The order of mutual generation of the five agents is as follows: Metal generates water; water generates wood; wood generates fire; fire generates soil; soil generates metal.

5.f *Nàn jīng* 難經
Sì shí jiǔ nàn 四十九難
The Forty-Ninth Difficult Issue

有正經自病。有五邪所傷。何以別之。然。經言憂愁思慮則傷心。形寒飲冷則傷肺。恚怒氣逆。上而不下則傷肝。飲食勞倦則傷脾。久坐濕地。强力入水則傷腎。是正經之自病也。何謂五邪。然。有中風。有傷暑。有飲食勞倦。有傷寒。有中濕。此之謂五邪。假令心病。何以知中風得之。然。其色當赤。何以言之。肝主色。自入爲青。入心爲赤。入脾爲黃。入肺爲白。入腎爲黑。肝爲心邪。故知當赤色。其病身熱。脇下滿痛。其脉浮大而弦。何以知傷暑得之。然。當惡臭。何以言之。心主臭。自入爲焦臭。入脾爲香臭。入肝爲臊臭。入腎爲腐臭。入肺爲腥臭。故知心病傷暑得之也。當惡臭。其病身熱而煩。心痛。其脈浮大而散。何以知飲食勞倦得之。然。當喜苦味也。虛爲不欲食。實爲欲食。何以言之。脾主味。入肝爲酸。入心爲苦。入肺爲辛。入腎爲鹹。自入爲甘。故知脾邪入心。爲喜苦味也。其病身熱而體重嗜臥。四肢不收。其脈浮大而緩。何以知傷寒得之。然。當譫言妄語。何以

言之。肺主聲。入肝爲呼。入心爲言。入脾爲歌。入腎爲呻。自入爲哭。故知肺邪入心。爲譫言妄語也。其病身熱。洒洒惡寒。甚則喘咳。其脈浮大而濇。何以知中濕得之。然。當喜汗出不可止。何以言之。腎主濕。入肝爲泣。入心爲汗。入脾爲涎。入肺爲涕。自入爲唾。故知腎邪入心。爲汗出不可止也。其病身熱而小腹痛。足脛寒而逆。其脉沉濡而大。此五邪之法也

有	yǒu	it may be that
正經	zhèng jīng	the regular conduits
自病	zì bìng	to fall ill by itself (as of a regular conduit, in contrast to a disease transmitted from another depot or conduit)
五邪	wǔ xié	the five evils
愁	chóu	anxiety
慮	lǜ	to consider
恚	huì	range
倦	juàn	fatigued; weary
坐	zuò	to sit
强力	qiáng lì	to force oneself; to exert one's strength
傷暑	shāng shǔ	to be harmed by summer-heat
中濕	zhōng shī	to be struck by dampness
假令	jiǎ lìng	suppose; if for example,...; take,for example, …
中風	zhòng fēng	to be struck by wind
焦	jiāo	burnt (breath odor)
臭	xiù	odor
香	xiāng	aromatic
臊	sāo	fetid
腐	fǔ	foul
腥	xīng	fishy

散	sàn	dispersed (movement in the vessels)
收	shōu	to contract (as one's limbs)
譫言	zhān yán	to speak incoherently
語	yǔ	to converse; language
呼	hū	to shout; to call
歌	gē	song; to sing
呻	shēn	to groan
哭	kū	to wail
洒洒	xiǎn xiǎn	to shiver
泣	qì	tears
涕	tī	snivel
唾	tuò	spittle
小腹	xiǎo fù	the lower abdomen
脛	jìng	the shinbone
沉	chén	in the depth (as a movement in the vessels)
濡	rú	soft (movement in the vessels)

Yǒu zhèng jīng zì bìng. yǒu wǔ xié suǒ shāng. hé yǐ bié zhī. rán. jīng yán yōu chóu sī lǜ zé shāng xīn. xíng hán yǐn lěng zé shāng fèi. huì nù qì nì. shàng ér bù xià zé shāng gān. yǐn shí láo juàn zé shāng pí. jiǔ zuò shī dì. qiáng lì rù shuǐ zé shāng shèn. shī zhèng jīng zhī zì bìng yě. hé wèi wǔ xié. rán. yǒu zhòng fēng. yǒu shāng shǔ. yǒu yǐn shí láo juàn. yǒu shāng hán. yǒu zhōng shī. cǐ zhī wèi wǔ xié. jiǎ lìng xīn bìng. hé yǐ zhī zhòng fēng dé zhī. rán. qí sè dāng chì. hé yǐ yán zhī. gān zhǔ sè. zì rù wéi qīng. rù xīn wéi chì. rù pí wéi huáng. rù fèi wéi bái. rù shèn wéi hēi. gān wéi xīn xié. gù zhī dāng chì sè. qí bìng shēn rè. xié xià mǎn tòng. qí mài fú dà ér xián. hé yǐ zhī shāng shǔ dé zhī. rán. dāng è xiù. hé yǐ yán zhī. xīn zhǔ xiù. zì rù wéi jiāo xiù. rù pí wéi xiāng xiù. rù gān wéi sāo xiù. rù shèn wéi fǔ xiù. rù fèi wéi xīng xiù. gù zhī xīn bìng shāng shǔ dé zhī yě. dāng è xiù. qí bìng shēn rè ér fán. xīn tòng. qí mài fú dà ér sàn. hé yǐ zhī yǐn shí láo juàn dé zhī. rán. dāng xǐ kǔ wèi yě. xū wéi bù yù shí. shí wéi yù shí. hé yǐ yán zhī. pí zhǔ wèi. rù gān wéi suān. rù xīn wéi kǔ. rù fèi wéi xīn. rù shèn wéi xián. zì rù wéi gān. gù zhī pí xié rù xīn. wéi xǐ kǔ wèi yě. qí bìng shēn rè ér tǐ zhòng shí wò. sì zhī bù shōu. qí mài fú dà ér huǎn. hé yǐ zhī shāng hán dé zhī. rán. dāng zhān yán wàng yǔ. hé yǐ yán zhī. fèi zhǔ shēng. rù gān wéi hū. rù xīn wéi yán. rù pí wéi gē. rù shèn wéi shēn. zì rù wéi kū. gù zhī fèi xié rù xīn. wéi zhān yán wàng yǔ yě. qí bìng shēn rè. xiǎn xiǎn wù hán. shèn zé chuǎn ké. qí mài fú dà ér sè. hé yǐ zhī zhōng shī dé zhī. rán. dāng xǐ hàn chū bù kě zhǐ. hé yǐ yán zhī. shèn zhǔ shī. rù gān wéi qì. rù xīn wéi hàn. rù pí wéi xián. rù fèi wéi tī. zì rù wéi tuò. gù zhī shèn xié rù xīn. wéi hàn chū bù kě zhǐ yě. qí bìng shēn rè ér xiǎo fù tòng. zú jìng hán ér nì. qí mài chén rú ér dà. cǐ wǔ xié zhī fǎ yě.

It happens that the regular conduits fall ill by themselves, or that one is harmed by one of the five evils. How can these [situations] be distinguished?
It is like this. The Classic states: Mourning and anxiety, thoughts and considerations harm the heart; a cold body and chilled drinks harm the lung; rage and anger let the qi flow contrary to their proper direction, they move upward but not downward. That harms the liver. Drinking and eating [without restraints], as well as taxation and weariness, harm the spleen. If one sits in a damp place for an extended period, or if one exerts one's strength and goes into water,[1] that harms the kidneys. These are [examples of a situation where] the regular conduits fall ill by themselves.
What is meant by "the five evils"?
It is like this. To be hit by wind, to be harmed by heat, to drink and eat [without restraints], as well as taxation and weariness, to be harmed by cold, to be struck by dampness, these [conditions] are called the five evils. Let us take a disease in the heart as an example.
How does one know that [the patient] has contracted it because he was struck by wind?
It is like this. His complexion should be red. Why do I say so? The liver rules the colors. [The color evil qi generates in the liver] itself is greenish-blue. [The color that is generated when it sends evil qi] into the heart is red. [The color that is generated when it sends evil qi] into the spleen is yellow. [The color that is generated when it sends evil qi] into the lung is white. [The color that is generated when it sends evil qi] into the kidneys is black. Hence, one knows from the red complexion [of a patient] that the liver has [sent evil qi] into the heart, causing the presence of evil [qi there]. [The patient] will suffer from a hot body, and [he will perceive] fullness and pain below his ribs. [The movement of the qi in] his vessels is at the surface, strong, and string[-like].
How does one know that [the patient has] contracted [his illness in the heart] because he was harmed by summer-heat?
It is like this. He should have a bad odor.[2] Why do I say so? The heart rules the odors. [The odor that is generated by the heart] itself is burnt. [The odor that is generated when the heart sends evil qi] into the spleen is aromatic. [The odor that is generated when the heart sends evil qi] into the liver is fetid. [The odor that is generated when it sends evil qi] into the kidneys is foul. [The odor that

is generated when it sends evil qi] into the lung is fishy. Hence, one knows if a disease in the heart has been contracted because of harm caused by heat, there should be a bad odor.[2] The patient will suffer from a hot body, and he will feel distressed. His heart aches, and [the movement in the] vessels is at the surface, strong, and dispersed.

How does one know that [the patient has] contracted [his disease in the heart] because of [unrestrained] drinking and eating, or because of taxation and weariness?

It is like this. He should prefer [to consume food with a] bitter flavor. [When one's spleen is] depleted, one will not wish to eat; [when one's spleen] is replete, one will wish to eat. Why do I say so? The spleen rules [one's preferences for a specific] flavor. [The flavor one prefers when the spleen sends evil qi] into the liver is sour. [The flavor one prefers when the spleen sends evil qi] into the heart is bitter. [The flavor one prefers when the spleen sends evil qi] into the lung is acrid. [The flavor one prefers when the spleen sends evil qi] into the kidneys is salty. [The flavor one prefers when the spleen keeps evil qi] within itself is sweet. Hence, one knows if evil [qi] from the spleen enter the heart, that causes a preference for bitter flavor. The patient will suffer from a hot body; [he will perceive] his body to be heavy, and he will have a desire to lie down. He cannot contract his four limbs. [The movement in] his vessels is at the surface, strong, and relaxed.

How does one know that [the patient has] contracted [his disease in the heart] because of harm caused of cold?

It is like this. He will talk incoherently and he will utter nonsense. Why do I say so? The lung rules the sounds. [The evil qi it sends] into the liver [cause one] to call. [The evil qi it sends] into the heart [cause one] to speak. [The evil qi it sends] into the spleen [cause one] to sing. [The evil qi it sends] into the kidneys [cause one] to groan. [The evil qi it keeps] within itself [cause one to wail]. Hence, one knows, if evil [qi] from the lung have entered the heart, they cause [the patient] to talk incoherently and to utter nonsense. The patient will suffer from a hot body, he will shiver, and he will dislike cold. In extreme cases, this leads to coughing. [The movement in] his vessels is at the surface, strong, and rough.

How does one know that [the patient has] contracted [his disease in the heart] because he was struck by dampness?

It is like this. He will have a tendency to sweat without end. Why do I say so? The kidneys rule the liquids. [The liquid that is generated when the kidneys send evil qi] into the liver are tears. [The liquid that is generated when the kidneys send evil qi] into heart is sweat. [The liquid that is generated when they send evil qi] into the spleen is saliva. [The liquid that is generated when they send evil qi] into the lung is snivel. [The liquid that is generated when they keep evil qi] within themselves is spittle. Hence, one knows, if evil [qi] from the kidneys have entered the heart, this causes [the patient] to sweat without end. He will suffer from a hot body and from pain in the lower abdomen; his feet and shinbones will be cold, and [the qi will] move contrary to their proper course. [The movement in] his vessels will be deep, soft, and strong. This is the pattern of the five qi.

Notes

[1] *Rù shuǐ* ("to enter water") has been interpreted by Lü Guang 呂廣 (3rd c.) and by Ding Deyong 丁德用 (fl. 1062) as "sexual intercourse before menstruation has come to an end". Lü Guang admitted, in addition, an interpretation of *rù shuǐ* as "to repeatedly sink down into water". The *Su wen* has the expression 以水爲事 *yǐ shuǐ wèi shì*, "one's work has to do with water".

[2] Some editions have the character 焦 *jiāo*, "burnt", here in addition to 惡 *è*, "bad". From the system outlined in the text, one would expect only 焦 *jiāo*, "burnt".

Lesson Six

Diagnostics: The Movement in the Vessels

Pulse-diagnosis is a characteristic aspect of Chinese traditional diagnostics; in fact, many contemporary teaching manuals of Traditional Chinese Medicine refer to the condition of the pulse as the most significant diagnostic parameter to be taken into account as a guideline for treatment. Originally, prior to the conceptualization of a circulatory system of conduits linking the entire organism, eleven separate vessels were described as penetrating the body in the so-called Mawangdui texts of ca. 200 BCE. These texts offer first hints that the vessels were examined for diagnostic purposes. In the *Su wen*, a text whose earliest historical layers were probably compiled during the first century CE on the basis of scriptures dating from the second and first centuries BCE, the states of repletion or depletion of the contents of the vessels, as well as their movement and further parameters, could signal illness, and had to be examined at locations in various parts of the body where the eleven vessels came close enough to the surface to be accessible to a palpating hand. The *Ling shu* and the *Nan jing*, two further medical texts compiled in the first or second centuries CE on the basis of writings from the preceding one or two hundred years, developed and systematized an approach to pulse diagnosis that appears to have emerged as a consequence of the assumption of a continuous flow of qi/vapors and blood through the body, either in the sense of a permanent multidirectional exchange among the individual functional units of the organism, or as a circulatory stream "in a ring without end". Similar to a Greek idea of air flowing through a system of channels (*aer-tereo*, "air holders", i.e. arteries), some Chinese authors conceptualized separate systems of conduits for qi and blood. Others recognized but one system where blood and qi shared the same conduits. The issue was never resolved, but despite these uncertainties the movements in the vessels that could be felt at various locations were an undisputed reality. The complexity of data presumably revealed through the movement in the vessels at the so-called inch-opening at the wrists, an approach developed most consistently in the *Nan jing*, is enormous. Based on the yinyang-doctrine (and, to a lesser extent, on the five-agents-doctrine), of systematic correspondence, numerous patterns of movements in the vessels were identified, and described in the literature, as indicating each detail a physician had to know of the origin, current status, and future course of a disease in the organism.

Key Terms Introduced in Lesson Six

三部	sān bù	three sections
三候	sān hòu	three indicators
額	é	the forehead
動脈	dòng mài	moving vessel
頰	jiá	a cheek
手太陰	shǒu tài yīn	the hand-major-yin (region)
手陽明	shǒu yáng míng	the hand-yang-brilliance (region)
大指	dà zhǐ	the thumb
手少陰	shǒu shào yīn	the hand-minor-yin (region)
銳[骨]	ruì(-gǔ)	the pointed (bone); i.e. the exterior tip of the ulna in the wrists
足厥陰	zú jué yīn	the foot-ceasing-yin (location)
毛際	máo jì	the (upper) border-line of the (pubic) hair
羊矢	yáng shǐ	sheep droppings (a term referring to the inguinal lymphatic glands palpable in the groins)
足少陰	zú shào yīn	the foot-minor-yin (location)
踝	huái	the ankle
跟	gēn	the heel
足太陰	zú tài yīn	the foot-major-yin (location)
魚腹	yú fù	the fish-belly (a term referring to a protuberance palpable in the upper thighs between the musculus sartorius and the musculus quadriceps femoris)
趨筋	qū jīn	the running sinews/muscles (a term referring to m. satorius and m. quadriceps femoris in the upper thighs)
頭角	tóu jiǎo	the temples
三部	sān bù	the three sections (at the wrists where the movement in the vessels can be felt; i.e. the inch, the gate, and the foot section)

三候	sān hòu	the three indicator (levels in each section at the wrists where the movement in the vessels can be felt; i.e. at the surface, in the center, in the depth)
寸	cùn	the inch (section of the wrists where the movement in the vessels can be felt)
關	guān	the gate (section of the wrists where the movement in the vessels can be felt)
正脈	zhèng mài	a regular (movement in the) vessels
重陰	chóng yīn	the doubling of yin (qi)
重陽	chóng yáng	the doubling of yang (qi)
七表	qī biǎo	the seven external (movements in the vessels)
八裏	bā lǐ	the eight internal (movements in the vessels)
數	shuò	frequent (movement in the vessels)
面	miàn	the face
肚	dù	the belly
動	dòng	excited (movement in the vessels)
微	wēi	feeble (movement in the vessels)
陽結	yáng jié	clottings of yang (qi)
陰結	yīn jié	clottings of yin (qi)
大便	dà biàn	stools
促	cù	hurried (movement in the vessels)
病脈	bìng mài	(a movement in the) vessels (indicating an) illness
緊	jǐn	tight (movement in the vessels)
太過	tài guò	great excess
不及	bù jí	insufficiency
覆	fù	turnover
溢	yì	overflow
關	guān	the gate(-line separating the inch and the foot sections at the wrist)
外關	wài guān	external closure
內關	nèi guān	internal closure
外格	wài gé	external obstruction
營	yíng	to circulate
魚際	yú jì	the fish-border (which separates the palm from the wrist)

大小便閉	dà xiăo biàn bì	constipation of s *Nei jing* tools and urine
厥冷	jué lĕng	cold (hands and feet) resulting from to receding (yang qi)
真藏	zhēn zàng	the true (qi of a) depot
虎口	hŭ kŏu	(the width of an opened) tiger mouth; i.e. the distance between the tip of one's thumb and the tip of one's index finger if spread apart from one hand
三關	sān guān	the three gate(-sections of the index fingers of small children)
疳	gān	the *gan*-illness
中惡	zhòng è	to be struck by the malevolent
風關	fēng guān	the wind-gate(-section; i.e. the section between the base fold, adjoining the palm, and the second fold on the inside of the index finger)
氣關	qì guān	the qi-gate(-section; i.e. the middle section of the inside of the index finger)
命關	mìng guān	the life-gate(-section; i.e. the uppermost of the three sections of the inside of the index finger)
乳癎	rŭ xián	convulsions (common in children that are still) breast(-fed)
風癎	fēng xián	convulsions (caused by) wind
牢	láo	firm (movement in the vessels)
便秘	biàn bì	constipation
細	xì	fine (movement in the vessels)
祟	suì	curse by evil spirits
宿食	sù shí	food remaining (in the stomach without being digested)
化	huà	to digest
變蒸	biàn zhēng	the transformation and steaming (of newly-borns)
單	dān	thin (movement in the vessels)
痘	dòu	pox (in modern medical literature: small pox)
斑	bān	streak(-like skin rash)
疹	zhĕn	pustules; eruptions

6.a *Huáng dì nèi jīng, Sù wèn* 20
黃帝內經·素問
Sān bù jiŭ hòu lùn 三部九候論
On the Three Sections and Nine Indicators

天地之至數。始於一。終於九焉。一者天。二者地。三者人。因而三之。三三者九。以應九野。故人有三部。部有三候。以決死生。以處百病。以調虛實。而除邪疾。帝曰。何謂三部。岐伯曰。有下部。有中部。有上部。部各有三候。三候者。有天有地有人也。必指而導之。乃以爲真。上部天。兩額之動脈。上部地。兩頰之動脈。上部人。耳前之動脈。中部天。手太陰也。謂肺脉也。在掌後寸口中。中部地。手陽明也。謂大腸脉也。在手大指次指歧骨間。中部人。手少陰也。謂心脉也。在掌後銳之端。下部天。足厥陰也。謂肝脉也。在毛際外羊矢下一寸半陷中。下部地。足少陰也。謂腎脉也。在足內踝後跟骨上陷中。下部人。足太陰也。謂脾脉也。在魚腹上趨筋間。故下部之天以候肝。地以候腎。人以候脾胃之氣。帝曰。中部之候奈何。岐伯曰。亦有天。亦有地。亦有人。天以候肺。地以候胸中之氣。人以候心。帝曰。上部以何候之。岐伯曰。亦有天。亦有地。

亦有人。天以候頭角之氣。地以候口齒之氣。人以候耳目之氣。

數	shù	a number
至數	zhì shù	the perfect numbers
野	yě	field
三部	sān bù	three sections
三候	sān hòu	three indicators
決	jué	to decide
處	chù	to manage
額	é	the forehead
動脈	dòng mài	moving vessel
頰	jiá	a cheek
手太陰	shǒu tài yīn	the hand-major-yin (region)
手陽明	shǒu yáng míng	the hand-yang-brilliance (region)
大指	dà zhǐ	the thumb
歧	qí	a fork; forked
手少陰	shǒu shào yīn	the hand-minor-yin (region)
銳[骨]	ruì(-gǔ)	the pointed (bone); i.e. the exterior tip of the ulna in the wrists
足厥陰	zú jué yīn	the foot-ceasing-yin (location)
毛際	máo jì	the (upper) border-line of the (pubic) hair
羊矢	yáng shǐ	sheep droppings (a term referring to the inguinal lymphatic glands palpable in the groins)
足少陰	zú shào yīn	the foot-minor-yin (location)
踝	huái	the ankle
跟	gēn	the heel
足太陰	zú tài yīn	the foot-major-yin (location)
魚腹	yú fù	the fish-belly (a term referring to a protuberance palpable in the upper thighs between the musculus sartorius and the musculus quadriceps femoris)

趨筋	qū jīn	the running sinews/muscles (a term referring to m. satorius and m. quadriceps femoris in the upper thighs)
候	hòu	to examine
頭角	tóu jiǎo	the temples

Tiān dì zhī zhì shù. shǐ yú yī. zhōng yú jiǔ yān. yī zhě tiān. èr zhě dì. sān zhě rén. yīn ér sān zhī. sān sān zhě jiǔ. yǐ yìng jiǔ yě. gù rén yǒu sān bù. bù yǒu sān hòu. yǐ jué sǐ shēng. yǐ chù bǎi bìng. yǐ tiáo xū shí. ér chú xié jí. dì yuē. hé wèi sān bù. qí bó yuē. yǒu xià bù. yǒu zhōng bù. yǒu shàng bù. bù gè yǒu sān hòu. sān hòu zhě. yǒu tiān yǒu dì yǒu rén yě. bì zhǐ ér dǎo zhī. nǎi yǐ wéi zhēn. shàng bù tiān. liǎng é zhī dòng mài. shàng bù dì. liǎng jiá zhī dòng mài. shàng bù rén. ěr qián zhī dòng mài. zhōng bù tiān. shǒu tài yīn yě. wèi fèi mài yě. zài zhǎng hòu cùn kǒu zhōng. zhōng bù dì. shǒu yáng míng yě. wèi dà cháng mài yě. zài shǒu dà zhǐ cì zhǐ qí gǔ jiān. zhōng bù rén. shǒu shào yīn yě. wèi xīn mài yě. zài zhǎng hòu ruì zhī duān. xià bù tiān. zú jué yīn yě. wèi gān mài yě. zài máo jì wài yáng shǐ xià yí cùn bàn. xià bù dì. zú shào yīn yě. wèi shèn mài yě. zài zú nèi huái hòu gēn gǔ shàng xiàn zhōng. xià bù rén. zú tài yīn yě. wèi pí mài yě. zài yú fù shàng qū jīn jiān. gù xià bù zhī tiān yǐ hòu gān. dì yǐ hòu shèn. rén yǐ hòu pí wèi zhī qì. dì yuē. zhōng bù zhī hòu nài hé. qí bó yuē. yì yǒu tiān. yì yǒu dì. yì yǒu rén. tiān yǐ hòu fèi. dì yǐ hòu xiōng zhōng zhī qì. rén yǐ hòu xīn. dì yuē. shàng bù yǐ hé hòu zhī. qí bó yuē. yì yǒu tiān. yì yǒu dì. yì yǒu rén. tiān yǐ hòu tóu jiǎo zhī qì. dì yǐ hòu kǒu chǐ zhī qì. rén yǐ hòu ěr mù zhī qì.

The perfect numbers of heaven and earth, they begin with one and they end with nine. One is heaven; two is the earth; three is man. Subsequently they are multiplied by three – three [times] three is nine – to correspond to the nine fields.[1]Hence, man has three sections. [Each] section has three indicators. They serve to decide about death or survival. They serve to manage the one hundred diseases. They serve to regulate [states of] depletion and repletion and to eliminate evil and disease.

[Huang] Di: What is that so say "three sections"?

Qi Bo: [Man] has a lower section, has a central section, and has an upper section. Each section has three indicators. The three indicators: there is heaven, there is earth, and there is man. One must [use] one's finger to point them out [on the body] and then accept them as real. The heaven [indicator] of the upper section: the moving vessels on the two [sides of the] forehead. The earth [indicator] of the upper section: the moving vessels on the two [sides of the] cheeks. The man [indicator] of the upper section: the moving vessels in front of the ears. The heaven [indicator] of the central section: the major yin [locations] of the hands. The earth [indicator] of the central section: the yang brilliance [locations] of the hands. The man [indicator] of the central section: the minor yin [locations] of the hands. The heaven [indicator] of the lower section: the ceasing yin [locations] of the feet. The earth [indicator] of the lower section: the minor yin [locations] of the feet. The man [indicator] of the lower section: the major yin [locations] of the feet. Hence, in the lower section, the heaven [indicator] serves to examine the liver. The earth [indicator] serves to examine the kidneys. The man [indicator] serves to examine the qi of spleen and stomach.

[Huang] Di: How about the indicators of the central section?

Qi Bo: It, too, has a heaven [indicator]; it, too, has an earth [indicator]; it, too, has a man [indicator]. The heaven [indicator] serves to examine the lung. The earth [indicator] serves to examine the qi in the chest. The man [indicator] serves to examine the heart.

[Huang] Di: What is examined through the upper section?

Qi Bo: It, too has a heaven [indicator]; it, too, has an earth [indicator]; it, too, has a man [indicator]. The heaven [indicator] serves to examine the qi at the corners of the head. The earth [indicator] serves to examine the qi of mouth and teeth. The man [indicator] serves to examine the qi of ears and eyes.

Note

[1] A reference to an ancient Chinese notion dividing the earth into nine fields.

6.b *Shòu shì bǎo yuán* 1 壽世保元 Zhěn mài 診脈 Examination of the [Movement in the] Vessels

---

人之四肢。各有脈也。一脈三部。一部三候。以應天數也。一脈三部。寸關尺也。一部三候。浮中沉也。所以應之九數也。愚謂脈之理亦微矣。人有四時之正脈。有平生之常脈。有內傷之變脈。有外感之邪脈。有重陰之脈。有重陽之脈。有陽虛而陰乘之脈。有陰虛而陽乘之脈。有陽極而陰生之脈。有陰極而陽生之脈。有獨見之脈。有兼見之脈。有初病之脈。有久病之脈。有可治之脈。有不治之脈。有左右上下表裏之間。有餘不足。惟在乎分別陰陽。能分別陰陽。斯可以識脈之體。劉復真曰。昔王叔和以七表八裏脉。決人之生死。然又文理浩繁。今撮其樞要。以浮沉遲數四脈爲宗。知風氣冷熱主病。且浮而有力者爲風。浮而無力爲虛。沉而有力爲積。沉而無力爲氣。遲而有力爲痛。遲而無力爲冷。數而有力爲熱。數而無力爲瘡。更分三部。在何部得之。若在寸部。主上焦頭面胸膈之疾。關部。主中焦肚腹脾胃之疾。尺部。主下焦小腹腰足之疾。診

其五臟。何臟得之。六腑亦然。學者又當以意會而加精別。庶不致按寸握尺之誚云。

三部	sān bù	the three sections (at the wrists where the movement in the vessels can be felt; i.e. the inch, the gate, and the foot section)
三候	sān hòu	the three indicator (levels in each section at the wrists where the movement in the vessels can be felt; i.e. at the surface, in the center, and in the depth)
寸	cùn	the inch (section of the wrists where the movement in the vessels can be felt)
關	guān	the gate (section of the wrists where the movement in the vessels can be felt)
愚	yú	ignoramus. Here, a term of self-depreciation: I; myself
正脈	zhèng mài	a regular (movement in the) vessels
重陰	chóng yīn	the doubling of yin (qi)
重陽	chóng yáng	the doubling of yang (qi)
間	jiān	to divide; to distinguish
體	tǐ	the essentials
劉復真	liú fù zhēn	Liu Fuzhen, honorary style-name of Liú Kāi 劉開, author of a book on pulse-lore of the 14th century
昔	xī	formerly
王叔和	wáng shū hé	Wang Shuhe, style-name of Wáng Xī 王熙 (210-285), author of the *Mài jīng* 脉經, the classic of pulse-lore
七表	qī biǎo	the seven external (movements in the vessels; i.e. 浮 *fú* [at the surface], 芤 *kōu* [hollow], 滑 *huá* [smooth], 實 *shí* [replete], 弦 *xián* [string-like], 緊 *jǐn* [tight], and 洪 *hóng* [vast])

八裏	bā lǐ	the eight internal (movements in the vessels; i.e. 微 *wéi* [feeble], 沉 *chén* [in the depth], 緩 *huǎn* [relaxed], 濇 *sè* [rough], 遲 *chí* [slow], 伏 *fú* [hidden], 濡 *rú* [soft], and 弱 *ruò* [weak])
文理浩繁	wén lǐ hào fán	complicated textual structure
撮	cuō	to gather; to pick
樞要	shū yào	of central importance; essential
數	shuò	frequent (movement in the vessels)
宗	zōng	the most important
積	jī	accumulation
面	miàn	the face
肚	dù	the belly
意會	yì huì	to reach a comprehensive understanding
庶	shù	it is to be hoped; possibly
握	wò	to hold fast; to grasp
誚	qiào	to blame; to ridicule

Rén zhī sì zhī. gè yǒu mài yě. yí mài sān bù. yí bù sān hòu. yǐ yìng tiān shù yě. yí mài sān bù. cùn guān chǐ yě. yí bù sān hòu. fú zhōng chén yě. suǒ yǐ yìng zhī jiǔ shù yě. yú wèi mài zhī lǐ yì wēi yǐ. rén yǒu sì shí zhī zhèng mài. yǒu píng shēng zhī cháng mài. yǒu nèi shāng zhī biàn mài. yǒu wài gǎn zhī xié mài. yǒu chóng yīn zhī mài. yǒu chóng yáng zhī mài. yǒu yáng xū ér yīn chéng zhī mài. yǒu yīn xū ér yáng chéng zhī mài. yǒu yáng jí ér yīn shēng zhī mài. yǒu yīn jí ér yáng shēng zhī mài. yǒu dú jiàn zhī mài. yǒu jiān jiàn zhī mài. yǒu chū bìng zhī mài. yǒu jiǔ bìng zhī mài. yǒu kě zhì zhī mài. yǒu bù zhì zhī mài. yǒu zuǒ yòu shàng xià biǎo lǐ zhī jiān. yǒu yú bù zú. wéi zài hū fēn bié yīn yáng. néng fēn bié yīn yáng. sī kě yǐ shí mài zhī tǐ. liú fù zhēn yuē. xī wáng shū hé yǐ qī biǎo bā lǐ mài. jué rén zhī shēng sǐ. rán yòu wén lǐ hào fán. jīn cuō qí shū yào. yǐ fú chén chí shuò sì mài wéi zōng. zhī fēng qì lěng rè zhǔ bìng. qiě fú ér yǒu lì zhě wéi fēng. fú ér wú lì wéi xū. chén ér yǒu lì wéi jī. chén ér wú lì wéi qì. chí ér yǒu lì wéi tòng. chí ér wú lì wéi lěng. shuò ér yǒu lì wéi rè. shuò ér wú lì wéi chuāng. gèng fēn sān bù. zài hé bù dé zhī. ruò zài cùn bù. zhǔ shàng jiāo tóu miàn xiōng gé zhī jí. guān bù. zhǔ zhōng jiāo dù fù pí wèi zhī jí. chǐ bù. zhǔ xià jiāo xiǎo fù yāo zú zhī jí. zhěn qí wǔ zàng. hé zàng dé zhī. liù fǔ yì rán. xué zhě yòu dāng yǐ yì huì ér jiā jīng bié. shù bù zhì àn cùn wò chǐ zhī qiào yún.

All four limbs of the human [body] have [locations where the movement in the] vessels [can be felt]. Each [of these locations where the movement in the] vessels [can be felt is divided into] three sections. And each of these three sections has three indicator [levels] in order to correspond to the numbers of heaven. The three sections of each [of the locations where the movement in the] vessels [can be felt] are the inch, the gate, and the foot [section]. And the three indicator [levels] of each section are at the surface, in the center, and in the depth. Thusly a correspondence to the number nine is reached. In my opinion, the principles of the [movement in the] vessels are similarly sophisticated. [That is,] man may have a regular [movement in the] vessels that [corresponds to the] four seasons, and he may have a normal [movement in the] vessels that [corresponds to a] balanced life. He may have a changed [movement in the] vessels [that corresponds to an] internal harm, and he may have [a movement in the] vessels [indicating the presence of] evil [qi resulting] from an external assault. He may have [a movement in the] vessels [corresponding to a] doubling of the yin [qi], and he may have [a movement in the] vessels [corresponding to a] doubling of the yang [qi]. He may have [a movement in the] vessels [indicating a] depletion of yang [qi] and the seizure [of the depleted region] by yin [qi], and he may have [a movement in the] vessels [indicating a] depletion of yin [qi], and the seizure [of the depleted region] by yang [qi]. He may have [a movement in the] vessels [corresponding to an] extreme [development] of yang [qi], and the emergence of yin [qi], and he may have [a movement in the] vessels [corresponding to an] extreme [development] of yin [qi], and the emergence of yang [qi]. There are [movements in the] vessels that appear by themselves, and there are [movements in the] vessels that appear jointly with others. There are [movements in the] vessels [indicating a] new illness, and there are [movements in the] vessels [indicating an] illness that has existed over a long time already. There are [movements in the] vessels [corresponding to diseases] that can be cured, and there are [movements in the] vessels [corresponding to diseases] that are incurable. One has to distinguish between left and right, above and below, external and internal, and there may be superabundance or insufficiency. [To recognize all these different states] depends on nothing but [one's ability] to distinguish between yin and yang [phenomena]. With the ability to distinguish between yin and yang [phenomena], it is possible to recognize the essentials of the [movement in the] vessels. Liu Fuzhen has said: Formerly, Wang Shuhe decided about a person's survival or [impending] death [due to disease] on the basis of the seven external and eight internal [movements in the] vessels. However, the structure of his text was complicated, and I have picked from it now only the most essential [elements]. I consider the four [movements in the] vessels at the surface, in the depth, slow, and frequent as the most important to recognize [the abnormal presence of] wind, qi, cold, and heat as the diseases responsible [for such movements]. That is to say, [a movement that is] at the surface and shows strength is [caused by a disease resulting from] wind. [A movement that is] at the surface and shows no strength is [caused by a disease resulting from] depletion [of qi. A movement in the vessels that is] in the depth and shows strength is [caused by an] accumulation [of qi]. [A movement that is] in the depth and shows no strength [indicates a depletion of] qi. [A movement that is] slow and shows strength [indicates] pain. [A movement that is] slow and shows no strength [indicates] cold. [A movement that is] frequent and shows strength [indicates] heat. [A movement that is] frequent and shows no strength [indicates the presence of] sores. Furthermore, one should distinguish among the three sections [at the wrists in order to find out] which section [of the body] has been affected [by a disease]. That is, the inch section is responsible for [providing evidence of] diseases affecting the upper [section of the triple] burner, head, face, chest, and diaphragm. The gate section is responsible for [providing evidence of] diseases affecting the central [section of the triple] burner, the belly, the abdomen, the spleen, and the stomach. The foot section [at the wrists] is responsible for [providing evidence of] diseases affecting the lower [section of the triple] burner, the lower abdomen, the waist, and the feet. One examines [the movement in the vessels corresponding to] the five depots [in order to find out] which of the depots has been affected by a [disease]. The same applies to the palaces. Students [of this kind of patient examination] should acquire a comprehensive understanding and add [an ability to] distinguish among the finest details, and it is to be hoped that they will not be ridiculed for [only] pressing the inch [section] and grasping the foot [section].

6.c *Zhù jiě shāng hán lùn* 1
註解傷寒論
Biàn mài fǎ 辨脈法
Patterns to Distinguish the [Movement in the] Vessels

問曰。脈有陰陽者何謂也。答曰。凡脈大。浮。數。動。滑。此名陽也。脈沉。濇。弱。弦。微。此名陰也。凡陰病見陽脈者生。陽病見陰脈者死。問曰。脈有陽結陰結者。何以別之。答曰。其脈浮而數。能食。不大便者。此爲實。名曰陽結也。期十七日當劇。其脈沉而遲。不能食。身體重。大便反鞕。名曰陰結也。期十四日當劇。結者。氣偏結固。問曰。病有灑淅惡寒而復發熱者何。答曰。陰脈不足。陽往從之。陽脈不足。陰往乘之。曰。何謂陽不足。答曰。假令寸口脈微。名曰陽不足。陰氣上入陽中。則灑淅惡寒也。曰。何謂陰不足。答曰。假令尺脈弱。名曰陰不足。陽氣下陷入陰中。則發熱也。陽脈浮陰脈弱者。則血虛。血虛則筋急也。其脈沉者。榮氣微也。其脉浮而汗出如流珠者。衛氣衰也。..。脈來緩。時一止復來者。名曰結。脈來數。時一止復來者。名曰促。脈陽盛則促。陰盛則結。此

皆病脈。脈一息四至曰平。一息三至曰遲。小駃於遲曰緩。一息六至曰數。時有一止者。陰陽之氣不得相續也。陰陽相搏名曰動。陽動則汗出。陰動則發熱。...。若數脈見於關上。上下無頭尾。如豆大。厥厥動搖者。名曰動也。脈浮而緊者。名曰弦也。弦者狀如弓弦。按之不移也。脈緊者。如轉索無常也。

動	dòng	excited (movement in the vessels)
微	wēi	feeble (movement in the vessels)
陽結	yáng jié	clottings of yang (qi)
陰結	yīn jié	clottings of yin (qi)
大便	dà biàn	stools
期	qí	a period; a fixed time
劇	jù	a crisis
硬	yìng	hard
偏	piān	onesided; unilateral
結固	jié gù	conglomeration
灑淅	xiǎn xī	shivering
往	wǎng	to proceed to
陷	xiàn	to sink
珠	zhū	a pearl
時	shí	occasionally
促	cù	hurried (movement in the vessels)
病脈	bìng mài	(a movement in the) vessels (indicating an) illness
息	xí	breath; to breathe
駃	kuài	fast; swift
續	xù	to succeed to; to follow
尾	wěi	tail; end
豆	dòu	a bean
搖	yáo	to shake; to agitate
緊	jǐn	tight (movement in the vessels)

弓弦	gōng xián	a bow-string
索	suǒ	a large rope; to bind
無常	wú cháng	abnormal

Wèn yuē. mài yǒu yīn yáng zhě hé wèi yě. dá yuē. fán mài dà. fú. shuò. dòng. huá. cǐ míng yáng yě. mài chén. sè. ruò. xián. wēi. cǐ míng yīn yě. fán yīn bìng xiàn yáng mài zhě shēng. yáng bìng xiàn yīn mài zhě sǐ. wèn yuē. mài yǒu yáng jié yīn jié zhě. hé yǐ bié zhī. dá yuē. qí mài fú ér shuò. néng shí. bù dà biàn zhě. cǐ wéi shí. míng yuē yáng jié yě. qí shí qī rì dāng jù. qí mài chén ér chí. bù néng shí. shēn tǐ zhòng. dà biàn fǎn yìng. míng yuē yīn jié yě. qí shí sì rì dāng jù. jié zhě. qì piān jié gù. wèn yuē. bìng yǒu xiǎn xī wù hán ér fù fā rè zhě hé. dá yuē. yīn mài bù zú. yáng wǎng cóng zhī. yáng mài bù zú. yīn wǎng chéng zhī. yuē. hé wèi yáng bù zú. dá yuē. jiǎ lìng cùn kǒu mài wēi. míng yuē yáng bù zú. yīn qì shàng rù yáng zhōng. zé xiǎn xī wù hán yě. yuē. hé wèi yīn bù zú. dá yuē. jiǎ lìng chǐ mài ruò. míng yuē yīn bù zú. yáng qì xià xiàn rù yīn zhōng. zé fā rè yě. yáng mài fú yīn mài ruò zhě. zé xuě xū. xuě xū zé jīn jí yě. qí mài chén zhě. róng qì wēi yě. qí mài fú ér hàn chū rú liú zhū zhě. wèi qì shuāi yě. .... mài lái huǎn. shí yì zhǐ fù lái zhě. míng yuē jié. mài lái shuò. shí yì zhǐ fù lái zhě. míng yuē cù. mài yáng shèng zé cù. yīn shèng zé jié. cǐ jiē bìng mài. mài yì xí sì zhì yuē píng. yì xí sān zhì yuē chí. xiǎo kuài yú chí yuē huǎn. yì xí liù zhì yuē shuò. shí yǒu yì zhǐ zhě. yīn yáng zhī qì bù dé xiāng xù yě. yīn yáng xiāng bó míng yuē dòng. yáng dòng zé hàn chū. yīn dòng zé fā rè. .... ruò shuò mài xiàn yú guān shàng. shàng xià wú tóu wěi. rú dòu dà. jué jué dòng yáo zhě. míng yuē dòng yě. mài fú ér jǐn zhě. míng yuē xián yě. xián zhě zhuàng rú gōng xián. àn zhī bù yí yě. mài jǐn zhě. rú zhuǎn suǒ wú cháng yě.

Question: There are yin and yang [movements in the] vessels. What does that mean?
Answer: All [movements in the] vessels that are strong, at the surface, frequent, excited, or smooth, they are called yang [movements. Movements in the] vessels that are in the depth, rough, weak, string[-like], and feeble, they are called yin [movements]. Whenever a yang [movement in the] vessels occurs in case of a yin disease, [the patient will] survive. In case a yin [movement in the] vessels occurs together with a yang disease, [the patient will] die.
Question: In the [movements in the] vessels, there are yang-clottings and yin-clottings. How are they distinguished?
Answer: When the [movement in the] vessels is at the surface and frequent, when [the patient] can eat, but passes no stools, that is a case of repletion; it

is called clotting of yang [qi]. A crisis will occur on the seventeenth day. A [movement in the] vessels that is in the depth and slow, and if [that person] cannot eat, if his body [appears to be] heavy, and if his stools are hard, in contrast to what they should be, that is called a clotting of yin [qi]. A crisis will occur on the fourteenth day. Clottings are unilateral conglomerations of [either yin or yang] qi. [1]

Question: A patient shivers; he hates cold and also develops heat. What is that?

Answer: [In this case] the yin [qi in the] vessels are insufficient, and yang [qi] proceed to follow them on their heels, or the yang [qi in the] vessels are insufficient, and yin [qi] proceed to seize their [location].

[Question:] What does it mean: the yang [qi] are insufficient?

Answer: If, for example, the [movement in the] vessels at the inch-opening is feeble, that is called 'the yang [qi] are insufficient'. [In this case] the yin qi move upwards and enter into the [region of the] yang qi. As a result, one shivers and hates cold.

[Question:] What does 'the yin [qi] are insufficient' mean?

Answer: If, for example, the [movement in the] vessels in the foot-section is weak, that is called 'the yin [qi] are insufficient'. [In this case] the yang qi move downwards and sink into the [region of the] yin [qi]. As a result, one develops heat. If the [movement of] yang [qi in the] vessels is at the surface, while [the movement of the] yin [qi in the] vessels is weak, [that indicates a] depletion of blood. When the blood is depleted, the sinews are tense. If the [movement in the] vessels is in the depth, the camp qi are feeble; if the [movement in the] vessels is at the surface, and if sweat leaves [the body] like a flow of pearls, [that indicates a] weakness of the guardian qi. ... If the [movement in the] vessels comes relaxedly, stops once in a while and then comes again, that is called 'clotting'. If the [movement in the] vessels comes frequently, stops once in a while and then comes again, that is called 'hurried' [movement in the] vessels. An abundance of yang [qi] causes a clotting [in the vessels]. All of these are [movements in the] vessels [indicating a] disease.

If the [movement in the] vessels arrives four times during one period of breathing, that is called normal. Three arrivals during one period of breathing is called slow. A little faster than slow is called relaxed. Six arrivals during one period of breathing is called frequent.If [the movement in the vessels] stops once in a while, [that indicates that] the yin and yang qi cannot follow each other.

If yin and yang [qi] strike at each other, that is called excitement. When the yang [qi] are excited, sweat leaves [the body]; when the yin [qi] are excited, one develops heat. ... If a frequent [movement in the] vessels is apparent above the gate, [2] and has neither head nor tail on top or at the bottom, and if it has the size of a bean, and if [the qi] recede and recede and are agitated in excitement, that is called excited. If the [movement in the] vessels is at the surface and tight, that is called string[-like]. A string[-like movement in the vessels] is shaped like a bow-string. It does not move under pressure. Tight [movements in the] vessels resemble an extremely twisted rope.

Note

[1] Main text by the later Han dynasty author Zhang Ji 張機 (ca. 200 CE). The commentary was added by Cheng Wuji 成無已 during the Song dynasty.

[2] The "gate" is an imaginary line or section in the lower arms (see Text 6.b) near the wrist. If one holds one's lower arm in an upright position, wrist and hand are "above" the gate.

6.d *Tú zhù bā shí yī nàn-jīng* 圖註八十一難經 Sān nàn 三難 The Third Difficult Issue

脉有太過。有不及。有陰陽相乘。有覆有溢。有關有格。何謂也。然關之前者。陽之動也。脉當九分而浮。過者法曰太過。減者法曰不及。遂上魚爲溢。爲外關內格。此陰乘之脉也。關以後者。陰之動也。脉當見一寸而沉。過者法曰太過。減者法曰不及。遂入尺爲覆。爲內關外格。此陽乘之脉也。

太過不及。脉見本位而言。陰陽相乘。脉越本位而言。九分者。陽之位。一寸者。陰之位。浮者。陽脉也。沉者。陰脉也。法者。診之法也。遂者。徑行也。關前爲陽脉。當見九分而浮。關後爲陰脉。當見一寸而沉。若太過不及。則陰陽偏勝矣。甚則覆溢關格見焉。覆者自上之下。溢者自下之上。關則無出之由。格則無入之理。脉度篇曰。關者陰氣太盛。陽氣不能營也。格者陽氣太盛。陰氣不能營也。陽氣不得營於陰。陰遂上出而溢于魚際。爲外關內格也。外關內格者。乃陰脉乘陽。陽外閉而不下。陰內出以格拒之也。其爲病外熱而液汗不通。內寒而胸滿吐食。陰氣不得營於陽。陽遂下陷而覆於尺部。爲內關外格也。內關外格者。乃陽脉乘陰。陰內閉而不上。陽從外入以格拒之也。其爲病內熱而大小便閉。外寒而手足厥冷。

故曰覆溢。是其真藏之脉。人不病而死也。

覆則內關外格。如物從上之下。溢則外關內格。如水由內溢外。診而得此。此係孤陰獨陽。乃真藏之脉。無胃氣以和者也。雖不病。其死也。豈能逃哉。

太過	tài guò	great excess
不及	bù jí	insufficiency
覆	fù	turnover
溢	yì	overflow
關	guān	the gate(-line separating the inch and the foot sections at the wrist)
減	jiǎn	to be reduced; to fall short of
遂	suí	to extend
魚	yú	the fish(-line separating the palm from the wrist)
外關	wài guān	external closure
內關	nèi guān	internal closure
外格	wài gé	external obstruction
張世賢	zhāng shì xián	Zhang Shixian, a renowned 16th c. medical author and editor of the *Nan jing*
註	zhù	to comment; commentary
越	yuè	to exceed
徑	jìng	a short-cut; direct
脉度篇	mài dù piān	the treatise "Mai du" (of the *Ling shu*)
營	yíng	to circulate
魚際	yú jì	the fish-border (which separates the palm from the wrist)
閉	bì	closure
格拒	géjù	to meet with obstruction; to ward off
以	yǐ	and
大小便閉	dà xiǎo biàn bì	constipation of stools and urine
厥冷	jué lěng	cold (hands and feet) due to ceasing (yang)

孤	gū	solitary
真臟	zhēn zàng	the true (qi of a) depot
和	hé	to mix; to blend

Mài yǒu tài guò. yǒu bù jí. yǒu yīn yáng xiāng chéng. yǒu fù yǒu yì. yǒu guān yǒu gé. hé wèi yě. rán guān zhī qián zhě. yáng zhī dòng yě. mài dāng jiǔ fēn ér fú. guò zhě fǎ yuē tài guò. jiǎn zhě fǎ yuē bù jí. suí shàng yú wéi yì. wéi wài guān nèi gé. cǐ yīn chéng zhī mài yě. guān yǐ hòu zhě. yīn zhī dòng yě. mài dāng jiàn yí cùn ér chén. guò zhě fǎ yuē tài guò. jiǎn zhě fǎ yuē bù jí. suí rù chǐ wéi fù. wéi nèi guān wài gé. cǐ yáng chéng zhī mài yě. tài guò bù jí. mài xiàn běn wèi ér yán. yīn yáng xiāng chéng. mài yuè běn wèi ér yán. jiǔ fēn zhě. yáng zhī wèi. yí cùn zhě. yīn zhī wèi. fú zhě. yáng mài yě. chén zhě. yīn mài yě. fǎ zhě. zhěn zhī fǎ yě. suí zhě. jìng xíng yě. guān qián wéi yáng mài. dāng jiàn jiǔ fēn ér fú. guān hòu wéi yīn mài. dāng jiàn yí cùn ér chén. ruò tài guò bù jí. zé yīn yáng piān shèng yǐ. shèn zé fù yì guān gé jiàn yān. fù zhě zì shàng zhī xià. yì zhě zì xià zhī shàng. guān zé wú chū zhī yóu. gé zé wú rù zhī lǐ. mài dù piān yuē. guān zhě yīn qì tài shèng. yáng qì bù néng yíng yě. gé zhě yáng qì tài shèng. yīn qì bù néng yíng yě. yáng qì bù dé yíng yú yīn. yīn suí shàng chū ér yì yú yú jì. wéi wài guān nèi gé yě. wài guān nèi gé zhě. nǎi yīn mài chéng yáng. yáng wài bì ér bù xià. yīn nèi chū yǐ gé jù zhī yě. qí wéi bìng wài rè ér yè hàn bù tōng. nèi hán ér xiōng mǎn tù shí. yīn qì bù dé yíng yú yáng. yáng suí xià xiàn ér fù yú chǐ bù. wéi nèi guān wài gé yě. nèi guān wài gé zhě. nǎi yáng mài chéng yīn. yīn nèi bì ér bù shàng. yáng cóng wài rù yǐ gé jù zhī yě. qí wéi bìng nèi rè ér dà xiǎo biàn bì. wài hán ér shǒu zú jué lěng. gù yuē fù yì. shī qí zhēn zàng zhī mài. rén bù bìng ér sǐ yě. fù zé nèi guān wài gé. rú wù cóng shàng zhī xià. yì zé wài guān nèi gé. rú shuǐ yóu nèi yì wài. zhěn ér dé cǐ. cǐ xì gū yīn dú yáng. nǎi zhēn zàng zhī mài. wú wèi qì yǐ hé zhě yě. suī bù bìng. qí sǐ yě. qǐ néng táo zāi.

The [movement in the] vesels may have [the following conditions:] great excess and insufficiency, mutual seizure [of territory] by yin and yang [qi], turnover, and overflow, closure, and obstruction. What does that mean?
It is like this. [The section] in front of the gate, that is where the yang [qi] move. [The movement in] the vessels should [appear here] over a distance of nine *fen*, and it should occur at the surface. [If that movement] exceeds [the nine-*fen* section], that is a pattern indicating great excess. [If the movement] falls short [of covering the entire nine-*fen* section], that is a pattern indicating insufficiency. [If the movement] extends upwards to the fish[-border], that

constitutes an overflow. It signals external closure and internal obstruction. That is a [movement in the] vessels [which indicates that] the yin [qi] have seized [that section where normally only yang qi should be. The section] behind the gate, that is where the yin [qi] move. [The movement in] the vessels should appear here over a distance of one inch, and it should occur in the depth. [If that movement] exceeds [the one-inch section], that is a pattern indicating great excess. [If the movement] falls short of [covering the entire one-inch section], that is a pattern indicating insufficiency. [If the movement] extends downwards into the foot[-long section towards the elbow], that constitutes a turnover. It signals internal closure and external obstruction. That is a [movement in the] vessels [which indicates that] the yang [qi] have seized [that section where normally only yin qi should be].

(Zhang Shixian's commentary:) "Great excess" and "insufficiency" refer to [movements] apparent in the vessels at their original location; "mutual seizure" [of territory] by yin and yang [qi]" refers to [movements] exceeding their original location. The nine-fen [section] is the location of the yang [movement in the vessels]; the one-inch [section] is the location of the yin [movement in the] vessels. Near the surface is the yang [movement in the] vessels; in the depth is the yin [movement in the] vessels. "Pattern" means here "diagnostic pattern"; "extend" stands for "proceed directly". The [section] in front of the gate is the yang [section]; the [movement in the] vessels should appear here over a distance of nine tenths [of an inch], and it should occur on the surface. The [section] behind the gate is the yin [section]; the [movement in the] vessels should appear here over a distance of one inch, and it should be in the depth. In case of great excess or insufficiency, either the yin or the yang [qi] dominate onesidedly. In extreme cases, turnover and overflow, closure and obstruction [conditions may] appear. Turnover is a movement from above downwards; overflow is a movement from below upwards. Closure means there is nothing from where to move out; obstruction means there is no structure to move in. In the treatise "Mai du" [of the Ling shu] it is stated: "In case of closure, yin qi are present in great abundance, and the yang qi cannot circulate. In case of obstruction, yang qi are present in great abundance, and the yin qi cannot circulate." If the yang qi cannot circulate through the yin [sections], the yin [qi] will ascend, leaving [their original location], and flow over the fish-border. That constitutes external closure and internal obstruction. In case of external closure and internal obstruction, the [qi from the] yin vessels have availed themselves of yang [territory]. The yang [qi suffer from] external closure and cannot move downwards as the yin [qi] come out from inside and meet them with obstruction. The resulting illness is external heat, with liquids and sweat being unable to pass. There is internal cold with fullness in the chest, and vomiting of food. When the yin qi cannot circulate through the yang [section], the yang [qi] will move down directly and turn into the foot section. That constitutes internal closure and external obstruction. In case of internal closure and external obstruction, the [qi from the] yang vessels have availed themselves of yin [territory]. The yin [qi suffer from] internal closure and cannot move upwards; the yang [qi] enter from outside and meet them with obstruction. The resulting illness is internal heat and constipation of both urine and stool together with external cold and a cooling of hands and feet resulting from recession. Hence, one speaks of turnover and overflow. This is [a movement in] the vessels of the true [qi of the] conduits. Without having felt ill that person will die.

Hence one speaks of turnover and overflow. This [reflects a movement in the] vessels of the true [qi of the] depots [themselves]. The [afflicted] person [perceives] no illness, and yet he will die.

(Zhang Shixian's commentary:) Turnover, then, [is a condition of] internal closure and external obstruction. This is like something moving downwards from above. Overflow, then, [represents a condition of] external closure and internal obstruction; as if there were water flowing from within [a container] outwards over [the rim of that container] If, in an examination [of a patient], one gets a hold of such a [movement, then] this [movement] is a [movement of] solely yin or only yang [qi;] that is, it is a [movement in the] vessels of the true [qi of the] depots, with no qi from the stomach blended into them. Although [the patient] does not feel ill, how could he escape his death?

6.e *Xú líng tāi xiān sheng yī shū quán jí, juan* 3/10 徐靈胎先生醫書全集 (Huí xī mài xué 洄溪脉學) Mài wú gēn yǒu liǎng shuō 脈無根有兩說 On Two [Different Meanings of the] Statement "The [Movement in the] Vessels has no Root"

天下之醫籍多矣。或者各持一論。而讀者不能融會。漫無可否。則不見書之益。而徒見書之害矣。又何貴乎博學者。即如脈之無根。便有兩說。一以尺中爲根。脈之有尺。猶樹之有根。叔和曰。寸關雖無。尺猶不絕。如此之流。何憂殞滅。蓋因其有根也。若腎脈獨敗。是無根矣。安望其有發生乎。一以沉候爲根。經曰。諸浮脈無根者皆死。是謂有表無裏。孤陽不生。夫造化之所以亘萬古而不息者。一陰一陽。互爲其根也。使陰既絕矣。孤陽豈能獨存乎。二說似乎不同。久而虛心討論。實無二致也。蓋尺爲腎部。而沉候之六脈皆腎也。要知兩尺之無根。與沉取之無根。總爲腎水涸竭而乏資始之源。宜乎病之重困矣。王宗正曰。診脈之法。當從心肺俱浮。肝腎

俱沉。脾在中州。則與叔和之守寸關尺部位以候五臟六腑之脈。大相徑庭矣。知宗正亦從經文諸浮脈無根者皆死之句悟入。遂謂本乎天者親上。本乎地者親下。心肺居於至高之分。故應乎寸。腎肝處乎至陰之位。故應乎尺。脾胃在中。故應乎關。然能以叔和之法。參而用之。正有相成之妙。淺工俗學。此則疑彼者。皆不肯深思古人推本之說。所以除一二師家授受之外。盡屬擬臆。許學士之不肯著書以示後來。乃深鑒于此弊也夫。

天下	tiān xià	under heaven; the world; the empire
醫籍	yī jí	medical literature
持	chí	to hold; to grasp
論	lùn	argument; view
融會	róng huì	a comprehensive understanding
漫	màn	ubiquitous
可否	kě foǔ	what is right and what is wrong; what can be and what cannot be
徒	tú	only
害	hài	harm
貴	guì	to value
樹	shù	a tree
叔和	shū hé	Shuhe, style-name of Wáng Xī 王熙 (3rd c.), author of the *Mai jing* 脈經
殞滅	yǔn miè	to die; to perish
敗	bài	to become eliminated; to vanish
望	wàng	to look forward to; to hope
造化	zào huà	the process of creation
亘	gèn	to revolve
息	xí	to rest; to stop

一	yì	all
互	hù	mutually; reciprocal
虛心	xū xīn	open-minded; without prejudice
討論	tǎo lùn	to debate; to discuss
涸	hé	dried up; exhausted
乏	fá	to be in want of
困	kùn	difficult; critical
王宗正	wáng zōng zhèng	Wang Zongzheng, a 12th c. author of medical texts
守	shǒu	to focus on
徑庭	jìng tíng	a narrow track and a wide hall; very unlike
文	wén	literature; text
句	jù	a sentence
悟入	wù rù	to enter into a perfect understanding of reality
親	qīn	to approach; to be near to
參	cān	to combine; to mix
妙	miào	subtle; subtlety
則	zé	a rule
疑	yí	to doubt; to suspect
此則疑彼	cǐ zé yí bǐ	to consider this (which is near) as a rule and doubt that (which is distant)
肯	kěn	to consent; to be willing
推	tuī	to investigate
除…外	chú…wài	except for
師	shī	a teacher
授	shòu	to transmit
擬	nì	to make propositions
膺	yīng	to oppose
許	xǔ	perhaps; it may be
學士	xué shì	a scholar
深鑒	shēn jiàn	to be deeply concerned
弊	bì	narrow-mindedness

Tiān xià zhī yī jí duō yǐ. huò zhě gè chí yí lùn. ér dú zhě bù néng róng huì. màn wú kě foǔ. zé bù jiàn shū zhī yì. ér tú jiàn shū zhī hài yǐ. yòu hé guì hū bó xué zhě. jí rú mài zhī wú gēn. biàn yǒu liǎng shuō. yī yǐ chǐ zhōng wéi gēn. mài zhī yǒu chǐ. yóu shù zhī yǒu gēn. shū hé yuē. cùn guān suī wú. chǐ yóu bù jué. rú cǐ zhī liú. hé yōu yǔn miè. gài yīn qí yǒu gēn yě. ruò shèn mài dú bài. shī wú gēn yǐ. ān wàng qí yǒu fā shēng hū. yī yǐ chén hòu wéi gēn. jīng yuē. zhū fú mài wú gēn zhě jiē sǐ. shī wèi yǒu biǎo wú lǐ. gū yáng bù shēng. fū zào huà zhī suǒ yǐ gèn wàn gǔ ér bù xí zhě. yì yīn yì yáng. hù wéi qí gēn yě. shǐ yīn jì jué yǐ. gū yáng qǐ néng dú cún hū. èr shuō sì hū bù tóng. jiǔ ér xū xīn tǎo lùn. shí wú èr zhì yě. gài chǐ wéi shèn bù. ér chén hòu zhī liù mài jiē shèn yě. yào zhī liǎng chǐ zhī wú gēn. yǔ chén qǔ zhī wú gēn. zǒng wéi shèn shuǐ hé jiē ér fá zī shǐ zhī yuán. yí hū bìng zhī zhòng kùn yǐ. wáng zōng zhèng yuē. zhěn mài zhī fǎ. dāng cóng xīn fèi jù fú. gān shèn jù chén. pí zài zhōng zhōu. zé yǔ shū hé zhī shǒu cùn guān chǐ bù wèi yǐ hòu wǔ zàng liù fǔ zhī mài. dà xiāng jìng tíng yǐ. zhī zōng zhèng yì cóng jīng wén zhū fú mài wú gēn zhě jiē sǐ zhī jù wù rù. suí wèi běn hū tiān zhě qīn shàng. běn hū dì zhě qīn xià. xīn fèi jū yú zhì gāo zhī fēn. gù yìng hū cùn. shèn gān chù hū zhì yīn zhī wèi. gù yìng hū chǐ. pí wèi zài zhōng. gù yìng hū guān. rán néng yǐ shū hé zhī fǎ. cān ér yòng zhī. zhèng yǒu xiāng chéng zhī miào. qiǎn gōng sú xué. cǐ zé yí bǐ zhě. jiē bù kěn shēn sī gǔ rén tuī běn zhī shuō. suǒ yǐ chú yī èr shī jiā shǒu shòu zhī wài. jìn shǔ nì yīng. xǔ xué shì zhī bù kěn zhù shū yǐ shì hòu lái. nǎi shēn jiàn yú cǐ bì yě fū.

There are many medical texts under heaven. Some of them cling to only one view, and those who read [only these texts] will not be able to achieve a comprehensive understanding. They have absolutely no [basis to decide] what is right and wrong, and thus, rather than experiencing a benefit from reading books, they only experience harm from reading books. Furthermore, what is more valuable than extensive studies? For instance, [in the literature one may find] two different statements concerning "the absence of a root in the [movement in the] vessels." One of them identifies the [movement] in the foot[-section] as "root". [In this perspective, the movement in] the vessels has a foot[-section], just as a tree has a root. [Wang] Shuhe has said: Even if no [movement in the vessels can be felt at the] inch- and gate[-sections], as long as the foot[-section] has not been cut off [from the movement in the vessels], why should such a flow [of the qi cause one to] mourn about death? The reason, of course, [for such a statement] is that the [movement still] has its root. If, however, nothing but the [movement in the] vessels [associated with the] kidneys has vanished, that is a case where no root exists any longer. How could anybody hope here that new life emerges? The other [statement referred to initially] considers a [movement in the vessels] indicating depth as root. The classic states: "All [movements in the] vessels at the surface that have no root, [signal impending] death."[1] That is to say, [these are situations] where external [movements] occur but no internal [movements]. The solitary yang [qi] cannot exist in isolation. The fact that the creative [process] revolves through all ages since remotest antiquity, and never stops, is based on the fact that all yin and all yang constitute each other's roots. If, therefore, one allows the yin [qi] to be cut off, how could the solitary yang [qi] exist solely by themselves? The two statements [outlined above] appear to be very different. I have considered them without any prejudice for a long time, [and I have reached the conclusion that] they, in fact, do not diverge. The fact is, the foot[-section] is the section [associated with] the kidneys, and when the six vessels exhibit [movements in the] depth, [then] they [too] are all [associated with] the kidneys. One should know [therefore,] that the absence of a root [movement in the vessels at] the two foot[-sections at the wrists] and the absence of a root [movement] that could be felt in the depth, both indicate a source in which the water of the kidneys has dried up and which lacks any provisions to [serve as the continous] beginning [of man's life]. This, then, should certainly be a serious and critical illness. [A further statement comes from] Wang Zongzheng, who said: "The pattern of examining the [movement in the] vessels is such that one should start from [the fact that] heart and lung [movements occur] both near the surface, while liver and kidneys' [movements occur] in the depth, and the [movement associated with the] spleen occupies the central region. This [statement] is very different from [the view offered by Wang] Shuhe, who focussed his attention on the inch-, the gate-, and the foot-section in order to analyse the [movements in the] vessels [associated with the] five depots and six palaces." Obviously, [Wang] Zongzheng based his understanding on the basis of the sentence in the text of the classic: "All [movements in the] vessels at the surface that have no root, [signal impending] death." After all, it is said: That which has its basis in heaven is near the top, that which has its basis on earth is near the bottom. Heart and lung reside both in the top-most section [of the body], hence [the movements in the vessels associated with them] are reflected at the inch[-section]. The kidneys and the liver both occupy an extreme yin position, hence [the movements in the vessels associated with them] are reflected at the foot[-section]. Spleen and stomach are in the center, hence they correspond to the gate[-section]. This [view], then, can be applied together with the pattern advocated by [Wang] Shuhe, and a subtlety emerges that is really the result of the mutual supplementation [of both views]. Practitioners with shallow [knowledge], and [people with a] vulgar learning – who accept as a rule only what lies right in front of them while they doubt what is far away

– they all are unwilling to consider thoroughly the doctrine of the ancients and to search for the basis. Hence, except for one or two teacher-families transmitting [true learning from generation to generation], all [practitioners today] may be counted among those who propose [new thoughts] and oppose [tradition]. The unwillingnesss of scholars to write books and instruct posterity may result from their deep concern with this narrow-mindedness.

Note

[1] "Classic" refers here to the *Maijing* 脈經. However, the textus receptus of the *Maijing* has a statement that is only faintly reminiscent of the wording here. The citation quoted here appears for the first time in the *Leijing* 類經 compiled by Zhang Jingyue 張景岳 during the Ming dynasty.

6.f *Yī xué liù yào* 醫學六要
Xiǎo ér mài 小兒脈
The [Movement in the] Vessels of Small Children

小兒三歲以下。看虎口三關紋。紫熱。紅傷寒。青驚。白色疳。黑紋知中惡。黃色應脾端。大抵黃色隱隱。淡紅爲吉。黑色凶。其他紋色。在風關爲輕。氣關漸重。命關尤重也。及三歲以上。乃以一指按其寸關尺。當以六七至爲率。添則爲熱。減則爲寒。若脉浮數表熱。爲乳癇風熱。五臟壅。虛濡爲驚風。緊實爲風癇。緊弦爲腹痛。弦急爲氣不和。牢實爲便秘。沉細爲寒。大小不勻爲祟。或小或緩。或沉或短。皆爲宿食不化。脈亂身熱。汗出不食。食則吐。此爲變蒸也。浮爲風。伏沉皆爲物聚。單細爲疳勞。小兒但見增寒壯熱。即問曾出痘否。或時候發斑疹及痘。須防之。

小兒	xiǎo ér	small children
以下	yǐ xià	… and below
虎口	hǔ kǒu	(the width of an opened) tiger mouth; i.e. the distance between the tip of one's thumb and the tip of one's index finger if spread apart from one hand

關	guān	the gate(-sections of the index fingers of small children)
三關	sān guān	the three gate(-sections of the index fingers of small children)
紋	wén	(skin-)lines
疳	gān	the *gan*-illness
中惡	zhòng è	to be struck by the malevolent
大抵	dà dǐ	generally speaking
隱隱	yǐn yǐn	scarcely visible
淡	dàn	light, in color
風關	fēng guān	the wind-gate(-section; i.e. the section between the base fold, adjoining the palm, and the second fold on the inside of the index finger)
氣關	qì guān	the qi-gate(-section; i.e. the middle section of the inside of the index finger)
命關	mìng guān	the life-gate(-section; i.e. the uppermost of the three sections of the inside of the index finger)
以上	yǐ shàng	... and above
率	shuài	standard
添	tiān	to add to; to increase
乳癎	rǔ xián	convulsions (in children that are still) breast(-fed)
壅	yōng	to stop up; to obstruct
風癎	fēng xián	convulsions (caused by) wind
牢	láo	firm (movement in the vessels)
便秘	biàn bì	constipation
細	xì	fine (movement in the vessels)
勻	yún	even; uniform
祟	suì	curse by evil spirits
宿食	sù shí	food remaining (in the stomach without being digested)
化	huà	to digest
變蒸	biàn zhēng	the transformation and steaming (of newly-borns)
單	dān	singular (movement in the vessels)

但	dàn	only
痘	dòu	pox (in modern medical literature: small pox)
或時	huò shí	occasionally
斑	bān	streak(-like skin rash)
疹	zhěn	pustules; eruptions
防	fáng	to prevent

Xiǎo ér sān suì yǐ xià. kàn hǔ kǒu sān guān wén. zǐ rè. hóng shāng hán. qīng jìng. bái sè gān. hēi wén zhī zhòng è. huáng sè yìng pí duān. dà dǐ huáng sè yǐn yǐn. dàn hóng wéi jí. hēi sè xiōng. qí tā wén sè. zài fēng guān wéi qīng. qì guān jiàn zhòng. mìng guān yóu zhòng yě. jí sān suì yǐ shàng. nǎi yǐ yì zhǐ àn qí cùn guān chǐ. dāng yǐ liù qī zhì wéi lǜ. Tiān zé wéi rè. jiǎn zé wéi hán. ruò mài fú shuò biǎo rè. wéi rǔ xián fēng rè. wǔ zàng yōng. xū rú wéi jìng fēng. jǐn shí wéi fēng xián. jǐn xián wéi fù tòng. xián jí wéi qì bù hé. láo shí wéi biàn mì. chén xì wéi hán. dà xiǎo bù yún wéi suì. huò xiǎo huò huǎn. huò chén huò duǎn. jiē wéi sù shí bù huà. mài luàn shēn rè. hàn chū bù shí. shí zé tù. cǐ wéi biàn zhēng yě. fú wéi fēng. fú chén jiē wéi wù jù. dān xì wéi gān láo. xiǎo ér dàn jiàn zēng hán zhuàng rè. jí wèn cēng chū dòu foǔ. huò shí hòu fā bān zhěn jí dòu. xū fáng zhī.

[When examining] small children of the age of three years or younger, one inspects the tiger's mouth and the lines in the three gate[-sections of the index-fingers].[1] If they are purple, [that indicates] heat; if they are red, [that indicates] harm caused by cold. If they are blue, [that indicates that the respective child] has beeen frightened; if they are of white color, [that indicates the child suffers from] *gan*-illness.[2] Black lines indicate [the child] has been struck by the malevolent.[3] A yellow color corresponds to a beginning in the spleen. Generally speaking, a yellow color and a scarcely visible or light red are auspicious signs, while a black color is an inauspicious sign. All other colors of the [skin-]lines [in the gate-sections of the index-fingers] indicate a minor [illness] if they appear in the wind-gate, a slightly more serious [illness] if they appear in the life-gate. [When the child to be examined is] three years or older, one uses [only] one finger to press its inch, gate- and foot[-sections at the wrists]. The [movement in the vessels] should arrive six or seven times [during one breathing period] as a standard; an increased [speed] signals heat; a decreased [speed] signals cold. If the [movement in the] vessels is at the surface and frequent, and if [the child suffers from] external heat, that indicates convulsions [as they are common in children that are still] breast-fed, [and also] heat caused by wind, and obstructions in the five depots. [If the movement in the vessels is] depleted and soft, that indicates [that the child suffers from] fright and wind. A tight and replete [movement in the vessels] indicates convulsions caused by wind. A tight and string[-like movement in the vessels] indicates abdominal pain. [If the movement is] string[-like] and tense, the [yin and yang] qi are not harmoniously blended. A firm and replete [movement] indicates constipation. A [movement] in the depth that is fine indicates cold; and an uneven [movement that changes between] strong and minor, indicates a curse by an evil spirit. Minor and relaxed [movements], as well as [movements that are] in the depth or short, they all indicate that food has remained [in the stomach for too long] without digestion. If the [movement in the] vessels is chaotic, and if [at the same time] the body is hot, and if [the child] perspires and does not eat, or eats and vomits afterwards, these [are symptoms of the stages of] transformation and steaming [of newly borns].[5] [A movement in the vessels that is] at the surface indicates wind; one that is hidden or in the depth signals that something has become accumulated [somewhere in the body]. A singular and a fine [movement in the vessels] indicate *gan*-illness and taxation. If a child shows only an increased cold or strong heat, then one should ask whether it has already brought forth pox. Occasionally this is an indication that [a child] is about to develop rashes, pustules, or pox, and this should be prevented.

Notes

[1] These are the small vessels discernible in the three sections on the inside of the index finger.

[2] The term 疳 *gān* refers to pediatric diseases; symptoms associated traditionally with *gān* resemble those attributed to malnutrition today. The *Zhu bing yuan hou lun* 諸病源侯論 by Chao Yuanfang 巢元方 of CE 610 offers in ch. 18 a definition of *gān* based on the segments "illness" and "sweet" that constitute the written character. Accordingly, a consumptiom of sweet food in excessive quantities will excite the worms inhabiting stomach and intestines to enter and eat away the internal organs, and to cause, among other signs, ulcers and tooth decay. Hence the term *gān* might be rendered literally as "illness caused by sweetness". A thousand years later, the author of the Korean medical work *Dong yi bao jian* 東醫寶鑑 of 1611 offered a different etymology by linking the sound of 疳 *gān* to the sound of 乾 *gān*, "dry", "exhausted", and defining the 疳 *gān*-illness as "emaciation, weariness, and paucity of blood". The *Dong yi bao jian* added that what is called 疳 *gān* in youths under the age of twenty, is called 癆 *lǎo*, "consumption", in persons older than twenty.

[3] "Malevolent" is a general designation of "demons".

[4] According to Chinese traditional pediatrics, a newly born child is far from being complete yet. An internal fire causes an infant to undergo, counted from the day of its birth, a basic developmental transformation every 32nd day, accompanied by a period of steaming every 64th day. An increased heat of an infant's body during these short periods was considered normal. Altogether, ten such transformations and five steamings occur within the first 320 days after birth. Some authors claimed an even longer continuation of these processes.

Lesson Seven

Treatment: General Principles

Traditional Chinese health care relied on a wide scope of therapeutic means. The earliest texts available already show an astonishing broadness of therapies employed in cases of illness. The so-called Mawangdui manuscripts, compiled around 200 BCE, contain, in addition to demonological practices, references to massage and petty surgery, to gymnastics and cauterization, and in particular detail, to pharmaceutics. (See Donald Harper, *Early Chinese Medical Literature, The Mawangdui Medical Manuscripts*, London and New York, 1998, for a complete translation and thorough analysis). Acupuncture, or needling, was not mentioned in these early texts and appears to have been developed only one or two centuries later. Beginning with the Han dynasty, conceptualized Chinese health care was characterized by two antagonistic traditions. These were, first, the continuation of non-medical health care untouched by the yinyang- and five-agents doctrines of systematic correspondences, and mainly documented in materia medica texts and prescription works. Second, the tradition of medical health care with acupuncture and dietetics at its center. While the former included a use of substances to treat manifest ailments; classic Chinese medicine, at least in its beginning, relied on acupuncture to prevent the outbreak of disease in the first place. After an early isolated attempt by Zhang Ji 張機 to link materia medica and the doctrine of systematic correspondences, it was only in the course of the Song-Jin-Yuan medicine between the 12th and the 15th centuries that the two traditions merged and various attempts at creating a pharmacology of systematic correspondences were untertaken. However, no unified system adhered to by a majority of practitioners was agreed upon. Subsequently, an ever greater diversity of conceptual approaches at treating diseases was propagated by an ever increasing number of schools.

Beginning with the first millennium, specialized literature appeared with works focussing on dietetics, drugs and needling, on orthopedics, gymnastics and massage, as well as on the use of spells and amulets, talismans and exorcistic rites. It was recognized early that children and women had special health care problems, and the treatment of these problems received attention in specialized works as did the treatment of some very common diseases, including smallpox, leprosy, and others. In general, the treatment advocated in the literature was designed to be carried out by educated laymen as well as medical specialists.

The texts selected for Lesson Seven offer some insights into the general values explicitly or implicitly recorded in traditional Chinese medical literature. We witness attempts at drawing a borderline between health care informed by Chinese natural sciences and earlier demonological practices, and we may follow the arguments employed in the persistent controversy between the adherents of aggressive treatments supposed to attack an evil directly, and others advocating changes in a patient's basic condition, changes that make it impossible for any evil to stay. Chinese traditional therapy followed many directions, and guiding principles were offered by numerous contradictory schools, especially so during the second millennium CE. Most sources, however, leave us with the impression that Chinese physicians were quite pragmatic in their therapies, and selected what they or their patients perceived as useful rather than what a specific theory prescribed.

Key Terms Introduced in Lesson Seven

標	biāo	tip (of a disease); sign; secondary location of a disease
劑	jì	a formula; a prescription
麻痹	má bì	numbness
癢	yǎng	to itch
拘攣	jū luán	cramps
上脘	shàng wǎn	the upper (opening of the) duct (passing through the stomach)
發散	fā sàn	to stimulate dispersion; to dissipate
臨診	lín zhěn	clinical diagnosis
鬱	yù	obstruction
祝由	zhù yóu	to invoke the origin (a term used to denote therapeutic exorcism)
八風	bā fēng	the eight winds (i.e. the winds from the eight cardinal points East, West, South, North, East-South, East-North, West-South, West-North)

六合	liù hé	the six [cardinal points] uniting [the world] East, West, South, North, Above, Below; i. e. "the world"
五痺	wǔ bì	the five blocks (i.e. of skin, flesh, sinews, bones, and vessels)
疏理	shū lǐ	open skin structures
癰瘍	yōng yáng	welling abscess
緻理	zhì lǐ	to have tight [skin] structures
攣	luán	cramp
九鍼	jiǔ zhēn	the nine [types of] needles [used in acupuncture]
導引	dǎo yǐn	guiding-pulling (a type of physical exercises)
按蹻	àn jiāo	pressing-lifting (a type of physical exercises)
庸醫	yōng yī	common physician
名醫	míng yī	renowned physician
立方	lì fāng	to compose a prescription
癆	láo	wasting; consumption
時醫	shí yī	physicians (who follow only the trends of their own time)

7.a *Xú líng tāi xiān sheng yī shū quán jí* 1/2
徐靈胎先生醫書全集
(Yī xué yuán liú lùn 醫學源流論)
Biǎo lǐ shàng xià lùn 表裏上下論
On Outside and Inner, Upper and Lower [Sections of the Body]

欲知病之難易。先知病之淺深。欲知病之淺深。先知病之部位。夫人身一也。實有表裏上下之別焉。何謂表。皮肉筋骨是也。何謂裏。臟腑精神是也。而經絡則貫乎其間。表之病易治而難死。裏之病難治而易死。此其大略也。而在表在裏者。又各有難易。此不可執一而論也。若夫病本在表。而傳於裏。病本在裏。而幷及于表。是爲內外兼病。尤不易治。身半已上之病。往往近於熱。身半已下之病。往往近於寒。此其大略也。而在上在下。又各有寒熱。此亦不可執一而論也。若夫病本在上。而傳於下。病本在下。而傳於上。是之謂上下兼病。亦不易治。所以然者。無病之處多。有病之處少。則精力猶可維持。使正氣漸充。而邪氣亦去。若夫一人之身。無處不病。則以何者爲驅病之本。而復其元氣乎。故善醫者。知病勢之盛而必傳也。豫爲之防。無使結

聚。無使泛濫。無使併合。此上工治未病之說也。若其已至於傳。則必先求其本。後求其標。相其緩急而施治之。此又桑榆之收也。以此决病之生死難易。思過半矣。

難	nán	difficult; hard
貫	guàn	to go through; to connect
大略	dà lüè	general rule
執一而論	zhí yī ér lùn	to treat all alike
已上	yǐ shàng	identical with 以上 *yǐ shàng*, "ascending from here"; "here and above"
往往	wǎng wǎng	often
近	jìn	to be close to; to accompany
所以然者	suǒ yǐ rán zhě	this being so; consequently
維持	wéi chí	to maintain
充	chōng	to reach one's fullest extent
驅	qū	to expel
復	fù	to restore
善醫	shàn yī	to be well versed in medicine; medical expert
豫	yù	beforehand
泛濫	fàn làn	to overflow
標	biāo	tip (of a disease); sign; secondary location of a disease
相	xiàng	to observe; to look at
桑榆	sāng yú	old age (lit.: mulberry and elm – trees whose tops are lit by the rays of the evening sun)
桑榆之收	sāng yú zhī shōu	the harvest of old age

Yù zhī bìng zhī nán yì. xiān zhī bìng zhī qiǎn shēn. yù zhī bìng zhī qiǎn shēn. xiān zhī bìng zhī bù wèi. fū rén shēn yī yě. shí yǒu biǎo lǐ shàng xià zhī bié yān. hé wèi biǎo. pí ròu jīn gǔ shī yě. hé wèi lǐ. zàng fǔ jīng shén shī yě. ér jīng luò zé guàn hū qí jiān. biǎo zhī bìng yì zhì ér nán sǐ. lǐ zhī bìng nán zhì ér yì sǐ. cǐ qí dà lüè yě. ér zài biǎo zài lǐ zhě. yòu gè yǒu nán yì. cǐ bù kě zhí yī ér lùn yě. ruò fū bìng běn zài biǎo. ér chuán yú lǐ. bìng běn zài lǐ. ér bìng jí yú biǎo. shī wéi nèi wài jiān bìng. yóu bù yì zhì. shēn bàn yǐ shàng zhī bìng. wǎng wǎng jìn yú rè. shēn bàn yǐ xià zhī bìng. wǎng wǎng jìn yú hán. cǐ qí dà lüè yě. ér zài shàng zài xià. yòu gè yǒu hán rè. cǐ yì bù kě zhí yī ér lùn yě. ruò fū bìng běn zài shàng. ér chuán yú xià. bìng běn zài xià. ér chuán yú shàng. shī zhī wèi shàng xià jiān bìng. yì bù yì zhì. suǒ yǐ rán zhě. wú bìng zhī chù duō. yǒu bìng zhī chù shǎo. zé jīng lì yóu kě wéi chí. shǐ zhèng qì jiàn chōng. ér xié qì yì qù. ruò fū yì rén zhī shēn. wú chù bù bìng. zé yǐ hé zhě wéi qū bìng zhī běn. ér fù qí yuán qì hū. gù shàn yī zhě. zhī bìng shì zhī shèng ér bì chuán yě. yù wéi zhī fáng. wú shǐ jié jù. wú shǐ fàn làn. wú shǐ bìng hé. cǐ shàng gōng zhì wèi bìng zhī shuō yě. ruò qí yǐ zhì yú chuán. zé bì xiān qiú qí běn. hòu qiú qí biāo. xiāng qí huǎn jí ér shī zhì zhī. cǐ yòu sāng yú zhī shōu yě. yǐ cǐ jué bìng zhī shēng sǐ nán yì. sī guò bàn yǐ.

If one likes to know whether a disease is difficult or easy [to cure], one should first know whether this disease is near the [body's] surface or in its depth. And if one likes to know whether a disease is near the [body's] surface or in its depth, one should first know which section [of the body] it occupies. The human body constitutes one single unit, and it has, indeed, different [sections of] outside and inside, upper and lower. What is meant by outside? [Outside includes] the skin, the flesh, the sinews, and the bones. What is meant by inside? [Inside includes] the depots, the palaces, the essence, and the spirit. And as far as the conduits and network [vessels] are concerned, they serve to connect [the body's outside and inside]. Diseases in the outside [sections of the body] are easy to cure, and one hardly dies of them. Diseases in the inside [sections of the body] are difficult to cure, and it is easy to die of them. But that is only a general rule, because [diseases] in both the outside and the inside [sections of the body] may be difficult or easy [to cure and to die of]. One cannot treat them all alike! If a disease was located originally in the outside [sections of the body] whence it was transmitted to the [body's] inside, or if a disease was located originally in the inside [sections of the body] whence it has spread now to the [body's] outside, [such cases] are joint diseases of the inside and outside [sections of the body]. They are particularly difficult to cure. Diseases in the upper half of the body are often accompanied by heat, while diseases in the lower half of the body are often accompanied by cold. But that is only a general rule, because cold and heat may occur [together with diseases affecting] the upper as well as the lower [half of the body]. They too cannot be treated all alike! If a disease was located originally in the upper [half of the body] whence it was transmitted to the lower [half], or if a disease was located originally in the lower [half] whence it was transmitted to the upper [half, such cases] are called joint diseases of the upper and lower [half of the body]. They, too, are not easy to cure. Consequently, if [a patient's body] has many areas that have not been affected by his disease, while those areas that have been affected by his disease are few, it will be quite possible to maintain his essence and strength, and to cause his regular qi to gradually reach their fullest extent again; the evil qi [that had invaded his body] will leave at the same time. If someone's body has been affected by a disease everywhere, where should one start from to expel this disease and to restore his original qi? Medical experts know therefore that if a disease reaches its full strength it will be transmitted [throughout the body] inevitably. That [transmission] is to be prevented beforehand, so that there may not be any clottings [of evil qi], any overflow [of a disease into neighboring areas], or any unions [between hitherto separate problems]. That is [meant by] the statement: The superior practitioner treats those that are not yet sick. If a [disease] has already reached a state of transmission, one must search first for its origin [and start a cure there], and then search for its secondary location [to complete the cure here]. One must observe whether it travels slowly or with great speed, and carry out one's treatment accordingly. The [necessary expertise] comes with old age. If one applies [these principles] to reach a decision whether a disease will result in survival or death, and whether it is difficult or easy [to cure], the major part [of the problem at hand] will have already been considered.

7.b *Rú mén shì qīn* 2 儒門事親 Hàn xià tù sān fǎ gāi jìn zhì bìng quán 汗下吐三法該盡治病詮 An Explanation of Why the Three Methods of Sweating, Purging, and Vomiting Should Suffice for the Treatment of Illness

---

夫病之一物。非人身素有之也。或自外而入。或由內而生。皆邪氣也。邪氣加諸身。速攻之可也。速去之可也。攬而留之。何也。雖愚夫愚婦。皆知其不可也。及其聞攻則不悅。聞補則樂之。今之醫者曰。當先固其元氣。元氣實。邪自去。世間如此妄人。何其多也。夫邪之中人。輕則傳久而自盡。頗甚則傳久而難已。更甚則暴死。若先論固其元氣。以補劑補之。真氣未勝。而邪已交馳橫騖而不可制矣。惟脈脫下虛。無邪無積之人。始可議補。其餘有邪積之人而議補者。皆鯀湮洪水之徒也。今予論吐。汗。下三法。先論攻其邪。邪去而元氣自復也。況予所論之法。識練日久。至精至熟。有得無失。所以敢爲來者言也。天之六氣。風暑火濕燥寒。地之六氣。霧露雨雹冰泥。人之六味。酸苦甘辛鹹淡。

故天邪發病。多在乎上。地邪發病。多在乎下。人邪發病。多在乎中。此爲發病之三也。處之者三。出之者亦三也。諸風寒之邪。結搏皮膚之間。藏於經絡之內。留而不去。或發疼痛走注。痲痹不仁。及四肢腫癢拘攣。可汗而出之。風痰宿食。在膈或上脘。可涌而出之。寒濕固冷。熱客下焦。在下之病。可泄而出之。內經散論諸病。非一狀也。流言治法。非一階也。...。其言補。時見一二。然其補非今之所謂補也。文具於補論條下。如辛補肝。鹹補心。甘補腎。酸補脾。苦補肺。若此之補。乃所以發腠理。致津液。通血氣。至其統論諸藥。則曰。辛甘淡三味爲陽。酸苦鹹三味爲陰。辛甘發散。淡滲泄。酸苦鹹涌泄。發散者歸於汗。涌者歸于吐。泄者歸于下。滲爲解表。歸於汗。泄爲利小溲。歸於下。殊不言補。乃知聖人止有三法。無第四法也。

物	wù	a thing; an entity
諸	zhū	fusion of 之於 *zhī yú*; "in it"; "to it"
速	sù	quickly
攻	gōng	to attack
攬	lǎn	to seize
何	hé	how?
樂	lè	to enjoy something; to be happy about something
固	gù	to strengthen
世間	shì jiān	in the world

何其多也	hé qí duō yě	what could be more numerous; innumerable
頗	pō	somewhat; a little
更	gèng	even more
甚	shèn	serious
暴	bào	sudden
先論	xiān lùn	previously mentioned
劑	jì	a formula; a prescription
交馳	jiāo chí	to move as fast as a horse
横騖	héng wù	to behave as wild as a duck
制	zhì	to restrain; to control
脱	tuō	to loose; loss
脱下	tuō xià	to sink down (of the surface of a structure); to shrink
始	shǐ	only if ..., then ...
鯀	gǔn	Gun, father of the legendary Yü the Great
湮	yān	to submerge; to drown
洪水	hóng shuǐ	a great flood
徒	tú	a follower
予	yú	I; myself
復	fù	to recover
練	liàn	to practice
日久	rì jiǔ	for a long time
熟	shú	mature
雹	báo	hail
泥	ní	mud
淡	dàn	weak in flavor; bland
出	chū	to make leave; to eliminate
搏	bó	to accumulate (something which is normally dissipated); used here for 摶 *tuán*
走	zǒu	to move
痳痺	má bì	numbness
拘攣	jū luán	cramps
上脘	shàng wǎn	the upper (opening of the stomach) duct
湧	yǒng	to [make] gush forth; to induce vomiting

固冷	gù lěng	constipation resulting from cold
客	kè	to reside
散	sǎn	diffuse
流言	liú yán	to speak (about something) at various occasions
階	jiē	class; standard
具	jù	to have
條	tiáo	a section; a paragraph
致	zhì	to make [something] reach [a certain destination]
統	tǒng	all; general
發散	fā sàn	to stimulate dispersion; to dissipate
歸	guī	to be counted as ...; to belong to ...
滲	shèn	to leak; to drain
小	xiǎo	short for 小便 *xiǎo biàn*, to urinate
溲	sōu	to urinate
第	dì	order; sequences; (with numbers: first, second, third, etc.)

Fū bìng zhī yí wù. fēi rén shēn sù yǒu zhī yě. huò zì wài ér rù. huò yóu nèi ér shēng. jiē xié qì yě. xié qì jiā zhū shēn. sù gōng zhī kě yě. sù qù zhī kě yě. lǎn ér liú zhī. hé yě. suī yú fū yú fù. jiē zhī qí bù kě yě. jí qí wén gōng zé bù yuè. wén bǔ zé lè zhī. jīn zhī yī zhě yuē. dāng xiān gù qí yuán qì. yuán qì shí. xié zì qù. shì jiān rú cǐ wàng rén. hé qí duō yě. fū xié zhī zhōng rén. qīng zé chuán jiǔ ér zì jìn. pō shèn zé chuán jiǔ ér nán yǐ. gèng shèn zé bào sǐ. ruò xiān lùn gù qí yuán qì. yǐ bǔ jì bǔ zhī. zhēn qì wèi shèng. ér xié yǐ jiāo chí héng wù ér bù kě zhì yǐ. wéi mài tuō xià xū. wú xié wú jī zhī rén. shǐ kě yì bǔ. qí yú yǒu xié jī zhī rén ér yì bǔ zhě. jiē yóu yān hóng shuǐ zhī tú yě. jīn yú lùn tù. hàn. xià sān fǎ. xiān lùn gōng qí xié. xié qù ér yuán qì zì fù yě. kuàng yú suǒ lùn zhī fǎ. shì liàn rì jiǔ. zhì jīng zhì shú. yǒu dé wú shī. suǒ yǐ gǎn wéi lái zhě yán yě. tiān zhī liù qì. fēng shǔ huǒ shī zào hán. dì zhī liù qì. wù lù yǔ báo bīng ní. rén zhī liù wèi. suān kǔ gān xīn xián dàn. gù tiān xié fā bìng. duō zài hū shàng. dì xié fā bìng. duō zài hū xià. rén xié fā bìng. duō zài hū zhōng. cǐ wéi fā bìng zhī sān yě. chǔ zhī zhě sān. chū zhī zhě yì sān yě. zhū fēng hán zhī xié. jié bó pí fū zhī jiān. cáng yú jīng luò zhī nèi. liú ér bù qù. huò fā téng tòng zǒu zhù. má bì bù rén. jí sì zhī zhǒng yǎng jū luán. kě hàn ér chū zhī. fēng tán sù shí. zài gé huò shàng wǎn. kě yǒng ér chū zhī. hán shī gù lěng. rè kè xià jiāo. zài xià zhī bìng. kě xiè ér chū zhī. nèi-jīng sǎn lùn zhū bìng. fēi yí zhuàng yě. liú yán zhì fǎ. fēi yì jiē yě. .... qí yán bǔ. shí jiàn yī èr. rán qí bǔ fēi jīn zhī suǒ wèi bǔ yě. wén jù yú bǔ lùn tiáo xià. rú xīn bǔ gān. xián bǔ xīn. gān bǔ shèn. suān bǔ pí. kǔ bǔ fèi. ruò cǐ zhī bǔ. nǎi suǒ yǐ fā còu lǐ. zhì jīn yè. tōng xuě qì. zhì qí tǒng lùn zhū yào. zé yuē. xīn gān dàn sān wèi wéi yáng. suān kǔ xián sān wèi wéi yīn. xīn gān fā sàn. dàn shèn xiè. suān kǔ xián yǒng xiè. fā sàn zhě guī yú hàn. yǒng zhě guī yú tù. xiè zhě guī yú xià. shèn wéi jiě biǎo. guī yú hàn. xiè wéi lì xiǎo sōu. guī yú xià. shū bù yán bǔ. nǎi zhī shèng rén zhǐ yǒu sān fǎ. wú dì sì fǎ yě.

A disease is something that the human body originally does not have. [A disease] may enter [the body] from outside of it, or it may emerge from inside of it. In each case, evil qi [are involved]. When evil qi attach themselves to the body, it is possible to quickly attack them, and it is possible to quickly eliminate them. But how [could it be possible] to seize and retain them? Even ignorant men and ignorant women know that this is impossible. And yet, when they hear of attacks, they are unhappy; when they hear that [one plans] to supplement [their regular qi], they like it. Today's physicians say: One must first strengthen [the patient's] original qi. Once the original qi are replete, the evil [qi] will leave by themselves. How can there be so many foolish people in the world? Now, when a person has been struck by evil [qi], in minor cases these [evil qi] are transmitted [in the body] for a long time until they have exhausted themselves. In more serious cases the [evil qi] are transmitted [in the body] for a long time and it is quite difficult to eliminate them. In extreme cases, they cause a sudden death. As for the above mentioned strengthening of the [patient's] original qi, the supplementing of the [original qi] with dosages designed to supplement [occurs at a moment] when the patient's true qi do not dominate, and when the evil [qi] move as fast as horses, and as wild as ducks, and cannot be brought under control. One should consider a supplementing [therapy] only for people whose [movement in the] vessels are sunk in and depleted, and [who show] no [signs of] evil [qi] and of accumulations. In all other cases, [physicians who] consider a supplementing [therapy] for persons who have been affected by evil [qi] accumulations [already] are followers of Gun who drowned in the great flood [because he applied the wrong method to drain it]. When I now talk of the three methods of [making a patient] vomit, [causing him to] perspire, or purging [him], I am speaking first of all of an attack against the evil [qi present in his body]. Once the evil [qi] have left, the original qi will recover by themselves. Moreover, these methods that I am speaking of are known and have been applied in practice for a long time already; they are extremely refined and extremely mature. They show success only, but no failure. Hence, I dare to explain them to those [practicing] in future The six qi [sent out] by heaven are wind, heat, fire, dampness, dryness, and cold. The six qi sent out by the earth are fog, dew, rain, hail, ice, and mud. The six flavors [consumed by] man are sour, bitter, sweet, acrid, salty, and bland. Hence, diseases resulting from evil [qi sent out by] heaven affect mostly the upper [sections of the body]; diseases resulting from evil [qi sent out by the] earth affect mostly the lower [sections of the body]; and diseases resulting from evil [qi invited by] man [through his living habits himself], mostly affect the central [section of his body]. These then are the three [possibilities] how a disease may emerge. Since they may be localized in three [sections], they can be driven out by three [methods] too. All evil [qi resulting from an impact of] wind or cold assemble in the skin; they are stored inside of the conduits and network [vessels]. When they remain [where they are] and do not leave [the body by themselves], in some cases they cause pain that moves [through the body], or numbness and loss of sensitivity, and also swelling, itching, and cramps in one's four limbs. [In all of these cases, the evil qi responsible] can be eliminated through [therapies causing] sweating. Phlegm caused by wind, and food that remains [in the body for too] long, either at the diaphragm or at the upper [opening of the stomach] duct, can be eliminated [from the body through induced] vomiting. Diseases in the lower [section of the body], such as cold and dampness, or constipation [of stools and urine] resulting from cold, as well as heat residing in the lower [section of the triple] burner, all can be eliminated [from the body through] discharging. The *Neijing* discusses diseases in many contexts; it does not [depict them] in a uniform manner. It variously speaks about the methods of treatment; it does not [present only] one standard! ... It talks about supplementation only occasionally, in one or two [passages], and that supplementation has nothing in common with the supplementation as it is understood today. In those paragraphs where the text has a discourse on supplementation, such as acrid supplements the liver; salty supplements the heart; sweet supplements the kidneys; sour supplements the spleen; and bitter supplements the lung, these supplementations are employed to open the skin structures, to make [the body's] liquids reach [their destination], or to cause the blood and the qi to penetrate [the body]. And in a general discussion of all the drugs, [the *Neijing* states:] "The three flavors acrid, sweet, and bland are yang; sour, bitter, and salty are yin. Acrid and sweet disperse; what is bland [causes] leakage and discharge; sour, bitter, and salty [cause] gushing forth and discharge." "Dispersion" is to be counted as [causing] sweating, "gushing forth" is to be counted as [causing] vomiting; and "discharge" is to be counted as [causing] downward passages [of stools and urine]. Leakage unties the outside [of the body] and is to be counted as [causing] sweating; discharge frees the passage of urine, and is to be counted as [causing] downward passages. [The *Nei jing*] does not refer to supplementation here at all! The Sages had only three methods [of treatment], and there was no fourth!

7.c *Dú yī suí bǐ* 4 讀醫隨筆 Fù guì pín jiàn gōng bǔ yì yí qí shuō yǒu biàn 富貴貧賤攻補異宜其說有辨 Statements [Concerning the Treatment of] Rich and Poor [People] by Attacking and Supplementing Distinguish Between Different [Approaches] Suitable [for these Two Groups of Patients]

前人皆謂。富貴之病利用補。貧賤之人利用攻。初未臨診之時。亦深以此語爲然。乃至今而覺其非也。富貴之人。安居厚奉。藏府經絡。莫不痰涎膠固。氣機凝滯。不能流通。故邪氣據之而不得去者。非正氣之不足。乃正氣之不運也。治之宜重用攻散。且氣血充裕。能任攻散者。正此輩也。若重之以補。是益之滯矣。貧賤之人。藜藿不充。敗絮不暖。四時力作。汗液常泄。榮虛衛散。經脈枯槁。及至有病。初起隱忍。勞役不輟。勢至重困。乃始求醫。故其邪氣之不去者。非正氣之不運。實正氣之不足也。治之須助正氣。正氣一充。其氣機之流利。自能鼓舞驅邪。非似富貴安逸者之氣滯。必待重施攻散也。

吾每診貧賤力食之人。病脈或粗大挺硬。或短弱細微。起伏總是無力。應指總是少神。求似富貴之脉之洪滑搏結者。殊不多覯也。蓋富病屬氣血之鬱滯。貧病屬氣血之匱乏。若謂筋骨柔脆與堅强之不同也。此在無病時則然耳。內經曰。形苦志樂。病生於筋。治之以熨引。是溫助其氣而運之。形已苦者。不得復開泄也。形樂志樂。病生於肉。治之以針石。形樂志苦。病生於脈。治之以灸刺。是形樂者。皆有血實。決之之義也。若攻苦之士。家徒四壁。謀道謀食。百計經營。此又不得與膏粱酣豢者同論矣。故形苦志苦。病生于困竭。治之以甘藥。謂表裏榮衛俱不足也。形苦宜補。形樂宜瀉。不校然可睹耶。

利用	lì yòng	to employ
初	chū	initially
臨	lín	in the face of
臨診	lín zhěn	clinical diagnosis
莫不	mò bù	no one not; all
膠固	jiāo gù	firm
機	jī	trigger; mechanics; movement
據	jù	to occupy; to take possession
裕	yù	abundant
輩	bèi	class; kind
藜藿	lí huò	coarse food; common vegetables
敗絮	bài xù	torn rags
力作	lì zuò	to exert one's strength
隱忍	yǐn rěn	to bear secretly

勞役	láo yì	to toil; to indulge in exhausting labor
輟	chuò	to rest
助	zhù	to assist; to support
鼓舞	gǔ wǔ	to stimulate
待	dài	must
重	zhòng	to treat as important; to emphasize
力食	lì shí	to toil physically to make a living
粗	cū	rough
挺	tǐng	rather; rigid
起伏	qǐ fú	emergence and disappearance
搏	bó	to beat
覯	gòu	to encounter
鬱	yù	obstruction
匱	kuì	failing; deficient; exhausted
柔	róu	soft
脆	cuì	fragile
引	yǐn	short for 導引 *dǎo yǐn*; (a qi) conducting (therapy); gymnastics
不得	bù dé	cannot; must not
士	shì	a person
壁	bì	the wall of a house
謀	móu	to devise; a plan
經營	jīng yíng	to engage in
膏粱	gāo liáng	rich; wealthy (lit.: fat meat and fine millet)
酣	hān	intoxicated; merry
豢	huàn	to feed
校	jiào	used here for 較 *jiào*: obvious; clear

Qián rén jiē wèi. fù guì zhī bìng lì yòng bǔ. pín jiàn zhī rén lì yòng gōng. chū wèi lín zhěn zhī shí. yì shēn yǐ cǐ yǔ wéi rán. nǎi zhì jīn ér jué qí fēi yě. fù guì zhī rén. ān jū hòu fèng. zàng fǔ jīng luò. mò bù tán xián jiāo gù. qì jī níng zhì. bù néng liú tōng. gù xié qì jù zhī ér bù dé qù zhě. fēi zhèng qì zhī bù zú. nǎi zhèng qì zhī bù yùn yě. zhì zhī yí zhòng yòng gōng sàn. qiě qì xuě chōng yù.

néng rèn gōng sàn zhě. zhèng cǐ bèi yě. ruò zhòng zhī yǐ bǔ. shì yì zhī zhì yǐ. pín jiàn zhī rén. lí huò bù chōng. bài xù bù nuǎn. sì shí lì zuò. hàn yè cháng xiè. róng xū wèi sàn. jīng mài kū gǎo. jí zhì yǒu bìng. chū qǐ yǐn rěn. láo yì bù chuò. shì zhì zhòng kùn. nǎi shǐ qiú yī. gù qí xié qì zhī bù qù zhě. fēi zhèng qì zhī bù yùn. shí zhèng qì zhī bù zú yě. zhì zhī xū zhù zhèng qì. zhèng qì yì chōng. qí qì jī zhī liú lì. zì néng gǔ wǔ qū xié. fēi sì fù guì ān yì zhě zhī qì zhì. bì dài zhòng shī gōng sàn yě. wū měi zhěn pín jiàn lì shí zhī rén. bìng mài huò cū dà tǐng yìng. huò duǎn ruò xì wēi. qǐ fú zǒng shī wú lì. yìng zhǐ zǒng shī shǎo shén. qiú sì fù guì zhī mài zhī hóng huá bó jié zhě. shū bù duō gòu yě. gài fù bìng shǔ qì xuě zhī yù zhì. pín bìng shǔ qì xuě zhī kuì fá. ruò wèi jīn gǔ róu cuì yǔ jiān qiáng zhī bù tóng yě. cǐ zài wú bìng shí zé rán ěr. nèi-jīng yuē. xíng kǔ zhì lè. bìng shēng yú jīn. zhì zhī yǐ yùn yǐn. shī wēn zhù qí qì ér yùn zhī. xíng yǐ kǔ zhě. bù dé fù kāi xiè yě. xíng lè zhì lè. bìng shēng yú ròu. zhì zhī yǐ zhēn shí. xíng lè zhì kǔ. bìng shēng yú mài. zhì zhī yǐ jiǔ cì. shī xíng lè zhě. jiē yǒu xuě shí. jué zhī zhī yì yě. ruò gōng kǔ zhī shì. jiā tú sì bì. móu dào móu shí. bǎi jì jīng yíng. cǐ yòu bù dé yǔ gāo liáng hān huàn zhě tóng lùn yǐ. gù xíng kǔ zhì kǔ. bìng shēng yú kùn jiē. zhì zhī yǐ gān yào. wèi biǎo lǐ róng wèi jù bù zú yě. xíng kǔ yí bǔ. xíng lè yí xiè. bù jiào rán kě dǔ yé.

People of former times said: [In treating] the illnesses of the rich, one employs a supplementing [therapy, and in treating] poor people, one employs an attacking [therapy]. Initially, before I had gained [experiences in] clinical diagnosis myself, I was deeply convinced of the accuracy of such statements. Now, however, I feel they are wrong. Rich people live comfortably and receive substantial incomes. All their [body's] depots and palaces, as well as their conduits and network [vessels] are [filled] with phlegm and saliva, and are stiff and firm. The mechanism triggering the [movement of] qi freezes and stagnates, and [the qi] are unable to flow and penetrate [the entire body]. As a result, evil qi take possession [of the regions not reached by one's regular qi], and the fact that one is unable to eliminate them does not result from an insufficiency of one's regular qi, but from a failure of the regular qi to move [through the entire body]. To treat such [conditions] one must assign an important role to the use of attacking and dispersing [remedies]. Also, it is exactly that kind [of people] whose qi and blood are present in abundance, who can stand attacking and dispersing [remedies]. If one adds to their [qi and blood] by applying a supplementing [therapy], one just adds to their stagnation. Poor people cannot even fill themselves with coarse vegetables. They wear rotten rags and do not feel warm. During all four seasons they exert all their strength, and they are regularly drained by perspiration and [the loss of bodily] liquid. Their camp

[qi] are depleted, and their guardian [qi] are dispersed. Their conduit vessels dry out, and when they reach a point where they are affected by a disease, they will bear it secretly in its initial stages, and they will not rest in their toil. Only when the strength of [the disease] has reached a serious and troublesome [stage], then they start to seek [the advice of] a physician. Hence, the fact that they [are affected by] evil qi which do not leave [the body again], is not the result of a failure of their regular qi to move; they really do not have enough regular qi. To treat such [conditions] one must support their regular qi. A soon as the regular qi are filled up, the mechanism triggering [the movement of] the qi is free and will itself be stimulated to push out the evil. This is quite different from the obstructions in the [flow of the] qi of the rich, who live in comfort and idleness, and [in whose treatment] one must place emphasis on attacking and dispersing [remedies]. Everytime I examine poor people who must work very hard physically to make a living, when they are ill the [movement in their] vessels is either rough, strong, rigid, and hard, or short, weak, fine, and feeble. Whether [the movement] emerges or disappears, it is always without strength; no matter how it responds to one's fingers, its spirits are always but few. If one were to search for such vast and soft, beating and clotting [movements in the] vessels as they characterize the rich, one would certainly not find them often. Now, the diseases of the rich belong to [the category of] obstructions and stagnation [in the flow] of the qi and of the blood. The diseases of the poor belong to [the category of] deficiency and want of qi and blood. If it is said that there are differences [between the rich and the poor] in that the sinews and bones [of the former] are soft and fragile, while those [of the latter] are firm and strong, that is the case as long as they are not ill. The *Neijing* states: "The diseases of those whose body suffers and whose mind is happy, they emerge from the sinews. One treats them by applying hot pressure or a conducting [therapy]." This way, warmth supports the movement of the qi. If someone's body suffers already, it would be wrong to open and drain it in addition. "The diseases of those whose body and whose mind is happy, they emerge from the flesh. One treats them with needles and [pointed] stones. The diseases of those whose body is happy and whose mind suffers, they emerge from the vessels. One treats them with cauterization and piercing." The reason is, whenever the body is happy one must dissolve a repletion of blood. Someone who suffers from hard labor, whose house consists of only four walls, who must carefully plan his way [in life] and who must carefully plan [how to earn his] food, and who is engaged in countless strategems, such [people] cannot, of course, be mentioned, in one breath, with those who are affluent, who have more than enough to eat and drink! Hence, [the statement] "diseases of those whose body and whose mind suffer, they emerge from exhaustion and are treated with sweet

drugs," is to say that their camp and guardian [qi] in the outside and inside [regions of the body] are insufficient. If the body suffers, one must fill; if the body is happy, one must drain. Is this not clearly recognizable?

7.d *Huáng dì nèi jīng, Sù wèn* 13
黃帝內經, 素問
Yí jīng biàn qì lùn 移精變氣論
On Changes in the [Assimilation of] Essence and on the Transformation of Qi

---

黃帝問曰。余聞古之治病。惟其移精變氣。可祝由而已。今世治病。毒藥治其內。鍼石治其外。或愈或不愈。何也。岐伯對曰。往古人居禽獸之間。動作以避寒。陰居以避暑。內無眷慕之累。外無伸官之形。此恬憺之世。邪不能深入也。故毒藥不能治其內。鍼石不能治其外。故可移精祝由而已。當今之世不然。憂患緣其內。苦形傷其外。又失四時之從。逆寒暑之宜。賊風數至。虛邪朝夕。內至五藏骨髓。外傷空竅肌膚。所以小病必甚。大病必死。故祝由不能已也。帝曰。善。余欲臨病人。觀死生。決嫌疑。欲知其要。如日月光。可得聞乎。岐伯曰。色脈者。上帝之所貴也。先師之所傳也。上古使僦貸季。理色脈而通神明。合之金木水火土。四時。八風。六合。不離其常。變化相移。以觀其妙。以知其要。欲知其要。則色脈是矣。色以應日。脈以應

月。常求其要。則其要也。夫色之變化。以應四時之脈。此上帝之所貴。以合于神明也。所以遠死而近生。生道以長。命曰聖王。中古之治病。至而治之湯液。十日以去八風五痺之病。十日不已。治以草蘇草荄之枝。本末爲助。標本已得。邪氣乃服。暮世之治病也則不然。治不本四時。不知日月。不審逆從。病形已成。乃欲微鍼治其外。湯液治其內。粗工兇兇。以爲可攻。故病未已。新病復起。

祝由	zhù yóu	to invoke the origin (a term used to denote therapeutic exorcism)
對	duì	to reply
往	wǎng	formerly; in the past
禽獸	qín shòu	animals
作	zuò	to act; to be active
避	bì	to avoid; to flee; to shun
陰	yīn	shade
眷慕	juàn mù	to think [of someone] with sentimental affection
累	lèi	to tie; to bind; entanglement
恬憺	tián dàn	peaceful and tranquil
緣	yuán	to affect
朝	zhāo	morning
夕	xī	evening
觀	guān	to observe
嫌疑	xián yí	suspicion; doubt
僦貸季	jiù dài jì	Jiu Daiji, legendary physician of ancient times
神明	shén míng	spirit brilliance

八風	bā fēng	the eight winds (i.e. the winds from the eight cardinal points East, West, South, North, East-South, East-North, West-South, West.North)
六合	liù hé	the six [cardinal points] uniting [the world]: East, West, South, North, Above, Below; i. e. "the world"
離	lí	to leave; to turn one's back to
常	cháng	permanently; constantly; regularly
五痺	wǔ bì	the five blocks (i.e. of skin, flesh, sinews, bones, and vessels)
草蘇	cǎo sū	*cao su*: name of a drug (?); herbal leaves (?)
草荄	cǎo gāi	*cao gai*: name of an herb or tree (?)
枝	zhī	a branch
標本	biāo běn	tip and root
服	fú	to yield
暮世	mù shì	later generations
兇兇	xiōng xiōng	to behave aggressively

Huáng-dì wèn yuē. yú wén gǔ zhī zhì bìng. wéi qí yí jīng biàn qì. kě zhù yóu ér yǐ. jīn shì zhì bìng. dú yào zhì qí nèi. zhēn shí zhì qí wài. huò yù huò bù yù. hé yě. qí bó duì yuē. wǎng gǔ rén jū qín shòu zhī jiān. dòng zuò yǐ bì hán. yīn jū yǐ bì shǔ. nèi wú juàn mù zhī lèi. wài wú shēn guān zhī xíng. cǐ tián dàn zhī shì. xié bù néng shēn rù yě. gù dú yào bù néng zhì qí nèi. zhēn shí bù néng zhì qí wài. gù kě yí jīng zhù yóu ér yǐ. dāng jīn zhī shì bù rán. yōu huàn yuán qí nèi. kǔ xíng shāng qí wài. yòu shī sì shí zhī cóng. nì hán shǔ zhī yí. zèi fēng shù zhì. xū xié zhāo xī. nèi zhì wǔ zàng gǔ suǐ. wài shāng kōng qiào jī fū. suǒ yǐ xiǎo bìng bì shèn. dà bìng bì sǐ. gù zhù yóu bù néng yǐ yě. dì yuē. shàn. yú yù lín bìng rén. guān sǐ shēng. jué xián yí. yù zhī qí yào. rú rì yuè guāng. kě dé wén hū. qí bó yuē. sè mài zhě. shàng dì zhī suǒ guì yě. xiān shī zhī suǒ chuán yě. shàng gǔ shǐ jiù dài jì. lǐ sè mài ér tōng shén míng. hé zhī jīn mù shuǐ huǒ tǔ. sì shí. bā fēng. liù hé. bù lí qí cháng. biàn huà xiāng yí. yǐ guān qí miào. yǐ zhī qí yào. yù zhī qí yào. zé sè mài shī yǐ. sè yǐ yìng rì. mài yǐ yìng yuè. cháng qiú qí yào. zé qí yào yě. fū sè zhī biàn huà. yǐ yìng sì shí zhī mài. cǐ shàng dì zhī suǒ guì. yǐ hé yú shén míng yě. suǒ yǐ yuǎn sǐ ér jìn shēng. shēng dào yǐ cháng. mìng yuē shèng wáng. zhōng gǔ zhī zhì bìng. zhì ér zhì zhī tāng yè shí rì. yǐ qù bā fēng wǔ bì zhī bìng. shí rì bù yǐ. zhì yǐ cǎo sū cǎo gāi zhī zhī. běn mò wéi zhù. biāo běn yǐ dé. xié qì nǎi fú. mù shì zhī zhì bìng yě zé bù rán. zhì bù běn sì shí. bù zhī rì yuè. bù shěn nì cóng. bìng xíng yǐ chéng. nǎi yù wēi zhēn zhì qí wài. tāng yè zhì qí nèi. cū gōng xiōng xiōng. yǐ wéi kě gōng. gù bìng wèi yǐ. xīn bìng fù qǐ.

Huang Di asked: I have heard that, when [the people] in antiquity treated a disease, they simply moved the essence and changed the qi. They were able to invoke the origin and [any disease] came to an end. When the people of nowadays treat a disease, [they employ] toxic drugs to treat their interior and [they employ] needles and [pointed] stones to treat their exterior. Some are healed; others are not healed. Why is this so?
Qi Bo responded: People in antiquity lived among their animals. They moved and were active and this way they avoided the cold. They resided in the shade and this way they avoided the summerheat. Internally, they knew no entanglements resulting from sentimental attachments; externally, they did not have the physical appearance of stretching towards officialdom. In this peaceful and tranquil world, the evil was unable to penetrate deeply. Hence toxic drugs were unsuited to treat their interior, and needles and [pointed] stones were unsuited to treat their exterior. Hence it was possible to move essence and invoke the origin and [any disease] came to an end. The people of today are different. Anxiety and suffering affect their interior; taxation of the physical appearance harms their exterior. Also, the [people] have lost [the knowledge how] to follow the four seasons and they oppose the requirements of cold and summerheat. The robber wind frequently reaches [them]. The depletion evil [is present] in the morning and in the evening; internally it reaches to the five depots, to the bones, and to the marrow; externally it harms the orifices, the muscles, and the skin. This is why minor diseases inevitably develop into serious [problems]; serious diseases inevitably result in death. Hence, invoking the origin cannot end [a disease any longer].
Huang Di: Good! When I attend a patient and when [I] observe [him to find out] whether [he must] die, or will survive, I should like to cast away all doubts. [I] should like to know the essentials – [they should be as clear] as the light of sun and moon. May [I] hear [of this]?
Qi Bo: Complexion and [movement in the] vessels, this is what the Lords on High valued and what the teachers of former times have transmitted. In high antiquity, Jiu Daiji was ordered to establish the structure of the complexions and the [movements in the] vessels, and to correspond to spirit brilliance. He matched them with [the five agents] metal, wood, water, fire, and soil, with the four seasons, the eight winds, and the six [cardinal points] uniting [the world]. He never left these regular [patterns], and their changes, transformations, and mutual shifts [of positions]. This way one can observe the mysteries and know

the essentials of [death and survival]. If one wishes to know the essentials of [death and survival], then it is in the complexion and the [movement in the] vessels that they are [to be found]. The complexion is that by which [a physician establishes] correspondences to the sun, the vessels are that by which [a physician establishes] correspondences to the moon. To permanently search for these essentials, this, then, is the essential in the [prediction of death and survival]. Now, the changes and transformations of the complexion, as they correspond to the [movements in the] vessels in the [course of the] four seasons, this is what was valued by the Lords on High, and [this is] by which they established links to spirit-brilliance. This way they kept death at a distance and remained close to life. It is therefore that they extended the Way of life, [and hence] they were called sage kings. When [the people] in middle antiquity treated a disease, once it had arrived, they treated it by means of decoctions. It took ten days to remove the diseases of the eight winds and five blocks. If they had not ended after ten days, they treated them with *cao su* [that is,] the branches of *cao gai*,[1] and supported this with roots and ends. When one has acquired a complete hold of tip and root, the evil qi will yield. When [the people of] later generations treated a disease, then this was different. The treatments were not based in the four seasons. They no longer knew of [the significance of] sun and moon. They did not investigate [whether the qi] moved contrary to or followed [its regular course]. When a disease had already assumed physical manifestation, they wished [to use] fine needles to treat the exterior of the [patient] and decoctions to treat his interior. Uneducated practitioners behave very aggressively, believing they can launch an attack. Before the old disease has ended, a new disease emerges in addition.

Note

1 For the time being, these pharmaceutical substances cannot be identified. The designations *cao su* 草蘇 and *cao gai* 草荄 are not documented in any other text.

7.e *Huáng dì nèi jīng, Sù wèn* 12
黃帝內經·素問
Yì fă fāng yí lùn 異法方宜論
On the Different Methods [of Treatment] That Suit the [Four Cardinal] Directions

黃帝問曰。醫之治病也。一病而治各不同。皆愈。何也。岐伯對曰。地勢使然也。故東方之域。天地之所始生也。魚鹽之地。海濱傍水。其民食魚而嗜鹹。皆安其處。美其食。魚者使人熱中。鹽者勝血。故其民皆黑色疏理。其病皆爲癰瘍。其治宜砭石。故砭石者。亦從東方來。西方者。金玉之域。沙石之處。天地之所收引也。其民陵居而多風。水土剛强。其民不衣而褐薦。其民華食而脂肥。故邪不能傷其形體。其病生於內。其治宜毒藥。故毒藥者。亦從西方來。北方者。天地所閉藏之域也。其地高陵居。風寒冰洌。其民樂野處而乳食。藏寒生滿病。其治宜灸焫。故灸焫者。亦從北方來。南方者。天地所長養。陽之所盛處也。其地下。水土弱。霧露之所聚也。其民嗜酸而食胕。故其民皆緻理而赤色。其病攣痺。其治宜微鍼。故九鍼者。亦從南方來。中央者。其地平以濕。天地所以生萬物也衆。其民食雜而不勞。故其病多痿厥寒熱。其治宜導引按蹻。故導引按蹻者。亦從中央出也。故聖人雜合以治。各得其所宜。故治所以異而病皆愈者。得病之情。知治之大體也。

勢	shì	a feature
域	yù	region
鹽	yán	salt
濱	bīn	a beach
傍	báng	to border on; by the side of
安	ān	to consider as comfortable
美	měi	delicious; beautiful
理	lǐ	the [skin] structures; short for: 腠理 *còu lǐ*
疏理	shū lǐ	open skin structures
癰瘍	yōng yáng	welling abscess
金	jīn	gold
玉	yù	jade
沙	shā	sand
收	shōu	to take in; to gather; to contract
陵	líng	earthen mound
剛	gāng	hard
衣	yī	clothes; to dress
褐	hè	serge; rough clothing; [garments of] hair
薦	jiàn	[garments of] grasses
華	huá	excellent; rich [food]
肥	féi	fat
乳	rǔ	milk
焫	ruò	to burn
胕	fū	to have a strong odor
緻理	zhì lǐ	to have tight [skin] structures
攣	luán	cramp

九鍼	jiǔ zhēn	the nine [types of] needles [used in acupuncture]
中央	zhōng yāng	center
平	píng	flat
濕	shī	damp
衆	zhòng	all; the whole of
雜	zá	diverse
導引	dǎo yǐn	guiding-pulling (a type of physical exercises)
按蹻	àn jiāo	pressing-lifting (a type of physical exercises)

Huáng dì wèn yuē. yī zhī zhì bìng yě. yí bìng ér zhì gè bù tóng. jiē yù. hé yě. qí bó duì yuē. dì shì shǐ rán yě. gù dōng fāng zhī yù. tiān dì zhī suǒ shǐ shēng yě. yú yán zhī dì. hǎi bīn páng shuǐ. qí mín shí yú ér shí xián. jiē ān qí chù. měi qí shí. yú zhě shǐ rén rè zhōng. yán zhě shèng xuě. gù qí mín jiē hēi sè shū lǐ. qí bìng jiē wéi yōng yáng. qí zhì yí biān shí. gù biān shí zhě. yì cóng dōng fāng lái. xī fāng zhě. jīn yù zhī yù. shā shí zhī chù. tiān dì zhī suǒ shōu yǐn yě. qí mín líng jū ér duō fēng. shuǐ tǔ gāng qiáng. qí mín bù yī ér hè jiàn. qí mín huá shí ér zhī féi. gù xié bù néng shāng qí xíng tǐ. qí bìng shēng yú nèi. qí zhì yí dú yào. gù dú yào zhě. yì cóng xī fāng lái. běi fāng zhě. tiān dì suǒ bì cáng zhī yù yě. qí dì gāo líng jū. fēng hán bīng liè. qí mín lè yě chǔ ér rǔ shí. zàng hán shēng mǎn bìng. qí zhì yí jiǔ ruò. gù jiǔ ruò zhě. yì cóng běi fāng lái. nán fāng zhě. tiān dì suǒ zhǎng yǎng. yáng zhī suǒ shèng chù yě. qí dì xià. shuǐ tǔ ruò. wù lù zhī suǒ jù yě. qí mín shí suān ér shí fǔ. gù qí mín jiē zhì lǐ ér chì sè. qí bìng luán bì. qí zhì yí wēi zhēn. gù jiǔ zhēn zhě. yì cóng nán fāng lái. zhōng yāng zhě. qí dì píng yǐ shī. tiān dì suǒ yǐ shēng wàn wù yě zhòng. qí mín shí zá ér bù láo. gù qí bìng duō wěi jué hán rè. qí zhì yí dǎo yǐn àn jiāo. gù dǎo yǐn àn jiāo zhě. yì cóng zhōng央 chū yě. gù shèng rén zá hé yǐ zhì. gè dé qí suǒ yí. gù zhì suǒ yǐ yī ér bìng jiē yù zhě. dé bìng zhī qíng. zhī zhì zhī dà tǐ yě.

Huang Di asked: When physicians treat diseases, one identical disease may be treated differently in each case, and is always healed. How is that?
Qi Bo responded: Physical features of the earth let it be this way. Now, the region of the East, this is where heaven and earth give life first. [This is] the land of fish and salt; of seacoast bordering on the water. Its people eat fish and crave for salty [meals]. All of them consider their place of residence as comfortable and they regard their food as delicious. As for the fish, it lets one develop a heated center; as for the salty [meals], they defeat the blood. Hence, its people all have a black complexion and open skin structure. Their illnesses

are always welling abscesses and ulcers. For their treatment, pointed stones are suitable. Hence, [the therapy with] pointed stones originated in the East, too. The West, this is the region of gold and jade. It is the location of sand and stones. It is where heaven and earth contract and pull [things together]. Its people live in earthen mounds and the winds are frequent. The water and the soil are hard and strong. Its people do not dress with clothes but wear [garments of] hair and grasses. Its people [enjoy] rich food and they are fat. Hence, [external] evil cannot harm their physical body; their diseases emerge from within. For their treatment, toxic drugs are appropriate. Hence, [the treatment with] toxic drugs originated in the West, too. The North, this is the region where heaven and earth secure and store. Its land lies at a high elevation, [its people] live in earthen mounds. Wind, cold, ice, and chilliness [dominate]. Its people find joy in living in the wilderness and in consuming milk. Their depots are cold and this generates diseases of fullness. For their treatment, moxa burning is appropriate. Hence, moxa burning originated in the North, too. The South, this is [the region] where heaven and earth bestow growth and nourishment; it is the place where yang [qi] is present in abundance. Its land lies low; water and soil are weak. It is [a region] where fog and dew assemble. Its people crave for sour [foods], and they eat [food of] a strong odor. Hence, its people all [have] tight [skin] structures and a reddish complexion. Their illnesses are cramps and blocks. For their treatment, fine needles are appropriate. Hence, the nine needles have originated in the South, too. The center, its land is flat and damp. It is here that heaven and earth give birth to the myriad beings in large numbers. Its people eat diverse [foods] and do not engage in heavy work. Hence, their diseases are often limpness, receding [qi], and [spells of] cold and heat. For their treatment, guiding-pulling and pressing-lifting are appropriate. Hence, guiding-pulling and pressing-lifting have originated in the center, too. Hence, the sages brought various [patterns] together in treatment; each [case] received what was appropriate for it. Hence, if what one uses for treatment is different, and the disease is healed in all [cases] nevertheless, [then this is because] one has grasped the nature of disease and knows the entire complex of treatment.

7.f *Chén xiū yuán yī shū wǔ shí zhǒng*
陳修園醫書五十種
(Cháng shā fāng gē kuò 長沙方歌括1)
Yī bìng shùn qí zì rán shuō
醫病順其自然說
Discourse on Treating a Disease by Following its Natural Course

---

病人之吉凶禍福。寄之於醫。醫者之任重。然權不操諸醫。而操諸用醫之人。何也。人有大病。庸醫束手無策。始求救於名醫。名醫入門診畢。告以病從何來。當從何去。得那一類藥而增劇者何故。得那一類藥除去那一病。而此外未能盡除者何故。病勢雖覺稍愈。逾一二日仍作。或逾一二日而更甚於前者又何故。一一爲病家說明。定其如此。救誤如此。溫清攻補如此。按法立方。服藥後必見出何證。又見出何證則向愈。預斷其愈于何日何時。病家能一一信其言而不疑。且架中不藏本草備要、醫方集解、萬病回春、本草綱目、東醫寶鑒、馮氏錦囊、赤水玄珠、薛氏醫案、景岳全書、石室秘錄、辨證奇聞、臨證指南之類。又無强不知以爲知之親友。與依阿兩可素稱果子藥之先生。朱紫不亂。則名醫得以盡其所

長。傷寒卒病二三日可愈。最遲亦不出十八日之外。風痨臌膈一月可愈。最遲亦不出三月之外。否則病家疑信參半。時醫猶可勉强從事。俟其病氣衰而自愈。若以名醫自命者。斷不可肩此重任。反致取怨敗名。

吉凶	jí xiōng	good or bad fortune
福	fú	happiness; prosperity
寄	jì	to entrust to
任	rèn	responsibility; burden
重	zhòng	heavy
權	quán	authority; responsibility
操	cāo	to hold; to lay into someone's hands; to burden on somebody.
庸醫	yōng yī	common physician
束手無策	shù shǒu wú cè	hands tied and without plan; helpless
救	jiù	to aid; help
名醫	míng yī	renowned physician
告	gào	to announce
那	nǎ	what? Which?
劇	jù	to add to; to increase
愈	yù	better
逾	yú	to exceed; to pass
家	jiā	a house; a family
說明	shuō míng	to explain
救誤	jiù wù	to save from the mistakes [committed by someone else]
清	qīng	cool
按	àn	according to
立方	lì fāng	to compose a prescription
向	xiàng	towards; in favor of
預	yù	beforehand

信	xìn	to believe; confidence
架	jià	shelf
本草備要	běn cǎo bèi yào	*Ben cao bei yao*, a popular *materia medica* of the late 17th century, by Wāng Áng 汪昂
醫方集解	yī fāng jí jiě	*Yi fang ji jie*, a popular collection of prescriptions of the late 17th century, by Wāng Áng 汪昂
萬病回春	wàn bìng huí chūn	*Wan bing hui chun*, a popular collection of prescriptions of the late 17th century, by Gōng Tíngxián 龔廷賢
本草綱目	běn cǎo gāng mù	*Ben cao gang mu*, an encyclopedic materia medica of the 16th century, by Lǐ Shízhēn 李時珍
東醫寶鑒	dōng yī bǎo jiàn	*Dong yi bao jian*, a Korean treatise on medicine of the early 17th century, by Xǔ Jùn 許浚
馮氏錦囊	féng shì jǐn náng	*Feng shi jin nang*, a medical work of the 17th century, by Féng Chǔzhán 馮楚瞻
赤水玄珠	chì shuǐ xuán zhū	*Chi shui xuan zhu*, a medical work of the 16th century, by Sūn Yīkuí 孫 一奎
薛氏醫案	xuē shì yī àn	*Xue shi yi an*, a collection of medical case histories of the 16th century, by Xuē Jǐ 薛己
景岳全書	jǐng yuè quán shū	*Jing yue quan shu*, the medical writings of Zhāng Jǐngyuè 張景岳 of the 17th century
石室秘錄	shí shì mì lù	*Shi shi mi lu*, a medical treatise of the 17th century, by Chén Shìduò 陳士鐸
辨證奇聞	biàn zhèng qí wén	*Bian zheng qi wen*, a medical treatise of the 17th century, by Chén Shìduò 陳士鐸
臨證指南	lín zhèng zhǐ nán	*Lin zheng zhi nan*, a medical treatise of the 18th century, by Yè Guì 葉桂
强	qiáng	definitely
親	qīn	relatives
友	yǒu	friend
依阿兩可	yī ē liǎng kě	to flatter with ambiguous statements
素稱	sù chēng	commonly called
果子	guǒ zǐ	fruits; berry
先生	xiān sheng	Mister

朱紫	zhū zǐ	(a hierarchy of different ranks characterized by) red and purple (seals); hierarchy
長	cháng	to excel
癆	láo	wasting; consumption
參半	cān bàn	half and half
時醫	shí yī	physicians (who follow only the trends of their own) time
從事	cóng shì	to perform one's duties
俟	sì	to wait; when
斷	duàn	definitely
肩	jiān	to shoulder
怨	yuàn	resentment

Bìng rén zhī jí xiōng huò fú. jì zhī yú yī. yī zhě zhī rèn zhòng. rán quán bù cāo zhū yī. ér cāo zhū yòng yī zhī rén. hé yě. rén yǒu dà bìng. yōng yī shù shǒu wú cè. shǐ qiú jiù yú míng yī. míng yī rù mén zhěn bì. gào yǐ bìng cóng hé lái. dāng cóng hé qù. dé nǎ yí lèi yào ér zēng jù zhě hé gù. dé nǎ yí lèi yào chú qù nǎ yí bìng. ér cǐ wài wèi néng jìn chú zhě hé gù. bìng shì suī jué shāo yù. yú yī èr rì réng zuò. huò yú yī èr rì ér gèng shèn yú qián zhě yòu hé gù. yī yī wéi bìng jiā shuō míng. dìng qí rú cǐ. jiù wù rú cǐ. wēn qīng gōng bǔ rú cǐ . àn fǎ lì fāng. fú yào hòu bì jiàn chū hé zhèng. yòu jiàn chū hé zhèng zé xiàng yù. yù duàn qí yù yú hé rì hé shí. bìng jiā néng yī yī xìn qí yán ér bù yí. qiě jià zhōng bù cáng běn cǎo bèi yào, yī fāng jí jiě, wàn bìng huí chūn, běn cǎo gāng mù, dōng yī bǎo jiàn, Féng shì jǐn náng, chì shuǐ xuán zhū, Xuē shì yī àn, jǐng yuè quán shū, shí shì mì lù, biàn zhèng qí wén, lín zhèng zhǐ nán zh ī lèi. yòu wú qiáng bù zhī yǐ wéi zhī zhī qīn yǒu . yǔ yī ē liǎng kě sù chēng guǒ zǐ yào zhī xiān sheng. zhū zǐ bù luàn. zé míng yī dé yǐ jìn qí suǒ cháng. shāng hán cù bìng èr sān rì kě yù. zuì chí yì bù chū shí bā rì zhī wài. fēng láo gǔ gé yí yuè kě yù. zuì chí yì bù chū sān yuè zhī wài. foǔ zé bìng jiā yí xìn cān bàn. shí yī yóu kě miǎn qiáng cóng shì. sì qí bìng qì shuāi ér zì yù. ruò yǐ míng yī zì mìng zhě. duàn bù kě jiān cǐ zhòng rèn. fǎn zhì qǔ yuàn bài míng.

A patient's good and bad fortune, his misery and his happiness are entrusted to his physician, and the burden that the physician carries is heavy. And still, the final responsibility [for the outcome of a treatment should] not be burdened on the physician, but on those people who employ the physician. Why is that so? When someone is very ill and a common physician [consulted first] has proven to be quite helpless, only then assistance will be sought from a renowned physician. A renowned physician enters the door, and as soon as he has finished his examination he will announce where the illness has originated from, and whence it will be eliminated. [He will state] which kinds of drugs, if employed, would only increase [the illness], and why this is so, and which kinds of drugs would eliminate this particular illness, but aside from this would not eliminate [the problem] entirely, and what the reasons are for this. [He will state further], why, while one my think that the strength of the illness has somewhat subsided, [the illness] will break out [again] after one or two days, or why it will turn even more serious than before after one or two days. One by one, [the physician] explains [all this] to the patient's family. He determines how he will save [the patient] from the [consequences of] mistakes [committed by the earlier healer], and how he will carry out an attack or fill [any depletion] with warming or cooling [remedies], and that he will compose a prescription in accordance with the [appropriate therapeutic] pattern. [He announces further] what kind of symptoms should appear after the drugs have been taken, and which symptoms, if they appear, indicate an improvement [in the condition of the patient; and, finally, the physician] will determine beforehand on what day and at what time the cure will be achieved. If the patient [and his] family can believe him word for word and harbor no doubt, and if [in the house of the patient] the shelves do not hold [books] such as the *Ben cao bei yao*, the *Yi fang ji jie*, the *Wan bing hui chun*, the *Ben cao gang mu*, the *Dong yi bao jian*, the *Feng shi jin nang*, the *Chi shu xuan zhu*, the *Xue shi yi an*, the *Jing yue quan shu*, the *Shi shi mi lu*, the *Bian zheng qi wen*, and the *Lin zheng zhi nan*, and if there are no relatives or friends who definitely know nothing but believe they are competent, or those who flatter with ambiguous statements and who are commonly called "Mr. Berry-Drug", that is, if the hierarchy [of expertise] is not disturbed, in that case a renowned physician may well reach the utmost of his abilities. A sudden illness resulting from harm caused by cold can then be cured within two or three days; at the most, [the cure] should not take longer than eighteen days. Consumption resulting from wind, bloating, and blockage can be cured within one month; at the most, [a cure] should not take longer than three months. If no [cure is achieved by that time], doubts will mix with confidence in the patient [and his] family. Physicians [who follow only the trends of their own] time may force [various interpretations on the patient's condition] until the qi [causing the] illness weaken, and a cure comes by itself. Those who name themselves renowned physicians will definitely not be able to shoulder this heavy burden; on the contrary, they will succeed only in becoming a target for resentment, and in destroying their name.

Lesson Eight

Pharmaceutics: General Principles

Apparently, Chinese traditional pharmaceutics originated from at least three sources. These included, first, attempts to treat wounds, boils, or simply pain by applying substances externally to the afflicted body parts; second, experiences with the ingestion of substances as food; and, third, a conscious search for substances that might provide man with long life without aging. While the first two of these origins date back to the remote past [and had led to a highly sophisticated materia medica as early as the third century BCE already], the quest for immortality may not have begun prior to the third century BCE. Among the Mawangdui manuscripts of the early 2nd century BCE is the so-called *Wushi'er bingfang* 五十二病方, a manual with prescriptions based on a total of more than two hundred pharmaceutical substances from plant, mineral, animal, and man-made sources. Also, the *Wushi'er bingfang* refers to a complex pharmaceutical technology designed to transform raw materials into refined drugs and various forms of medication. Throughout the two millennia of documented Chinese medical history, fixed formulas constituted the major basis of Chinese traditional pharmaceutical treatment. Physicians recorded tens of thousands of such recipes which appeared to have been effective in the treatment of an ailment and were believed to be effective again when applied to similar health problems. Until the twelfth century, the preoccupation with materia medica remained a domain of naturalists often inclined to Daoism. In contrast to acupuncture, and with the exception of the work of Zhang Ji 張機 (ca. 200 CE), the pharmaceutical approach was not integrated into the sciences of systematic correspondence. Only in the wake of Song Neo-Confucianism were the concepts of yinyang and of the five agents applied to drug use consistently, and several suggestions for creating a pharmacology of systematic correspondence were published. From now on, some physicians proposed the idea that identical diseases may appear in different symptoms, and that identical symptoms may be caused by different diseases. Consequently, they claimed, each prescription must be tailored to the individual requirements of a given patient. A compromise between this highly individualistic approach to pharmaceutical treatment on the one side, and the traditional use of fixed formulas on the other side resulted in the recommendation of core recipes to which were added (or from which were taken) specific components in accordance with the individual condition of a patient. During the Ming and Qing, the attempts at theorization initiated during the Song-Jin-Yuan dynasties received no new impulses, and arguments were voiced against some of its consequences, such as the idea that certain drugs were able to guide the effects of others to a desired region in the organism. Similar to Chinese traditional medical treatment in general, Chinese pharmaceutics split up into different schools during the second millennium CE. There were advocates of the classic, fixed formulas of the Han era, and others who claimed that the remedies of the past were unsuited to cure the illnesses of today. Some authors suggested the use of only one drug against a disease, while others preferred prescriptions comprising thirty to forty ingredients (and based on systematic correspondence), focusing on the needs of the individual patient.

Key Terms Introduced in Lesson Eight

藥品	yào pǐn	(pharmaceutical) drugs
純	chún	pure
厚	hòu	strongly developed (quality of a drug)
重	zhòng	pronounced (quality of a drug)
潤	rùn	to moisten
澀	sè	astringent
津	jīn	body liquid
君	jūn	ruler (drug in a prescription)
臣	chén	minister (drugs in a prescription)
製	zhì	to compound; to formulate (a prescription)
錠	dìng	an ingot; a cake
鎮	zhèn	to settle; to press down
生	shēng	fresh (drugs)
末	mò	powder
輕調	qīng tiáo	to regulate (a health problem by means of) light (drugs)
含	hán	to retain in one's mouth
食壓	shí yā	to press (drugs down in the body) by means of food

頓服	dùn fú	to take an entire dose of drugs at once
吞	tūn	to swallow
解	jiě	to dissolve
投	tóu	to add (to a prescription)
禀質	bǐng zhì	natural disposition
脫瀉	tuō xiè	loss (of qi) through drainage; diarrhea
藥蠱	yào gǔ	drug poisoning
四大	sì dà	the four elements (constituting the body)
少火	shào huǒ	the small fire (supposedly burning in the kidneys and being responsible for the maintenance of all physiological processes)
煩	fán	uneasiness; vexation
蒸髓	zhēng suǐ	(heat) steaming from the marrow (of one's bones). Equivalent to *gǔ zhēng* 骨蒸 in 9. b
發	fā	to stimulate (heat or perspiration)
劑	jì	a dose (of drugs)
佐	zuǒ	assistant (drugs in a prescription)
使	shǐ	aide (drugs in a prescription)
單行	dān xíng	(drugs which prefer) to act alone
相須	xiāng xū	(drugs which) depend on each other (in their effects)
相使	xiāng shǐ	(drugs which) reinforce each other (in their effects)
相畏	xiāng wèi	(drugs which) fear each other (i.e. suppress each other's effects)
相惡	xiāng wù	(drugs which) hate each other (i.e.; depotentiate each other)
相反	xiāng fǎn	(drugs which) are opposed to each other (in their effects)
相殺	xiāng shā	(drugs which) kill each other's (effects)
七情	qī qíng	the seven affects (which drugs harbor in their relations to each other)
病機	bìng jī	the movement of a disease (through the body); pathomechanism

消	xiāo	to digest
吐藥	tù yào	drugs causing vomiting; emetics
下藥	xià yào	drugs causing defecation; laxatives/purgatives
瘤	liú	tumor
發泄	fā xiè	to stimulate discharge
發熱	fā rè	to stimulate heat
湧泄	yǒng xiè	discharging through gushing forth (i.e. vomiting)
滲泄	shèn xiè	discharging through leakage (i.e. perspiration)
現成	xiàn chéng	ready-made (as of prescriptions)
通治	tōng zhì	cure-all
紫金錠	zǐ jīn dìng	the "dark-red golden ingot", a formula recommended to cure all possible eye afflictions
丹	dān	a small ball (formed to contain all the ingredients of a prescription)
至寶丹	zhì bǎo dān	the "extremely precious balls"
少陽	shào yáng	the minor-yang (conduit)
味	wèi	a (pharmaceutical) substance
胸	xiōng	the mind; lit.: the chest
辨證	biàn zhèng	to distinguish among patho-conditions (in order to apply a differential treatment)
陳方	chén fāng	age-old prescriptions
制	zhì	to formulate (a prescription), identical with 製
首	shǒu	numerary adjunct for prescriptions

8.a *Shòu shì bǎo yuán* 1 壽世保元 (Běn cǎo 本草) Yào lùn 藥論 On Drugs

---

夫藥者。天地間之萬物也。昔古神農憫蒼生之疾苦。格物理之精微。其用心可爲仁矣。故本草藥品雖多。然其味不過五。乃甘辛鹹苦酸是也。而其性不過六。溫涼補瀉升降是也。且甘辛溫補升者陽也。苦鹹涼瀉降者陰也。淡滲泄而屬陽。酸性陽而味陰。故藥有純陽者。有純陰者。有陰中之陽。有陽中之陰。有專用其氣者。有獨用其味者。大抵味之厚者必補。氣之重者必降。味淡則瀉。性輕則升。升者治在上在表之病。降者治在下在裏之疾。諸寒涼者治乎血熱。諸溫熱者治乎氣鬱氣虛。潤以濡燥。澀以收脫。又甘爲諸補之原。苦爲諸瀉之本。辛香者亦升瀉之類。酸鹹者皆補降之屬。所謂補者。性味各有所補。而其瀉者。亦各有所瀉。然補中有瀉。而瀉中有補。如酸入肝。生津以制燥。至苦入心。滋陰以降火。辛能溫肺以退寒。鹹可堅腎以禦熱。如欲去其邪。在使復其正。瀉陽有以補陰。瀉陰有以補陽。降則通其自升。升則欲其自降。惟病有兼

成。而法當合用。故方有奇偶。而藥有君臣。製之以散者散也。或成之以錠者鎮也。用湯者蕩也。取氣味蕩漾。而無所不至。用丸者緩也。取氣味緩達。而有所及遠。湯有生熟。瀉則宜生。補則宜熟。丸有大小。病在上者宜小。俱服於食後。或散末以輕調。或含丸以緩化。病在下者宜大。俱服於食前。或服後以食壓。或湯藥以頓服。吞補劑於蚤於未語之前。服疾藥當脫衣臨睡之際。凡用甘草者。解諸藥毒。取其甘以緩脾。劑投生薑者。行諸藥力。取辛以開胃。

萬物	wàn wù	the myriad things; everything
神農	shén nóng	Shen Nong, name of the legendary founder of Chinese materia medica; the “Divine Husbandman”
憫	mǐn	to pity; to grieve
蒼生	cāng shēng	the people
格	gé	to investigate
品	pǐn	thing
藥品	yào pǐn	(pharmaceutical) drugs
乃	nǎi	namely; that is to say
降	jiàng	to descend
純	chún	pure
厚	hòu	strongly developed (quality of a drug)
重	zhòng	pronounced (quality of a drug)
潤	rùn	to moisten
澀	sè	astringent
脫	tuō	to get lost; to go asunder
亦	yì	both
津	jīn	body liquid

禦	yù	to oppress
奇	jí	uneven (as numbers)
偶	ǒu	a pair; even (as numbers)
君	jūn	ruler (drug in a prescription)
臣	chén	minister (drugs in a prescription)
製	zhì	to compound; to formulate (a prescription)
錠	dìng	an ingot; a cake
鎮	zhèn	to settle; to press down
蕩	dàng	to excite; to agitate
蕩漾	dàng yàng	the rippling of water
生	shēng	fresh (drugs)
末	mò	powder
輕調	qīng tiáo	to regulate (a health problem by means of) light (drugs)
含	hán	to retain in one's mouth
食壓	shí yā	to press (drugs down in the body) by means of food
頓	dùn	a time; a turn
頓服	dùn fú	to take in one dose; to ingest together
吞	tūn	to swallow
蚤	zǎo	early
脫衣	tuō yī	to undress
睡	shuì	to sleep
甘草	gān cǎo	*gancao*, a drug prepared from Glycyrrhiza uralensis Fisch. and other Glycyrrhiza herbs
解	jiě	to dissolve
投	tóu	to add (to a prescription)
生薑	shēng jiāng	*shengjiang*, fresh ginger; a drug repared from Zingiber officinale Rosc. (mostly written: 生姜)

Fū yào zhě. tiān dì jiān zhī wàn wù yě. xī gǔ shén nóng mǐn cāng shēng zhī jí kǔ. gé wù lǐ zhī jīng wēi. qí yòng xīn kě wéi rén yǐ. gù běn cǎo yào pǐn suī duō. rán qí wèi bù guò wǔ. nǎi gān xīn xián kǔ suān shī yě. ér qí xìng bù guò liù.

wēn liáng bǔ xiè shēng jiàng shī yě. qiě gān xīn wēn bǔ shēng zhě yáng yě. kǔ xián liáng xiè jiàng zhě yīn yě. dàn shèn xiè ér shǔ yáng. suān xìng yáng ér wèi yīn. gù yào yǒu chún yáng zhě. yǒu chún yīn zhě. yǒu yīn zhōng zhī yáng. yǒu yáng zhōng zhī yīn. yǒu zhuān yòng qí qì zhě. yǒu dú yòng qí wèi zhě. dà dǐ wèi zhī hòu zhě bì bǔ. qì zhī zhòng zhě bì jiàng. wèi dàn zé xiè. xìng qīng zé shēng. shēng zhě zhì zài shàng zài biǎo zhī bìng. jiàng zhě zhì zài xià zài lǐ zhī jí. zhū hán liáng zhě zhì hū xuě rè. zhū wēn rè zhě zhì hū qì yù qì xū. rùn yǐ rú zào. sè yǐ shōu tuō. yòu gān wéi zhū bǔ zhī yuán. kǔ wéi zhū xiè zhī běn. xīn xiāng zhě yì shēng xiè zhī lèi. suān xián zhě jiē bǔ jiàng zhī shǔ. suǒ wèi bǔ zhě. xìng wèi gè yǒu suǒ bǔ. ér qí xiè zhě. yì gè yǒu suǒ xiè. rán bǔ zhōng yǒu xiè. ér xiè zhōng yǒu bǔ. rú suān rù gān. shēng jīn yǐ zhì zào. zhì kǔ rù xīn. zī yīn yǐ jiàng huǒ. xīn néng wēn fèi yǐ tuì hán. xián kě jiān shèn yǐ yù rè. rú yù qù qí xié. zài shì fù qí zhèng. xiè yáng yǒu yǐ bǔ yīn. xiè yīn yǒu yǐ bǔ yáng. jiàng zé tōng qí zì shēng. shēng zé yù qí zì jiàng. wéi bìng yǒu jiān chéng. ér fǎ dāng hé yòng. gù fāng yǒu qí ǒu. ér yào yǒu jūn chén. zhì zhī yǐ sǎn zhě sàn yě. huò chéng zhī yǐ dìng zhě zhèn yě. yòng tāng zhě dàng yě. qǔ qì wèi dàng yàng. ér wú suǒ bù zhì. yòng wán zhě huǎn yě. qǔ qì wèi huǎn dá. ér yǒu suǒ jí yuǎn. tāng yǒu shēng shú. xiè zé yí shēng. bǔ zé yí shú. wán yǒu dà xiǎo. bìng zài shàng zhě yí xiǎo. jù fú yú shí hòu. huò sǎn mò yǐ qīng tiáo. huò hán wán yǐ huǎn huà. bìng zài xià zhě yí dà. jù fú yú shí qián. huò fú hòu yǐ shí yā. huò tāng yào yǐ dùn fú. tūn bǔ jì yú zǎo yú wèi yǔ zhī qián. fú jí yào dāng tuō yī lín shuì zhī jì. fán yòng gān cǎo zhě. jiē zhū yào dú. qǔ qí gān yǐ huǎn pí. jì tóu shēng jiāng zhě. xíng zhū yào lì. qǔ xīn yǐ kāi wèi.

Everything between heaven and earth can serve as drug! In ancient times, Shennong pitied the illnesses and the suffering of the people, and he investigated the finest subtleties in the principles of things. The way how he put his mind into action may be considered as [an example of] humaneness. Hence, [his] *Ben cao* contains many drugs, but their flavors do not exceed [the number] five; they include sweet, acrid, salty, bitter, and sour. And their [different] natures do not exceed [the number] six, [namely] warming, cooling, supplementing, draining, ascending, and descending. Also, sweet, acrid, warming, supplementing, and ascending are yang [qualities]; bitter, salty, cooling, draining, and descending are yin [qualities]. What is weak in flavor drains and belongs to the yang. Sour is a yang nature but a yin flavor. That is to say, among the drugs are those that are pure yang, and others that are pure yin. There is also yang in yin, and yin in yang. In some cases, one makes special use of the [thermo-]qi of a [drug]; in other cases, one employs solely their flavor. In general, [drugs with] a strongly developed flavor will fill, while those with a pronounced [thermo-]qi will descend [in the body]. What is bland in flavor drains; what is light in nature ascends. [One makes use of] ascending [drugs] to treat diseases in the upper and in the external [sections of the body, and one makes use of drugs] descending [in the body] to treat diseases in the lower and in the internal [sections of the body]. All cold and cooling [drugs are used to] cure blood heat; all warm and heating [drugs are used to] treat qi obstructions and qi depletions. [One employs drugs that] moisten in order to moisten dryness, [and one employs drugs that are] astringent in order to gather what is going asunder. Also, sweet [flavor] is the source of all supplementation; bitter [flavor] is the basis of all draining. Acrid and aromatic are both [qualities indicating an] ascending and draining [nature]; sour and salty are both [qualities indicating a] supplementing and descending [nature]. As for supplementation, both nature and flavor [of a drug] may be suited to supplement and as far as draining is concerned, both [nature and flavor of a drug] may be suited to drain. However, an [ability to] supplement may also contain [an ability] to drain, and [an ability to] drain may also contain [an ability] to supplement. For instance, sourness enters the liver; it generates liquids in order to check dryness. Extreme bitterness enters the heart; it nourishes the yin [qi] in order to push down fire. Acrid [drugs] are able to warm the lung and push back cold; salty [drugs] are able to harden the kidneys and to oppress heat. If one wishes to expel evil [qi] from a specific [depot], it is important to let its regular [qi] recover. By draining yang [qi] one may supplement yin [qi], just as by draining yin [qi] one may supplement yang [qi. That is, one] makes use of [the fact that when yin qi] descend, [yang qi will] ascend by themselves, [and that when yang qi] ascend, [yin qi will] descend by themselves. Now, there are [different] diseases that emerge jointly. [In such cases] one must combine [different therapeutic] patterns. Hence, there are prescriptions [made up from] uneven or even [numbers of drugs], and among the drugs one distinguishes between rulers and ministers. Those [prescriptions] that are designed as powders, they disperse, and those that are prepared as ingots, they settle.[1] An application of hot liquids means agitation; one takes [advantage here of] the ripples [of liquids carrying the drugs' thermo-]qi and flavors in order to reach each and every [section of the body]. An application of pills [results in] slow [effects]; the slow penetration [of the body] by [thermo-]qi and flavor [if released from pills] is used here to reach [the most] distant locations. In hot liquids one may employ fresh or processed [substances]. Fresh [substances] are suitable for drainage; processed [substances] are suitable for supplementation. There are large and small pills. When a disease is located in the upper part [of the body], small [pills] are suitable. One should always take [such pills] after the meals. In some cases, one [crushes these pills with one's teeth into] powders, in this way regulating [a health problem by means of] light [drugs].[2] Or one keeps these pills in one's mouth [for an extended period] so that they dissolve only slowly. When a disease is located in the lower part [of the body], large [pills] are suitable. One should always take [such pills] before the meals. In some cases, after one has taken [such large pills] they are pressed [downward in the body] by one's meal. In some cases, drugs prepared as decoction are taken together [with a meal]. Prescriptions formulated to supplement are to be swallowed early in the morning before one has said a word; and drugs that [are supposed to] act quickly should be taken when one has undressed and goes to sleep. *Gan cao* is always employed to dissolve all possible poisonous [effects of] drugs; its sweetness is used here to slow down the [functions of the] spleen. Fresh ginger is added to prescriptions in order to pass the forces of all kinds of drugs [through the body]; its acrid [flavor] is used here to open the stomach.

Notes

[1] These statements are based on a word-play that is difficult to reproduce in an English translation. *Săn* 散 refers to both "powder" and "disperse" in Chinese. *Dìng* 錠, usually translated as "crisp cake" or "ingot" in a pharmaceutical context, has also the meaning of "anchor"; hence, such preparations serve to "settle" something that is unsteady. Further below, *tāng* 湯, "decoction", is equated with *dàng* 蕩, "agitated", "ripples"; *wán* 丸, "pills", is equated with the similarly sounding *huăn* 緩, "slow".

[2] Light-weight drugs are supposed to move upwards in the body, from the stomach, and to show their effects in the upper parts of the body.

8.b *Zhāng shì yī tōng* 9 張氏醫通
Yào gǔ 藥蠱
Drug Poisoning

近世豐裕之家。略有小病。即從事於醫藥。元氣堅固者。無論治之中窾與否。但得開通病氣。元神自復。若禀質素弱。及病後產後。亡血脫瀉之後。不能即愈。日以湯藥爲務。多致輕者重而重者劇。病氣日增。飲食日減。以致寒熱咳嗽。吐痰吐血。諸證百出。而猶以爲藥力未逮。邪熱未除。日以清火消痰爲務。遂成藥蠱之病矣。夫人之胃氣。全賴水穀滋養。胃氣旺。則諸病不生。縱有賊邪侵犯。氣復自已。原無急於調治也。嘗見世人不得盡其天年者。大都皆醫藥之誤耳。今既病之胃。轉爲藥力所侵。不至四大分崩不已。末流之挽。雖日事參。苓。芪。術。如以漏器承漿。漫無盈滿之期。况堪克任偏勝性味乎。凡虛羸之疾。治之不能即應。當暫爲休息。以俟胃氣之復。不特藥蠱爲然也。其藥蠱之患有三。一者胃氣爲藥所汩。飲食不爲肌膚。而骨不支床。一者藥毒流於坎陷。少火不能內藏。而煩蒸髓極。一者脾傷不能收精。藏氣固結不舒而羸瘦腹大。雖有脾胃之分。所重全在胃氣。胃爲五臟之本也。此惟膏粱豢養者有之。在藜藿勞勩之人。未之見也。其治藥蠱之病。當屏絕一切苦寒降泄。辛熱升發。氣味濃烈之藥。祗宜小劑參。耆。甘溫養胃之品。

近世	jìn shì	in recent times
豐裕	fēng yù	rich; wealthy
略	lüè	a little; minor
從事	cóng shì	to deal with
醫藥	yī yào	medication
無論	wú lùn	no matter; regardless of
中窾	zhòng kuǎn	to hit the mark
通	tōng	passage
稟質	bǐng zhì	natural disposition
亡	wáng	to lose
脫瀉	tuō xiè	loss (of qi) through drainage; diarrhea
務	wù	obligation; [to consider] necessary
日	rì	day by day; each day
吐	tù	to spit
逮	dǎi	to reach; to be sufficient
消	xiāo	to disperse
藥蠱	yào gǔ	drug poisoning
旺	wàng	to prosper; to be present in abundance
縱	zòng	even if
侵	qīn	to intrude
原	yuán	originally; basically
急	jí	to hurry
嘗	cháng	indication of past tense
大都	dà dū	for the most part
誤	wù	to commit a mistake
轉	zhuǎn	in turn; in addition; on top of
四大	sì dà	the four elements (constituting the body)

分崩	fēn bēng	to fall apart; to disintegrate
末流	mò liú	mediocre [physicians]
挽	wǎn	to save; to rescue
事	shì	to employ; to resort to
參	shēn	the pharmaceutical drug *rénshēn* 人參, i.e. ginseng, prepared from Panax Ginseng C.A. Meyer
苓	líng	the pharmaceutical drug *fúlíng* 茯苓, prepared from Poria cocos Wolf
耆	qí	the pharmaceutical drug *huángqí* 黃耆, prepared from Astragalus membranaceus Fisch. and others
术	zhú	the pharmaceutical drug *báizhú* 白术, prepared from Atractylodes macrocephala Koidzumi
漏器	lòu qì	a funnel
承	chéng	to contain; to collect
漿	jiāng	broth; liquid
漫	màn	to overflow; everywhere
盈	yíng	full; overflowing
堪克	kān kè	able for
勝	shèng	superior
偏勝	piān shèng	to be unilaterally dominant
性	xìng	thermo-quality of a pharmaceutical drug
羸	léi	emaciated
暫	zàn	for a time
特	tè	alone; only
汩	gǔ	to throw into disorder
支	zhī	to prop up
床	chuáng	a frame
坎陷	kǎn xiàn	the "cave at the bottom" (where all the liquids gather); identified here as a designation of the kidneys
少火	shào huǒ	the small fire (supposedly burning in the kidneys and being responsible for the maintenance of all physiological processes)

煩	fán	uneasiness; vexation
蒸髓	zhēng suǐ	(heat) steaming from the marrow (of one's bones). Equivalent to 骨蒸 *gǔ zhēng* in 9.b
舒	shū	to expand; to dissipate
豢養	huàn yǎng	to nourish
勞勩	láo yì	to toil
屏絕	píng jué	to put aside; to do away with
發	fā	to stimulate (heat or perspiration)
濃	nóng	viscous; strong
烈	liè	violent; fierce
祗	zhǐ	only
劑	jì	a dose (of drugs)
品	pǐn	a substance

Jìn shì fēng yù zhī jiā. lüè yǒu xiǎo bìng. jí cóng shì yú yī yào. yuán qì jiān gù zhě. wú lùn zhì zhī zhòng kuǎn yǔ foǔ. dàn dé kāi tōng bìng qì. yuán shén zì fù. ruò bǐng zhì sù ruò. jí bìng hòu chǎn hòu. wáng xuě tuō xiè zhī hòu. bù néng jí yù. rì yǐ tāng yào wéi wù. duō zhì qīng zhě zhòng ér zhòng zhě jù. bìng qì rì zēng. yǐn shí rì jiǎn. yǐ zhì hán rè ké sòu. tù tán tù xiě. zhū zhèng bǎi chū. ér yóu yǐ wéi yào lì wèi dǎi. xié rè wèi chú. rì yǐ qīng huǒ xiāo tán wéi wù. suí chéng yào gǔ zhī bìng yǐ. fū rén zhī wèi qì. quán lài shuǐ gǔ zī yǎng. wèi qì wàng. zé zhū bìng bù shēng. zòng yǒu zèi xié qīn fàn. qì fù zì yǐ. yuán wú jí yú tiáo zhì yě. cháng jiàn shì rén bù dé jìn qí tiān nián zhě. dà dū jiē yī yào zhī wù ěr. jīn jì bìng zhī wèi. zhuǎn wéi yào lì suǒ qīn. bù zhì sì dà fēn bēng bù yǐ. mò liú zhī wǎn. suī rì shì shēn. líng. qí. shù. rú yǐ lòu qì chéng jiāng. màn wú yíng mǎn zhī qí. kuàng kān kè rèn piān shèng xìng wèi hū. fán xū léi zhī jí. zhì zhī bù néng jí yìng. dāng zàn wéi xiū xí. yǐ sì wèi qì zhī fù. bù tè yào gǔ wéi rán yě. qí yào gǔ zhī huàn yǒu sān. yī zhě wèi qì wéi yào suǒ mì. yǐn shí bù wéi jī fū. ér gǔ bù zhī chuáng. yī zhě yào dú liú yú kǎn xiàn. shào huǒ bù néng nèi cáng. ér fán zhēng suǐ jí. yī zhě pí shāng bù néng shōu jīng. zàng qì gù jié bù shū ér léi shòu fù dà. suī yǒu pí wèi zhī fēn. suǒ zhòng quán zài wèi qì. wèi wéi wǔ zàng zhī běn yě. cǐ wéi gāo liáng huàn yǎng zhě yǒu zhī. zài lí huò láo yì zhī rén. wèi zhī jiàn yě. qí zhì yào gǔ zhī bìng. dāng píng jué yí qiè kǔ hán jiàng xiè. xīn rè shēng fā. qì wèi nóng liè zhī yào. zhǐ yí xiǎo jì shēn. qí. gān wēn yǎng wèi zhī pǐn.

In recent times, rich families, when they suffer from only a minor illness, they deal with it by means of medication. [If the patient's] original qi are firm and strong, it does not really matter whether the treatment hits the mark or not; all that is needed is to open a passage for the qi causing the illness [to leave the body], and the original spirit will recover by itself. If, however, [the patient] basically has a weak constitution, he is unable to recover by himself after an illness, after delivery, after a loss of blood, or [after] some diarrhea. If it is considered necessary [in such a situation that he] takes decoctions and [other] drugs day by day, this will often cause minor [ailments] to become serious [diseases], and serious [diseases] to turn into critical [problems]. The illness qi will increase each day, and one's intake of beverages and food will decrease each day, until all kinds of symptoms appear, such as [fits of] cold and heat, coughing, spitting of phlegm, and spitting of blood. And yet, [the people] assume that the strength of the drugs was insufficient, and that the evil heat has not yet been eliminated. Day after day they consider it necessary to [apply drugs that] cool the fire and disperse the phlegm, and as a result the disease of drug poisoning emerges. Man's stomach qi depend entirely upon nourishment by [the intake of] water and grain. As long as there is an abundance of stomach qi, no illness whatsoever will emerge. Even if a robber evil were able to intrude and attack, the [regular] qi would recover by themselves, and basically there would be no [need to] hurry and start a harmonizing treatment. I have observed, though, that most of the people who do not reach the age allotted to them by heaven, [succumb because of] the mistaken application of medication. Now, if a stomach that is sick already, on top of this is invaded by the force of drugs, a complete disintegration of the four elements [constituting the body][1] will be unavoidable. Even if a mediocre [physician attempting] to save [a patient] were to resort to [drugs as] *shen*, *ling*, *qi*, and *zhu* day after day, there would be no difference [between such activities and the attempt] to use a funnel in order to collect a liquid – it would never be filled! And how should [the stomach, in such a situation,] be able to endure [the impact of drugs with] unilaterally dominant thermo- and flavor qualities? All attempts to treat patients suffering from depletion or emaciation [with drugs] will remain without response; all that is necessary is to [let the patient] rest for a while until the stomach qi have recovered. This does not only apply to drug poisoning. There are three [possibilities how one may come to] suffer from drug poisoning. First, the stomach qi are thrown into disorder by drugs, and [, as a result,] food and beverages will no longer be transformed into flesh and skin, and the bones will no longer be the [firm] framework propping up [the body]. Second, the poison inherent in [some] drugs flows into the kidneys. [As a result, the water stored in the kidneys dries up, and] the small fire [that burns in the kidneys] can no longer be kept inside [the kidneys. The patient] has an extreme [feeling of] uneasiness because the marrow [of his bones] is steamed [by the fire].

Third, the spleen is harmed and can no longer receive the essence [qi of food and beverages; as a result], the qi in the depots will form firm clottings, unable to dissipate again. [That, in turn, leads to] emaciation and abdominal swelling. Although one distinguishes between stomach and spleen [in these processes], the qi of the stomach are the most important [factor involved]. The stomach is the basis of the five depots! This [problem of drug poisoning] occurs only among the wealthy;[2] I have not observed it among the poor and toiling people yet. To treat this disease of drug poisoning, one must do away with all bitter, cold, descending, draining, acrid, hot, ascending, and stimulating drugs, as well as with those that have strong and violent [thermo-]qi and flavors. Only small doses of substances that warm and nourish the stomach, such as *shen* and *qi*, are appropriate.

Notes

[1] This is a reference to the Buddhist/Indian notion holding soil, water, fire, and wind as constituting the human body.

[2] Literally: those nourished with fat meat and fine millet.

8.c *Xīn xiū běn cǎo* 1 新修本草 Shén-nóng běn cǎo jīng神農本草經 Excerpt From General Introduction Based on the Text of the *Shen nong ben cao jing* of the First Century

上藥一百二十種爲君。主養命以應天。無毒。多服久服不傷人。欲輕身益氣。不老延年者。本上經。中藥一百二十種爲臣。主養性以應人。無毒。有毒。斟酌其宜。欲遏病補虛羸者。本中經。下藥一百二十五種爲佐使。主治病以應地。多毒。不可久服。欲除寒熱邪氣。破積聚。愈疾者。本下經。三品合三百六十五種。法三百六十五度。一度應一日。以成一歲。藥有君臣佐使。以相宣攝。合和宜用一君。二臣。三佐。五使。又可一君。三臣。九佐使也。藥有陰陽配合。子母兄弟。根葉華實。草石骨肉。有單行者。有相須者。有相使者。有相畏者。有相惡者。有相反者。有相殺者。凡此七情。合和當視之。相須相使者良。勿用相惡相反者。若有毒宜制。可用相畏相殺。不爾。勿合用也。凡欲治病。先察其源。先候病機。五臟未虛。六腑未竭。血脈未亂。精神未散。食藥必活。若病已成。可得半愈。病勢已過。命將難全。若毒藥治病。先起如黍粟。病去即止。不去倍之。不去十之。取去爲度。治寒以熱藥。治熱以寒藥。飲食不消。以吐下藥。鬼疰蠱毒以毒藥。癰腫瘡瘤以瘡藥。風濕以風藥。各隨其所宜。

輕身	qīng shēn	to take the material weight from the body
延年	yán nián	to prolong the years of life
斟酌	zhēn zhuó	to consider
遏	è	to check; to prevent
佐	zuǒ	assistant (drugs in a prescription)
使	shǐ	aide (drugs in a prescription)
度	dù	degree
宣	xuān	to spread
合和	hé hé	to combine (drugs in a) balanced (prescription)
配合	pèi hé	to join (drugs) together (in a prescription)
兄弟	xiōng dì	elder brother and younger brother
華	huá	flowers
單行	dān xíng	(drugs which prefer) to act alone
相須	xiāng xū	(drugs which) depend on each other (in their effects)
相使	xiāng shǐ	(drugs which) reinforce each other (in their effects)
相畏	xiāng wèi	(drugs which) fear each other (i.e. suppress each other's effects)
相惡	xiāng wù	(drugs which) hate each other (i.e.; depotentiate each other)
相反	xiāng fǎn	(drugs which) are opposed to each other (in their effects)
相殺	xiāng shā	(drugs which) kill each other's (effects)
七情	qī qíng	seven natures (of behavior shown by drugs in their interactions)

不爾	bù ěr	otherwise; if not so
病機	bìng jī	the trigger of a disease; the movement of a disease (through the body); pathomechanism
食	shí	to eat; to take in
黍粟	shǔ sù	millet
倍	bèi	to double
十	shí	to increase tenfold
度	dù	to measure; standard
消	xiāo	to digest
吐藥	tù yào	drugs causing vomiting; emetics
下藥	xià yào	drugs causing defecation; laxatives/purgatives
蠱毒	gǔ dú	the poison of *gu*
瘤	liú	tumor

Shàng yào yì bǎi èr shí zhǒng wéi jūn. zhǔ yǎng mìng yǐ yìng tiān. wú dú. duō fú jiǔ fú bù shāng rén. yù qīng shēn yì qì. bù lǎo yán nián zhě. běn shàng jīng. zhōng yào yì bǎi èr shí zhǒng wéi chén. zhǔ yǎng xìng yǐ yìng rén. wú dú. yǒu dú. zhēn zhuó qí yí. yù è bìng bǔ xū léi zhě. běn zhōng jīng. xià yào yì bǎi èr shí wǔ zhǒng wéi zuǒ shǐ. zhǔ zhì bìng yǐ yìng dì. duō dú. bù kě jiǔ fú. yù chú hán rè xié qì. pò jī jù. yù jí zhě. běn xià jīng. sān pǐn hé sān bǎi liù shí wǔ zhǒng. fǎ sān bǎi liù shí wǔ dù. yí dù yìng yí rì. yǐ chéng yí suì. yào yǒu jūn chén zuǒ shǐ. yǐ xiāng xuān shè. hé hé yí yòng yì jūn. èr chén. sān zuǒ. wǔ shǐ. yòu kě yì jūn. sān chén. jiǔ zuǒ shǐ yě. yào yǒu yīn yáng pèi hé. zǐ mǔ xiōng dì. gēn yè huá shí. cǎo shí gǔ ròu. yǒu dān xíng zhě. yǒu xiāng xū zhě. yǒu xiāng shǐ zhě. yǒu xiāng wèi zhě. yǒu xiāng wù zhě. yǒu xiāng fǎn zhě. yǒu xiāng shā zhě. fán cǐ qī qíng. hé hé dāng shì zhī. xiāng xū xiāng shǐ zhě liáng. wù yòng xiāng wù xiāng fǎn zhě. ruò yǒu dú yí zhì. kě yòng xiāng wèi xiāng shā. bù ěr. wù hé yòng yě. fán yù zhì bìng. xiān chá qí yuán. xiān hòu bìng jī. wǔ zàng wèi xū. liù fǔ wèi jiē. xuě mài wèi luàn. jīng shén wèi sàn. shí yào bì huó. ruò bìng yǐ chéng. kě dé bàn yù. bìng shì yǐ guò. mìng jiāng nán quán. ruò dú yào zhì bìng. xiān qǐ rú shǔ sù. bìng qù jí zhǐ. bù qù bèi zhī. bù qù shí zhī. qǔ qù wéi dù. zhì hán yǐ rè yào. zhì rè yǐ hán yào. yǐn shí bù xiāo. yǐ tù xià yào. guǐ zhù gǔ dú yǐ dú yào. yōng zhǒng chuāng liú yǐ chuāng yào. fēng shī yǐ fēng yào. gè suí qí suǒ yí.

The upper [rank of] drugs comprises 120 kinds [of substances]. They are the rulers. They govern the nourishment of life and correspond to heaven. They are not toxic. To consume a lot [of these substances] or consume [them] over an extended period of time is not harmful to Man. If one wishes to take the material weight from the body, to supplement the qi, and to prolong the years of life without aging, one should base [one's efforts] on [drugs listed in] the upper [section of this] classic. The middle [rank of] drugs comprises 120 kinds [of substances]. They are the ministers. They govern the nourishment of one's nature and correspond to Man. Some of them are toxic, others not. [For every application,] the choice of a suitable [substance] should be considered carefully. If one wishes to prevent illness and to supplement depletions and emaciations, one should base [one's efforts] on [substances listed in] the middle [section of this] classic. The lower [rank of] drugs comprises 125 kinds [of substances]. They are the assistants and aides.[1] They master the treatment of illnesses and correspond to earth. They are toxic and must not be taken over a long period of time. If one wishes to remove cold, heat, and [other] evil qi [from the body], to break accumulations, and to cure illnesses, one should base [one's efforts] on [substances listed in] the lower [section of this] classic. The three ranks together are composed of 365 kinds [of substances. This corresponds to] the pattern of 365 degrees. One degree corresponds to one day. Together that makes one year. Among the drugs are rulers, ministers, assistants, and aides. They assist each other in spreading [their effects]. In combinations one should use one ruler [drug], two minister [drugs], three assistant [drugs], and five aides [drugs], or one may [use] one ruler [drug], three minister [drugs], and nine assistant and aides [drugs. In prescriptions,] drugs are matched in accordance with their yin and yang [categorization].There are mother/child and older/younger brother [relationships]. There are also root, stalk, blossom, and fruit drugs, as well as herbal, mineral, bone, and flesh drugs. There are those [drugs which prefer to] act alone, others whose [effects] depend [on one or more other drugs]. There are those which reinforce each other [in their effects], and those which fear each other. Some [drugs] hate each other, and others are directly opposed to each other [in their effects. Finally, there are drugs] which kill each other. All these seven natures must be observed when combining [drugs]. The application of [drugs] which depend upon and reinforce each other is fine. One should by no means use those which directly oppose or hate each other. If there are toxic [drugs in a prescription], it is advisable to restrain them. [For this purpose one] can use [drugs which] fear or kill each other. Otherwise [such substances] should not be used together. Whenever one intends to treat an illness, one [should] first examine the origin and investigate the movement of the disease. As long as the five depots are not yet depleted, as long as the six palaces are not yet exhausted, as long as the [movements in the] blood vessels are not yet disturbed, and as long as one's essence and spirit are not yet dispersed, the intake of drugs will keep [the patient] alive! If the disease has become manifest already, a cure can be affected in half [of all cases]. If the strength of the disease has progressed too far, it will be difficult to restore [the patient's existence]. In treating illnesses with toxic drugs, one should first start with [a dosage of the size of] a millet [seed]. As soon as the illness has been eliminated one stops [the administration of the drugs]. If [the illness] persists, the [amount of the dosage should] be doubled. If the [illness continues even then, the dosage should] be increased ten times. One should take the elimination [of an illness] as a stardard [for the dosage. Illnesses due to the intrusion of] cold should be treated with drugs of a hot [qi. Illnesses due to the intrusion of] heat should be treated with drugs of a cold [qi]. If food and beverages are not digested, emetics and laxatives should be used. Against demonic possessions and the poison of *gu*[2], poisonous drugs should be used. For welling abscesses, swelling, sores, and tumors, sore drugs should be taken. [Illnesses caused by the intrusion of] wind and dampness should be treated with wind drugs. In each case, one should follow a suitable course.

Notes

[1] In the hierarchy of *jūn* 君, *chén* 臣, *zuǒ* 佐, *shǐ* 使 drugs, the terms *zuǒ* 佐 and *shǐ* 使 refer to subordinate officials. It was only beginning with the Song-Jin-Yuan era that the term *shǐ* 使 was understood as referring to "messenger" drugs in the sense of fulfilling a function of conducting the effects of other drugs to a desired destination. To point out this historical development, *shǐ* 使 is rendered here, in a Han text, as "aide", and in 8.d, a text of the Song-Jin-Yuan tradition, as "messenger". One might even speculate that the term *shǐ* 使 was added to the Han text only later, and that the original hierarchy comprised only *jūn* 君, *chén* 臣, and *zuǒ* 佐.

[2] *Gǔ dú* 蠱毒 is a term of demonologic origin (see 4.c) and refers – among other conditions – to abdominal bloating. *Gǔ dú* 蠱毒 may therefore occasionally be interpreted as "toxic bloating" but should be rendered as "poison of *gǔ* 蠱" in an explicitly demonologic context as indicated here by the preceding term "demonic possession."

8.d *Tāng yè běn cǎo* 1 湯液本草 Zhì fāng zhī fǎ 制方之法 Patterns in the Formulation of Prescriptions

夫藥有寒熱溫涼之性。酸苦辛鹹甘淡之味。各有所能。不可不通也。藥之氣味。不比同時之物。味皆鹹。其氣皆寒之類是也。凡同氣之物必有諸味。同味之物必有諸氣。互相氣味。各有厚薄。性用不等。製其方者。必且明其爲用。經曰。味爲陰。味厚爲純陰。味薄爲陰中之陽。氣爲陽。氣厚爲純陽。氣薄爲陽中之陰。然味厚則泄。薄則通。氣薄則發泄。厚則發熱。又曰。辛甘發散爲陽。酸苦涌泄爲陰。鹹味涌泄爲陰。淡味滲泄爲陽。凡此之味。各有所能。然辛能散結潤燥。苦能燥濕堅軟。鹹能軟堅。酸能收緩收散。甘能緩急。淡能利竅。故經曰。肝苦急。急食甘以緩之。心苦緩。急食酸以收之。脾苦濕。急食苦以燥之。肺苦氣上逆。急食苦以泄之。腎苦燥。急食辛以潤之。開腠理。致津液。通其氣也。肝欲散。急食辛以散之。心欲軟。急食鹹以軟之。脾欲緩。急食甘以緩之。肺欲收。急食酸以收之。腎欲堅。急食苦以堅之。凡此者。是明其氣味之用也。若用其味。必明其氣之可否。用其氣。必明其味之所宜。識其病之標本。臟腑。寒熱。虛實。微甚。緩急。而用其藥之氣味。隨其證而製其方也。是故方有君臣佐使。輕重緩急。大小。反正逆從之制也。主治病者爲君。佐君者爲臣。應臣者爲使。用此隨病之所宜。

比	bǐ	to compare
互相	hù xiāng	vice versa
等	děng	equal
用	yòng	usage
爲用	wéi yòng	function
發泄	fā xiè	to stimulate discharge
發熱	fā rè	to stimulate heat
湧泄	yǒng xiè	discharging through gushing forth (i.e. vomiting)
滲泄	shèn xiè	discharging through leakage (i.e. perspiration)
軟	ruǎn	soft; to soften
收	shōu	to pull together (what is relaxed)
反	fǎn	short for 反治 *fǎn zhì*: a treatment in contrast to (what one should expect; i.e. a treatment which disregards misleading symptoms and is directed against the true nature of an illness)
正	zhèng	short for 正治 *zhèng zhì*: regular treatment (i.e. a treatment directed against the nature of a disease as it is apparent from its symptoms)
逆從	nì cóng	(therapies relying on drugs with a nature) opposite to or identical with (the nature of a patient's symptoms)
制	zhì	laws; regulations
使	shǐ	messenger (drug in a prescription)

Fū yào yǒu hán rè wēn liáng zhī xìng. suān kǔ xīn xián gān dàn zhī wèi. gè yǒu suǒ néng. bù kě bù tōng yě. yào zhī qì wèi. bù bǐ tóng shí zhī wù. wèi jiē xián. qí qì jiē hán zhī lèi shī yě. fán tóng qì zhī wù bì yǒu zhū wèi. tóng wèi zhī wù bì yǒu zhū qì. hù xiāng qì wèi. gè yǒu hòu bó. xìng yòng bù děng. zhì qí fāng zhě. bì qiě míng qí wéi yòng. jīng yuē. wèi wéi yīn. wèi hòu wéi chún yīn. wèi bó wéi yīn zhōng zhī yáng. qì wéi yáng. qì hòu wéi chún yáng. qì bó wéi yáng zhōng zhī yīn. rán wèi hòu zé xiè. bó zé tōng. qì bó zé fā xiè. hòu zé fā rè. yòu yuē. xīn gān fā sàn wéi yáng. suān kǔ yǒng xiè wéi yīn. xián wèi yǒng xiè wéi yīn. dàn wèi shèn xiè wéi yáng. fán cǐ zhī wèi. gè yǒu suǒ néng. rán xīn néng sàn jié rùn zào. kǔ néng zào shī jiān ruǎn. xián néng ruǎn jiān. suān néng shōu huǎn shōu sàn. gān néng huǎn jí. dàn néng lì qiào. gù jīng yuē. gān kǔ jí. jí shí gān yǐ huǎn zhī. xīn kǔ huǎn. jí shí suān yǐ shōu zhī. pí kǔ shī. jí shí kǔ yǐ zào zhī. fèi kǔ qì shàng nì. jí shí kǔ yǐ xiè zhī. shèn kǔ zào. jí shí xīn yǐ rùn zhī. kāi còu lǐ. zhì jīn yè. tōng qí qì yě. gān yù sàn. jí shí xīn yǐ sàn zhī. xīn yù ruǎn. jí shí xián yǐ ruǎn zhī. pí yù huǎn. jí shí gān yǐ huǎn zhī. fèi yù shōu. jí shí suān yǐ shōu zhī. shèn yù jiān. jí shí kǔ yǐ jiān zhī. fán cǐ zhě. shī míng qí qì wèi zhī yòng yě. ruò yòng qí wèi. bì míng qí qì zhī kě foǔ. yòng qí qì. bì míng qí wèi zhī suǒ yí. shí qí bìng zhī biāo běn. zàng fǔ. hán rè. xū shí. wēi shèn. huǎn jí. ér yòng qí yào zhī qì wèi. suí qí zhèng ér zhì qí fāng yě. shī gù fāng yǒu jūn chén zuǒ shǐ. qīng zhòng huǎn jí. dà xiǎo. fǎn zhèng nì cóng zhī zhì yě. zhǔ zhì bìng zhě wéi jūn. zuǒ jūn zhě wéi chén. yìng chén zhě wéi shǐ. yòng cǐ suí bìng zhī suǒ yí.

Drugs may have a cold, hot, warm, or cool nature, and they may have a sour, bitter, acrid, salty, sweet, or bland flavor. Each of these [qi and flavors] has its specific [therapeutic] ability, and it is imperative to know all [of them]. The qi and the flavors of the drugs are not like items that appear as identical [pairings] all the times, such as that all [drugs with a] salty flavor always have a cold qi. Substances with identical qi may have all [possible] flavors, and substances with identical flavor may have all [possible] qi. Qi and flavor may all be strongly or weakly developed, and vice versa, and their nature and usage differ accordingly. To prepare a prescription, one must understand in addition [to the drugs' qi and flavors] their functions. The Classic states: "The flavor is yin; if it is strongly developed it is pure yin; a flavor that is weak is yang in yin. The qi is yang; if it is strongly developed it is pure yang; a qi that is weak is yin in yang. This being so, if the flavor [of a drug] is strong, it will drain; if it is weak, it will penetrate. If the qi [of a drug] is weak, it will stimulate discharge; if it is strong, it will stimulate heat."[1] [The Classic] states further: "Acrid and sweet stimulate dispersion and are yang. Sour and bitter [cause] discharge that gushes forth and are yin. A salty flavor [causes] discharge that gushes forth and is yin; a bland flavor discharges through leakage and is yang."[2] All these flavors have their specific [therapeutic] abilities. This being so, acrid is able to disperse clottings and to moisten dryness. Bitter is able to dry out dampness and to harden what is soft. Salty is able to soften what is hard. Sour is able to pull together what is relaxed, and to pull together what is dispersed. Sweet is able to relax what is tense. Bland [flavor] is able to clear the passage through the orifices. Hence, the Classic states: "If the liver suffers from tension, quickly eat [something] sweet to relax these [tensions]. If the heart suffers from relaxation, quickly eat [something] sour to pull together [what is relaxed]. If the spleen suffers from dampness, quickly eat [something] bitter to dry this [dampness]. If the lung suffers from an upward movement of the qi, contrary [to their proper direction], quickly eat [something] bitter to drain these [qi]. If the kidneys suffer from dryness, quickly eat [something] acrid to moisten them. [The purpose is always] to open the skin structures, to cause the [body's] liquids to move, and to have the [body's] qi penetrate [all of its sections]. If the liver longs for dispersion, one should quickly eat [something] acrid to disperse there. If the heart longs for softening, one should quickly eat [something] salty to soften there. If the spleen longs for relaxation, one should quickly eat [something] sweet to cause relaxation there. If the lung longs for [something] pulling [things] together, one should quickly eat [something] sour to pull together. If the kidneys long for hardening, one should quickly eat [something] bitter to harden there."[3] All such [therapies] reflect an understanding of the [correct] use of qi and flavor. If one makes use of a specific flavor, he should know whether the qi of that [particular drug] is appropriate or not; and if one makes use of a specific qi, he should know whether the flavor of that [particular drug] fits [into the treatment or not]. In using the qi and flavors of specific drugs, one should know a disease's secondary location and its starting point, whether the depots and palaces have been affected by cold or heat, by depletion or repletion, whether [the disease] is minor or serious, and whether it moves slowly or quickly [in the body]; one formulates the prescription for a [disease] in accordance with its symptoms. For this reason, the structure of prescriptions follows [the hierarchy of] ruler, ministers, assistants, and messengers,[4] [and includes] light or heavy, slowly or quickly acting [drugs. Prescriptions may be] large or small,[5] [and a treatment may be] in contrast to [what one should expect from the nature of a patient's symptoms,[6] or it may be] regular.[7] [That is to say, the drugs employed may have a nature] opposite to or identical with [the nature of a patient's patho-conditions].[8] "Those [drugs] that master the treatment of a disease are the rulers; those that assist the rulers are the ministers; and those that respond to [the orders of] the ministers are the messengers."[9] One employs all of them in accordance with the requirements of the diseases.

Notes

[1] Quoted from *Huang Di Nei jing*, *Su wen*, treatise 5, Yin yang ying xiang da lun 陰陽影象大論. Wording not identical with *textus receptus*.

[2] Quoted from *Su wen*, treatise 74, Zhi zhen yao da lun 至真要大論.

[3] Quoted from *Su wen*, treatise 22, Cang qi fa shi lun 藏氣法時論.

[4] 使*shǐ* drugs were redefined, by authors of the Song-Jin-Yuan period (13th – 15th c.), as substances able to carry the effects of other drugs to a desired location in the body. The *Tang ye ben cao* is based on the theories of the Song-Jin-Yuan era marking the application of doctrines of systematic correspondences, expressed in the *Huang Di Nei jing*, to the realm of pharmaceutics.

[5] *Su wen* treatise 74 has the following definition. "One ruler, two ministers represent a small structure (*xiao zhi* 小制); one ruler, three ministers, and five assistants represent a medium structure (*zhong zhi* 中制); one ruler, three ministers, and nine assistants represent a large structure (*da zhi* 大制).

[6] If a physician diagnoses, in a patient with fever, a disease related to cold, he will prescribe, "in contrast to" what the fever might suggest, drugs with a hot qi.

[7] In case of symptoms indicating heat, a regular treatment resorts to drugs whose qi is cold.

[8] *Su wen* treatise 74 states: 逆者政治從者反治. That is: "[a treatment] opposite to [the nature of a disease's symptoms] is a proper therapy; [a treatment] identical with [the nature of a disease's symptoms] is a therapy in contrast to [a proper treatment]. "

[9] Quoted from *Su wen* treatise 74. Wording not identical with *textus receptus*.

8.e *Xú líng tāi xiān sheng yī shū quán jí* 1/2 徐靈胎先生醫書全集 (Yī xué yuán liú lùn 醫學源流論) Zhì bìng bù bì fēn jīng luò zàng fǔ lùn 治病不必分經絡臟腑論 [Situations] where it is not Necessary to Distinguish between the [Main] Conduits and Network [Vessels], the Depots and the Palaces in the Treatment of Illness

---

治病之法多端。有必求經絡臟腑者。有不必求經絡臟腑者。蓋人之氣血。無所不通。而藥性之寒熱溫涼。有毒無毒。其性亦一定不移。入於人身。其功能亦無所不到。豈有其藥止入某經之理。即如參耆之類。無所不補。砒鴆之類。無所不毒。幷不耑於一處也。所以古人有現成通治之方。如紫金錠。至寶丹之類。所治之病甚多。皆有奇效。蓋通氣者。無氣不通。解毒者。無毒不解。消痰者。無痰不消。其中不過略有專宜耳。至張潔古輩。則每藥註定云獨入某經。皆屬附會之談。不足徵也。曰。然則用藥竟不必分經絡臟腑耶。曰。此不然也。蓋人之病。各有所見

之處。而藥之治病必有專長之功。如柴胡治寒熱往來。能愈少陽之病。桂枝治畏寒發熱。能愈太陽之病。葛根治肢體大熱。能愈陽明之病。蓋其止寒熱。已畏寒。除大熱。此乃柴胡。桂枝。葛根專長之事。因其能治何經之病。後人即指爲何經之藥。孰知其功能。實不僅入少陽。太陽。陽明也。顯然者尙如此。餘則更無影響矣。故以某藥爲能治某經之病則可。以某藥爲獨治某經則不可。謂某經之病。當用某藥則可。謂某藥不復入他經則不可。故不知經絡而用藥。其失也泛。必無捷效。執經絡而用藥。其失也泥。反能致害。總之變化不一。神而明之。存乎其人也。

求	qiú	to take into account
功能	gōng néng	effects
到	dào	to reach
砒	pī	arsenic
鴆	zhèn	the Zhen-bird
耑	zhuān	only; exclusively; identical with 專 *zhuān*
現成	xiàn chéng	ready-made (as of medications)
通治	tōng zhì	cure-all
紫金錠	zǐ jīn dìng	the "dark-red golden ingot", a formula recommended to cure all possible eye afflictions
丹	dān	a small ball (formed to contain all the ingredients of a prescription)
至寶丹	zhì bǎo dān	the "extremely precious balls"; a formula recommended to treat a great number of illnesses with sudden onset

張潔古	zhāng jié gǔ	Zhang Jiegu, style Yuansu 元素, 12th c., was one of the theoreticians of the Song-Jin-Yuan era contributing to the development of a pharmacology of systematic correspondence.
附會	fù huì	to add and to assemble; farfetched
談	tán	ta talk; rhetoric
徵	zhēng	evidence
竟	jìn	finally; in the end
專長	zhuān cháng	special expertise; special abilities
柴胡	chái hú	*chaihu*, a drug prepared from Bupleurum chinense DC, and other Bupleurum herbs
少陽	shào yáng	the minor-yang (conduit)
桂枝	guì zhī	*guizhi*, a drug prepared from Cinnamomum cassia Presl.
葛根	gé gēn	*gegen*, a drug prepared from Pueraria lobata (Willd.) Ohwi
何	hé	specific
孰	shú	who?
僅	jǐn	merely
顯	xiǎn	evident; obvious
餘	yú	the remaining
影響	yǐng xiǎng	effect; trace
泛	fàn	superficial; superficiality
捷效	jié xiào	to be successful
泥	ní	narrow-minded
變化	biàn huà	variations
存乎其人	cún hū qí rén	to be up to a suitable person

Zhì bìng zhī fǎ duō duān. yǒu bì qiú jīng luò zàng fǔ zhě. yǒu bù bì qiú jīng luò zàng fǔ zhě. gài rén zhī qì xuě. wú suǒ bù tōng. ér yào xìng zhī hán rè wēn liáng. yǒu dú wú dú. qí xìng yì yí dìng bù yí. rù yú rén shēn. qí gōng néng yì wú suǒ bù dào. qǐ yǒu qí yào zhǐ rù mǒu jīng zhī lǐ. jí rú shēn qí zhī lèi. wú suǒ bù bǔ. pī zhèn zhī lèi. wú suǒ bù dú. bìng bù zhuān yú yí chù yě. suǒ yǐ gǔ rén yǒu xiàn chéng tōng zhì zhī fāng. rú zǐ jīn dìng. zhì bǎo dān zhī lèi. suǒ zhì zhī bìng shèn duō. jiē yǒu qí xiào. gài tōng qì zhě. wú qì bù tōng. jiē dú zhě. wú dú bù jiě. xiāo tán zhě. wú tán bù xiāo. qí zhōng bù guò lüè yǒu zhuān yí ěr. zhì Zhāng jié gǔ bèi. zé měi yào zhù dìng yún dú rù mǒu jīng. jiē shǔ fù huì zhī tán. bù zú zhēng yě. yuē. rán zé yòng yào jìng bù bì fēn jīng luò zàng fǔ yé. yuē. cǐ bù rán yě. gài rén zhī bìng. gè yǒu suǒ jiàn zhī chù. ér yào zhī zhì bìng bì yǒu zhuān cháng zhī gōng. rú chái hú zhì hán rè wǎng lái. néng yù shào yáng zhī bìng. guì zhī zhì wèi hán fā rè. néng yù tài yáng zhī bìng. gé gēn zhì zhī tǐ dà rè. néng yù yáng míng zhī bìng. gài qí zhǐ hán rè. yǐ wèi hán. chú dà rè. cǐ nǎi chái hú. guì zhī. gé gēn zhuān cháng zhī shì. yīn qí néng zhì hé jīng zhī bìng. hòu rén jí zhǐ wéi hé jīng zhī yào. shú zhī qí gōng néng. shí bù jǐn rù shào yáng. tài yáng. yáng míng yě. xiǎn rán zhě shàng rú cǐ. yú zé gèng wú yǐng xiǎng yǐ. gù yǐ mǒu yào wéi néng zhì mǒu jīng zhī bìng zé kě. yǐ mǒu yào wéi dú zhì mǒu jīng zé bù kě. wèi mǒu jīng zhī bìng. dāng yòng mǒu yào zé kě. wèi mǒu yào bù fù rù tā jīng zé bù kě. gù bù zhī jīng luò ér yòng yào. qí shī yě fàn. bì wú jié xiào. zhí jīng luò ér yòng yào. qí shī yě ní. fǎn néng zhì hài. zǒng zhī biàn huà bù yī. shén ér míng zhī. cún hū qí rén yě.

The treatment of a disease may follow many principles. It may well be that one has to take the conduits and the network [vessels], as well as the depots and palaces, into account. But it may also be that one does not have to take the conduits and the network [vessels], as well as the depots and palaces, into account. Now, man's qi and his blood penetrate every [region of his body]; similarly, whether the nature of a drug is cold or hot, warm or cool, whether it is toxic or not, is firmly determined and does not change; also, if [a drug] enters the human body, its effects will reach every [section of it]. How could there be a principle that a particular drug enters one particular conduit? For example, [drugs] like *shen* and *qi* exert their [ability to] fill everywhere [in the body], and [drugs] like arsenic or the *zhen*[-bird] distribute their poison everywhere [in the body] – certainly not only at one single location! It is for this reason that the people of ancient times had ready-made cure-all prescriptions, such as the "dark-red golden ingot" or the "extremely valuable pills", [prescriptions] that cured very many diseases and that achieved miraculous successes. The fact is, [drugs] that cause qi to move, they cause qi everywhere to move. Poison-neutralizing drugs [are able to] neutralize all poisons, and phlegm-dispersing drugs [are able to] disperse all [types of] phlegm. And among them are only a small number that are appropriate [to treat only very] specific [problems]. But beginning with people like Zhang Jiegu, each drug was given a commentary specifying that it would enter a particular conduit only. That, however, is nothing but farfetched rhetoric, not supported by any sufficient evidence. [Now, someone might] say: If that is so, is it absolutely unnecessary to distinguish between conduits and network [vessels] and between depots and palaces in the application of drugs? [My] answer would be: That is not the case, because man's diseases all appear at specific locations [in the body], and drugs, when they are used in the treatment of a disease, do of course show effects that are based on their specific abilities. For instance, *chaihu* [is used to] treat alternative fits of cold and heat; it cures diseases of the minor yang [conduits]. *Guizhi* [is used to] treat aversions to cold and the development of heat; it cures diseases of the major yang [conduits]. *Gegen* [is used to] treat great heat in one's limbs and body; it cures diseases of the yang brilliance [conduits]. That is to say, the halting of fits of cold and heat, the ending of an aversion to cold, and the elimination of great heat, these are the workings of the specific abilities of *chaihu*, *guizhi*, and *gegen*. Because these [drugs] are able to cure diseases in specific conduits, the people in later times pointed them out as drugs of specific conduits. Who would know that the effects of those [drugs], in reality, do not enter merely into the minor yang, the major yang, or the yang brilliance [conduits respectively]? There are some [drugs whose effects are] quite obvious [so that one may assume] it were like this. But all the remaining leave even less traces [of their paths of action]. Hence, it is quite possible to assume that a particular drug is capable of treating a disease in a particular conduit. But it is not possible to take a particular drug and think it [can be used] solely to treat [diseases] in a particular conduit. To say, for [the treatment of] a disease in a particular conduit one must use a particular drug, is quite possible. But to say a particular drug does not enter into other conduits also, that is impossible. Hence, if someone does not know about the conduits and the network [vessels] and makes use of drugs, his mistake is in his superficiality; and [his treatment] will definitely fail to have any good results. [On the other hand, regarding those] who cling only to the conduits and network [vessels] in their use of drugs, their mistake lies in their narrow-mindedness. Contrary [to their intentions] they may even cause harm. To sum up, there are many variations [in the effects of drugs, and in the locations of their effects]. To [employ one's] spirit to reach an understanding of all of this, that is up to capable individuals.

8.f *Xú líng tāi xiān sheng yī shū quán jí* 3/8
徐靈胎先生醫書全集
(Shèn jí chú yán 愼疾芻言)
Yòng yào 用藥
The Use of Drugs

醫道起於神農之著本草。以一藥治一病。但一病有數證。後之聖人取藥之對證者。合幾味而成方。故治病必先有藥而後有方。方成之後。再審其配合之法。與古何方相似。則云以某方加減。幷非醫者先有一六味。八味。理中等湯橫於胸中。而硬派人服之也。至其辨證用藥之法。如有人風寒痰食合而成病。必審其風居幾分。寒居幾分。痰食居幾分。而藥則隨其邪之多寡以爲增減。或一方不能兼治。則先治其最急者。所以無一味虛設之藥。無一分不斟酌之分兩也。況醫之爲道。全在自考。如服我之藥而病情不減。或反增重。則必深自痛懲。廣求必效之法而後已。則學問自能日進。若不論何病。總以幾味溫補投之。愈則以爲己功。死則以爲病本不治。毫無轉計。此則誤盡天下而終身不自知也。又其所名陳方者。用柴胡一味即名柴胡湯。用大黃一味即名承氣湯。於古人制方之義。全然不知。隨其口之

所指而已。其醫也。則襲幾句陰陽虛實。五行生尅籠統套語。以爲用溫補之地。而文人學士又最易欺。見有陰陽五行等說。即以爲有本之學。深信不疑。其人亦自詡爲得醫學之捷徑。將千古聖人窮思極想所製對症之方數千首。皆不必問。而已稱名醫矣！

對	duì	to direct against; to confront
味	wèi	a (pharmaceutical) substance
理	lǐ	to regulate
橫	héng	to harbor; to carry
胸	xiōng	the mind[1]
硬	yìng	rigid
派	pài	to send; to order someone to do something
辨證	biàn zhèng	to distinguish among patho-conditions (in order to apply a differential treatment)
幾分	jǐ fēn	what percentage; how much of it
寡	guǎ	few
虛	xū	void (of meaning); meaningless
分兩	fēn liǎng	candareens and taels; quantities
考	kǎo	thoughtful attention
我	wǒ	I; myself
懲	chéng	to reprimand; to exhort
學問	xué wèn	scholarship
進	jìn	to advance
論	lùn	to take into consideration
毫	háo	an intensive; especially before negatives
轉	zhuǎn	to change basically
終身	zhōng shēn	an entire lifetime
陳方	chén fāng	age-old prescriptions
大黃	dà huáng	*dahuang*, a drug prepared from Rheum palmatum L. (and other Rheum plants)
制	zhì	to formulate (a prescription), identical with 製

然	rán	particle added to an adjective to indicate adverbial use
襲	xí	to appropriate; to clad oneself with
籠統	lóng tǒng	general
套語	tào yǔ	conventional phrases
地	dì	a field; an arena
文人學士	wén rén xué shì	literati and learned scholars
詡	xǔ	to brag; to boast
捷徑	jié jìng	a short-cut
千古	qiān gǔ	ancient times
將	jiāng	to take into one's hands; particle preceding an object
想	xiǎng	to think
窮思極想	qióng sī jí xiǎng	thorough considerations and farreaching thoughts
首	shǒu	numerary adjunct for prescriptions

Yī dào qǐ yú shén nóng zhī zhù běn cǎo. yǐ yí yào zhì yí bìng. dàn yí bìng yǒu shù zhèng. hòu zhī shèng rén qǔ yào zhī duì zhèng zhě. hé jǐ wèi ér chéng fāng. gù zhì bìng bì xiān yǒu yào ér hòu yǒu fāng. fāng chéng zhī hòu. zài shěn qí pèi hé zhī fǎ. yǔ gǔ hé fāng xiāng sì. zé yún yǐ mǒu fāng jiā jiǎn. bìng fēi yī zhě xiān yǒu yī liù wèi. bā wèi. lǐ zhōng děng tāng héng yú xiōng zhōng. ér yìng pài rén fú zhī yě. zhì qí biàn zhèng yòng yào zhī fǎ. rú yǒu rén fēng hán tán shí hé ér chéng bìng. bì shěn qí fēng jū jǐ fēn. hán jū jǐ fēn. tán shí jū jǐ fēn. ér yào zé suí qí xié zhī duō guǎ yǐ wéi zēng jiǎn. huò yì fāng bù néng jiān zhì. zé xiān zhì qí zuì jí zhě. suǒ yǐ wú yí wèi xū shè zhī yào. wú yì fēn bù zhēn zhuó zhī fēn liǎng yě. kuàng yī zhī wéi dào. quán zài zì kǎo. rú fú wǒ zhī yào ér bìng qíng bù jiǎn. huò fǎn zēng zhòng. zé bì shēn zì tòng chéng. guǎng qiú bì xiào zhī fāng ér hòu yǐ. zé xué wèn zì néng rì jìn. ruò bù lùn hé bìng. zǒng yǐ jǐ wèi wēn bǔ tóu zhī. yù zé yǐ wéi jǐ gōng. sǐ zé yǐ wéi bìng běn bù zhì. háo wú zhuǎn jì. cǐ zé wù jìn tiān xià ér zhōng shēn bù zì zhī yě. yòu qí suǒ míng chén fāng zhě. yòng chái hú yí wèi jí míng chái hú tāng. yòng dà huáng yí wèi jí míng chéng qì tāng. yú gǔ rén zhì fāng zhī yì. quán rán bù zhī. suí qí kǒu zhī suǒ zhì ér yǐ. qí yī yě. zé xí jǐ jù yīn yáng xū shí. wǔ xíng shēng kè lóng tǒng tào yǔ. yǐ wéi yòng wēn bǔ zhī dì. ér wén rén xué shì yòu zuì yì qī. jiàn yǒu yīn yáng wǔ xíng děng shuō. jí yǐ wéi yǒu běn zhī xué. shēn xìn bù yí. qí rén yì zì xǔ wéi dé yī xué zhī jié jìng. jiāng qiān gǔ shèng rén qióng sī jí xiǎng suǒ zhì duì zhèng zhī fāng shù qiān shǒu. jiē bù bì wèn. ér jǐ chēng míng yī yǐ！

The doctrine of medicine emerged when Shennong wrote his *Ben cao*. [In his time,] one took one drug to treat one disease. But one disease may be associated with a number of patho-conditions. Hence, the Sages of later times selected from the drugs those which were opposed to the patho-conditions, and they combined several substances to form a prescription. To treat a disease, one should, therefore, have [an idea of which] drugs [to employ against the individual patho-conditions associated with this disease], and then one should have [an idea about how to combine these drugs to form a suitable] prescription. Once one has formed a prescription, one should investigate to which prescription of ancient times [one's own] pattern of the combination [of drugs] is similar. Then one may tell [the patient] one is going to use a particular prescription [of antiquity whose original ingredients, however,] should be expanded or diminished [in accordance with the requirements of his specific disease]. It would certainly be inappropriate for physicians to have, for example, one single "Center-Rectifying Decoction", made up from six or eight substances, in mind[1] and to rigidly ask the people to consume this [remedy]. As for the method to base an application of drugs on a differentiation of patho-conditions, for example, if there is a person in whom wind, cold, phlegm, and food have come together and generated a disease, one must find out how much [of the disease] is due to wind, how much is due to cold, and how much is due to phlegm and food. Then one increases or decreases the [proportions of the respective] drugs [in an ancient prescription] in accordance with the [respective] amounts of evil [qi present in the patient's body]. There are cases in which one single prescription cannot [be employed to] treat all [the patho-conditions of a disease] at the same time. In such situations one treats first the most urgent [aspect of the patient's illness]. Thus, there should be no medication that includes even a single substance arranged without meaning, and there should be no [advice on] quantities including a single weight that has not been considered carefully. Furthermore, the [perfect] practice of medicine depends entirely on one's own thoughtful attention. If someone takes my drugs, and the condition of his illness does not improve, or, on the contrary, increases in severity, that must cause deep pain in myself, and I shall feel exhorted to search for a truly effective [therapeutic] pattern everywhere until finally [the disease] is cured. As a result, [my] scholarship will advance by itself each day. If [a physician] does not care which disease [is involved], and always offers [the patients] only a few substances with a warming and supplementing [effect], he will consider a successful cure to be his personal achievement, and he will believe that a disease was basically incurable if [the patient] dies. [Hence,] he will not at all [feel motivated to introduce any] fundamental changes in his [therapeutic] scheme. His mistakes will fill the entire world, but he himself will remain unaware of this for his entire life. Also, as far as the so-called "age-old prescriptions" are concerned, if one takes just the one substance *chaihu* and calls this a "decoction with *chaihu*", or if one takes but the one substance *dahuang* and calls this a "decoction to contain qi",[2] [one demonstrates that] one has absolutely no understanding of the meaning behind the formulation of prescriptions by the people in ancient times. [Persons acting like this] follow but some oral instructions and nothing else. They clad their medical practice in a few general conventional phrases, such as depletion and repletion of yin or yang, or [mutual] generation and destruction of the five agents, and they assume that [medicine] is an arena to employ [nothing but] warming and supplementing [drugs]. The literati and learned scholars will be cheated most easily [by such an approach], because when they see that someone talks about yinyang and the five agents, they believe this to be a well-founded learning. Their confidence is deep, and they harbor no doubts. Such persons [as described above] will even boast themselves to have found a short-cut through the study of medicine. Although they do not take into consideration any of the many thousands of prescriptions formulated on the basis of comprehensive thoughts by the Sages of the remote past to confront the patho-conditions, they nevertheless call themselves "renowned physicians".

Notes

[1] A literal rendering of *xiōng* 胸 is "breast", "bosom". From the latter comes the meaning "mind".
[2] The technical meaning of *chéng qì* 承氣 is "to purge".

Lesson Nine

Drug Monographs

The mythical emperor Yandi 炎帝, also named Shennong 神農, is credited with the gift of materia medica to mankind, but the historical beginnings of specialized pharmaceutical, i.e. *ben cao* 本草, literature in China date back to the first century CE. Pharmaceutical literature is distinguished from prescription literature in that the former focusses on data on individual substances, i.e. their qualities, their effects, and their origins and modes of preparation. Until the sixteenth century, when the impressive *Ben cao gang mu* was compiled, Chinese materia medica and, hence, the literature conveying pharmaceutical knowledge, were expanded continuously. A steady flow of encyclopedic *ben cao* works gathered (occasionally, since 657 CE, on government initiative) all the available knowledge on drugs in China herself, but also from remote regions and overseas. These works provided information on names and the appearance of drugs (supplemented, beginning with the seventh century at the latest, by illustrations), on their flavor and their degree of effectiveness, on their indications, contraindications, and compatibilities, and other data as well. In addition, specialized *ben cao* works were published, focussing on one drug only or on drugs from specific regions, on drugs to be used under specific circumstances (such as in times of famine or to deal with the illnesses resulting from the luxuries at the court). Following the impact of Song Neo-Confucianism on medicine, the theories of yinyang and the five agents found their way into drug monographs, but pragmatic descriptions persisted as well.

Key Terms Introduced in Lesson Nine

聰耳	cōng ěr	to sharpen one's hearing
悸	jì	palpitations
發熱	fā rè	to develop heat (as a body); fits of heat; fever
瘟疫	wēn yì	warmth epidemics
噦	yuè	to belch; to vomit

淋瀝	lín lì	strangurious drip
紛紜	fēn yún	perturbation
離魂	lí hún	departure of one's *hun*(-soul)
慢	màn	slow; chronic
痘科	dòu kē	the branch of medicine concerned with pox
外科	wài kē	the branch of medicine concerned with external illnesses, including impact and other traumatic injuries, surgery, bone-setting, and skin diseases
陰毒	yīn dú	poisoning by (the presence of purely) yin (qi and the absence of yang qi)
煎	jiān	to decoct
進	jìn	to give (a drug to a patient)
痧	shā	illness with sand(-like skin eruptions)
瘢	bān	illness with streak(-like rashes)
鉛	qiān	lead (metal); grey
焙	bèi	to dry over a fire in a pan
金瘡	jīn chuāng	wounds caused by metal weapons; sword wounds
寸白蟲	cùn bái chóng	tape worm
蕎麥	qiáo mài	buckwheat
卵	luǎn	testicles
癇	xián	convulsions
癲疾	diān jí	the falling sickness
奔豚	bēn tún	running piglet (syndrom)
癃	lóng	blockages (in the path of urine and other body liquids)
攣縮	luán suō	bent and shrunk; cramps
痔	zhì	hemorrhoids
伏熱	fú rè	deep-lying heat
敗瘡	bài chuāng	badly (healing) wounds
肚	dù	the stomach; the entrails
利	lì	dysentery
骨蒸	gǔ zhēng	bone-steaming

霍	huò	violent (intestinal disturbance); short for 霍亂 *huò luàn* (often interpreted now as cholera)
脚氣	jiăo qì	(evil) qi (which have moved down into the) legs.
赤白	chì bái	red and white (colored stools)
腦	năo	the brain
少陰	shào yīn	the minor-yin (conduit)
淚	lèi	tears
豉	chǐ	salted beans
努肉	nŭ ròu	flesh(-like) growths (in one's eyes). Also written: 胬肉
平	píng	balanced (thermo-qualities of pharmaceutical drugs)
點	diăn	eye-drops; to drop (a liquid into the eyes)
月經	yuè jīng	a (woman's) monthly period
尸疰	shī zhù	corpse possession, i.e. possession by the *hun*-soul of an alien corpse
石蛔	shí huí	stone(-like) roundworms
疣	yóu	swelling
拭	shì	to wipe (the eyes)
爛	làn	brightness (of eyes)
盜汗	dào hàn	robber sweat; night sweat
瘥	chài	to recover; to get well
煮	zhŭ	to boil; to decoct
血室	xuĕ shì	the blood-chamber (of women; i.e. the womb)
胎前	tāi qián	pregnancy
五疳	wŭ gān	the five types of *gan*-illness
癉瘧	dăn nüè	the solitary (heat-)malaria
癰疽	yōng jū	welling and deep-seated abscesses
瘡瘍	chuāng yáng	open sores
五癆	wŭ láo	the five types of consumption
厥陰	jué yīn	the ceasing-yin (conduits)
錫	xī	tin
糊	hú	paste

鉛丹	qiān dān	Lead Balls (i.e. minium; lead tetroxide)
黃丹	huáng dān	Yellow Balls (i.e. minium; lead tetroxide)
硫黃	liú huáng	sulphur
雌黃	cí huáng	auripigment
螫	zhē	poison; poisonous
三蟲	sān chóng	the three worms (which inhabit the human body and may cause illness)
墮胎	duò tāi	to cause an abortion
食復	shí fù	recurrence (of an illness) due to (inappropriate) eating
勞復	láo fù	recurrence (of an illness) due to (physical) taxation
疥癬	jiè xuǎn	itching skin diseases, consisting of either eruptive, scattered, small patches (疥 *jiè*), or noneruptive, large patches (癬 *xuǎn*)
狐臭	hú xiù	fox odor (from under the arm-pits)
尸蟲	shī chóng	corpse worms (i.e. the three worms inhabiting the human body)

9.a *Běn cǎo cóng xīn* 本草從新
(Cǎo bù 草部)
Rén shēn 人參
Ginseng

【人參】甘溫微苦。大補肺中元氣。瀉火除煩。生津止渴。開心益智。聰耳明目。安精神。定魂魄。止驚悸。通血脈。破堅積。消痰水。氣壯而胃自開。氣和而食自化。治虛勞內傷。發熱自汗。虛咳喘促。心腹寒痛。傷寒瘟疫。嘔噦反胃。痎瘧瀉痢。淋瀝脹滿。多夢紛紜。離魂異疾。妊娠吐水。胎產諸虛。小兒慢驚。痘科險證。外科陰毒。因虛失血。氣虛甚者。濃煎獨參湯進之。挾寒者。稍加附子。按人參功能在諸藥之上。但閉氣。肺有火熱及肺氣不利者忌之。實表。表有邪者忌之。凡痧痘癍毒。欲出未出。但悶熱而不見點。若誤用之。以阻截其路。爲禍尤烈。產遼東寧古臺出者。光紅結實。船廠出者。空鬆鉛塞。幷有糙有熟。宜隔紙焙用。忌鐵。不宜見風日。茯苓爲使。畏五靈脂。惡皂角。黑大豆。紫石英。人溲。反藜蘆。

【參條】乃橫生蘆頭上者。其力甚薄。止可用以調理常病。及生津止渴。其性橫行手臂。凡指臂無力者。服之甚效。

【參鬚】亦橫生蘆頭上而更細者。其性與參條同。而力尤薄。要知參條參鬚。不過得參之餘氣。危險之證。斷難倚仗。

人參	rén shēn	*renshen*, ginseng; a drug prepared from Panax ginseng C.A. Meyer
智	zhì	wisdom; knowledge
聰耳	cōng ěr	to sharpen one's hearing
定	dìng	to fix; to keep in a position
悸	jì	palpitations
通	tōng	to make passable
發熱	fā rè	to develop heat (as a body); fits of heat; fever
瘟疫	wēn yì	warmth epidemics
噦	yuè	to belch
淋瀝	lín lì	strangurious drip
夢	mèng	dream
紛紜	fēn yún	perturbation
離魂	lí hún	departure of one's *hun*(-soul)
異	yì	strange
妊娠	rèn shèn	pregnant
慢	màn	slow; chronic
痘科	dòu kē	the branch of medicine concerned with pox
險	xiǎn	dangerous
外科	wài kē	the branch of medicine concerned with external illnesses, including impact and other traumatic injuries, surgery, bone-setting, and skin diseases
陰毒	yīn dú	poisoning by (the presence of purely) yin (qi and the absence of yang qi)
煎	jiān	to decoct
進	jìn	to give (a drug to a patient)

挾	xié	to carry; to include
附子	fù zǐ	*fuzi*, a drug prepared from Aconitum carmichaeli Debx.
按	àn	to examine; introductory particle to a commentary
痧	shā	illness with sand(-like skin eruptions)
瘢	bān	illness with streak(-like rashes)
點	diǎn	a dot
阻截	zǔ jié	to obstruct
遼東	liáo dōng	Liaodong, name of a region; Manchuria
寧古臺	níng gǔ tái	Ninggutai, a place-name
光	guāng	bare; shiny
結實	jié shí	firm
船廠	chuán chǎng	Chuanchang, a place-name
空鬆	kōng sōng	hollow and loose; soft
鉛	qiān	lead (metal); grey
塞	sè	speckled
糙	cāo	coarse; raw
隔	gé	to separate; to wrap
紙	zhǐ	paper
焙	bèi	to dry over a fire in a pan
茯苓	fù líng	*fuling*, a drug prepared from Poria cocos (Schw.) Wolf
五靈脂	wǔ líng zhī	*wulingzhi*, a drug prepared from the droppings of Trogopterus xanthipes Milne-Edwards
皂角	zào jiǎo	*zaojiao*, a drug prepared from Gleditsia sinensis Lam.
紫石英	zǐ shí yīng	*zishiying*, a mineral drug; fluorite
藜蘆	lí lú	*lilu*, a drug prepared from Veratrum nigrum L.
橫	héng	sideways; to all sides; laterally
蘆頭	lú tóu	the stalk on top (of the ginseng root)
鬚	xū	whiskers
危險	wēi xiǎn	dangerous
倚仗	yǐ zhàng	to rely on; to trust

【Rén shēn】 gān wēn wēi kǔ. dà bǔ fèi zhōng yuán qì. xiè huǒ chú fán. shēng jīn zhǐ kě. kāi xīn yì zhì. cōng ěr míng mù. ān jīng shén. dìng hún pò. zhǐ jìng jì. tōng xuě mài. pò jiān jī. xiāo tán shuǐ. qì zhuàng ér wèi zì kāi. qì hé ér shí zì huà. zhì xū láo nèi shāng. fā rè zì hàn. xū ké chuǎn cù. xīn fù hán tòng. shāng hán wēn yì. ǒu yuè fān wèi. jiē nüè xiè lì. lín lì zhàng mǎn. duō mèng fēn yún. lí hún yì jí. rèn shèn tù shuǐ. tāi chǎn zhū xū. xiǎo ér màn jìng. dòu kē xiǎn zhèng. wài kē yīn dú. yīn xū shī xuě. qì xū shèn zhě. nóng jiān dú shēn tāng jìn zhī. xié hán zhě. shāo jiā fù zǐ. àn rén shēn gōng néng zài zhū yào zhī shàng. dàn bì qì. fèi yǒu huǒ rè jí fèi qì bù lì zhě jì zhī. shí biǎo. biǎo yǒu xié zhě jì zhī. fán shā dòu bān dú. yù chū wèi chū. dàn mènrè ér bù xiàn diǎn. ruò wù yòng zhī. yǐ zǔ jié qí lù. wéi huò yóu liè. chǎn liáo dōng níng gǔ tái chū zhě. guāng hóng jié shí. chuán chǎng chū zhě. kōng sōng qiān sāi. bìng yǒu cāo yǒu shú. yí gé zhǐ bèi yòng. jì tiě. bù yí jiàn fēng rì. fù líng wéi shǐ. wèi wǔ líng zhī. wù zào jiǎo. hēi dà dòu. zǐ shí yīng. rén sōu. fǎn lí lú.

【shēn tiáo】 nǎi héng shēng lú tóu shàng zhě. qí lì shèn bó. zhǐ kě yòng yǐ tiáo lǐ cháng bìng. jí shēng jīn zhǐ kě. qí xìng héng xíng shǒu bì. fán zhǐ bì wú lì zhě. fú zhī shèn xiào.

【shēn xū】 yì héng shēng lú tóu shàng ér gèng xì zhě. qí xìng yǔ shēn tiáo tóng. ér lì yóu bó. yào zhī shēn tiáo shēn xū. bù guò dé shēn zhī yú qì. wēi xiǎn zhī zhèng. duàn nán yǐ zhàng.

Renshen: sweet, warm, slightly bitter. It has a great [ability to] supplement the original qi in the lung. It drains fire and eliminates [heat causing, in the chest, a feeling of] uneasiness. It generates [body] liquids and quenches thirst. It opens one's mind and improves one's wisdom. It sharpens one's hearing and brightens the eyes. It calms down one's spirit, and fixes *hun* and *po*. It ends fright and palpitations. It makes the blood-vesels passable, and breaks through hardenings and accumulations. It disperses phlegm and water. When [a person's] qi is strengthened [by *renshen*, his] the stomach will open. When [a person's] qi is harmonized [by *renshen*, his] food will be transformed. It cures depletions and taxation, internal damage, fits of heat, spontaneous sweating, depletion and coughing, hasty panting, cold and pain in one's heart and abdomen, harm caused by cold, warmth epidemics, vomiting and belching due to one's stomach's turning back [the food it receives], *jie* and malaria, diarrhea and stranguríous drip, swelling and fullness, frequent dreams and perturbation, departure of one's *hun* and [further] strange illnesses, vomiting of water during pregnancy, all types of depletions after delivery, chronic fright in children, dangerous symptoms related to pox, poisoning by [the presence of purely] yin [qi – a problem belonging to] the branch of external [medicine], and loss of blood following depletion. In cases of extreme depletion of one's qi, one prepares a strong decoction of nothing but [*ren*]*shen*, and gives it [to the patient]. If [additional] cold is involved, add a little *fuzi*.

In my opinion, the effects of *renshen* are superior to all other drugs. However, in case of a closure of one's qi, if there is fire in the lung with heat, and if the qi in the lung have lost their free passage, one must not take this [drug]. It replenishes the external [sections of the body]. If evil [qi have settled] in the external [sections of the body], one must not take this [drug]. In all cases where the poison causing a disease with sand[-like skin eruptions,] pox, or a disease with streak[-like rashes] is about to break out but has not yet broken out, where [patients experience a] pressing sensation in the chest and heat, but where no dots have appeared yet, if this [drug] is used erroneously, it will block the way of these [poisons to leave the body], and cause greatest misery. [Specimens] originating from Ninggutai in Liaodong are shiny red and firm. Those originating from Chuanchang are soft, grey, and speckled. Both have those that are raw, and those that have been processed [when they reach the market. Before] using [this drug] one must wrap it in paper and dry it over fire in a pan. [Contact with] iron must be avoided. [*Renshen*] should not see wind or the sun. *Fuling* acts as its messenger. [*Renshen*] fears *wulingzhi*; it hates *zaojiao*, large black beans, *zishiying*, and human urine. It is directly opposed to *lilu*.

[*Ren*] *shen* twigs: These grow sideways from the stalk on top [of the *renshen* root]. Their strength is extremely weak. They can be used only to achieve some harmonizing and regulating effects in cases of common illnesses. Also, they generate [body] liquid and quench thirst. Because their nature is directed laterally, they move into hands and arms. Whenever one's fingers and arms are weak, the intake of these [twigs] will show great results.

[*Ren*]*shen* whiskers: They, too, grow sideways from the stalk on top [of the *renshen* root] but they are much finer. Their nature is identical with that of the [*ren*]*shen* twigs, and their strength is even weaker. One should know that [*ren*]*shen* twigs and [*ren*]*shen* whiskers contain only surplus qi of [*ren*]*shen*. In cases of dangerous patho-conditions, it would be very difficult to rely on [their use].

9.b *Shí wù běn cǎo yuē yán* 4
食物本草約言
(Shòu bù liù 獸部六)
Zhū ròu 猪肉
Pork

猪肉。味苦。微寒。主閉血脈。弱筋骨。發痰。令人少子。食之暴肥。以其風虛故也。瘧病金瘡勿食。不可同牛肉食。生寸白蟲。同蕎麥食。患熱風。脫鬚眉。豚卵。味甘。溫。無毒。主驚癇癲疾。鬼疰蠱毒。除寒熱奔豚。五癃邪氣攣縮。懸蹄。主五痔。伏熱在腸。腸癰內蝕。四足。主傷撻諸敗瘡。下乳汁。心。主驚邪憂恚。血不足。補虛劣。多食耗心氣。不可同茱萸食。肚。微溫。補中益氣。止渴利。主骨蒸熱勞。殺勞蟲。補羸。助血脈。止痢。四季宜食。肺。微寒。能補肺。不可同白華菜食。令滯氣。發霍。肝。溫。主脚氣。冷洩赤白臟虛。不可同魚子食。腎。冷。和理腎氣。通利膀胱。補虛勞。消積滯。冬不可食。損真氣。發虛擁。脾。主脾胃虛熱。舌。健脾。補不足。令人能食。頭。補虛乏。去驚癇五痔。煮極熟食之。腦。不可食。鬐脂。主生髮。脂膏。主惡瘡。利血脈。解風熱。

皮膚風。潤肺。解斑猫。芫青毒。臘月者。殺蟲。忌食烏梅。皮。味甘。寒。猪。水畜。其氣先入腎。解少陰客熱。加白蜜食。潤燥除煩。加米粉。益氣斷痢。腸臟。主下焦虛竭。大小腸風熱。宜食之。

猪	zhū	a hog
肉	ròu	meat
虛	xū	to loosen
金瘡	jīn chuāng	wounds caused by metal weapons; sword wounds
牛肉	niú ròu	beef
寸白蟲	cùn bái chóng	tape worm
蕎麥	qiáo mài	buckwheat
豚	tún	a sucking pig; piglet
卵	luǎn	testicles
癎	xián	convulsions
癲疾	diān jí	the falling sickness
奔豚	bēn tún	running piglet (syndrom)
癃	lóng	protuberance ill; blockages (in the path of urine and other body liquids)
五癃	wǔ lóng	the five protuberance ills; the five blockages (in the paths of liquids through the body)
攣縮	luán suō	bent and shrunk; cramps
懸蹄	xuán tí	the (rear) suspended toes (of artiodactyles)
痔	zhì	piles
伏熱	fú rè	deep-lying heat
蝕	shí	to “eat-away”
撻	tà	to flog
敗瘡	bài chuāng	badly (healing) wounds
乳汁	rǔ zhī	(human) milk sap
劣	liè	want of strength; weakness

茱萸	zhū yú	*zhuyu*, a drug prepared from Evodia rutaecarpa (Juss.) Benth.
肚	dù	the stomach; the entrails
利	lì	dysentery
骨蒸	gŭ zhēng	bone-steaming
勞	láo	wasting
季	jì	a season
白華菜	bái huá cài	*baihuacai*, a drug prepared from Cleome gynandra L.
霍	huò	violent (intestinal disturbance); short for 霍亂 *huò luàn* (often interpreted now as cholera)
脚氣	jiăo qì	(evil) qi (which have moved down into the) legs. This term is used in modern medicine to refer to the disease of beri-beri. In Chinese traditional medicine, the term included a wide range of different syndromes.
洩	xiè	to leak
赤白	chì bái	red and white (colored stools)
魚子	yú zĭ	fish roe
擁	yōng	to block; to obstruct
健	jiàn	to strengthen
腦	năo	the brain
鬐	qí	a mane
脂	zhī	lard
斑猫	bān māo	*banmao*, a drug prepared from Mylabris phalerata Pall., and M. Cichorii L.; the cantharides flies
芫青	yuán qīng	*yuanqing*, a drug prepared from the beetle Lytta caraganae Pallas
臘月	là yuè	the twelfth lunar month
烏梅	wū méi	black plums
畜	chù	domestic animal
少陰	shào yīn	the minor-yin (conduit)
蜜	mì	honey
米粉	mĭ fĕn	rice flour

Zhū ròu. wèi kǔ. wēi hán. zhǔ bì xuě mài. ruò jīn gǔ. fā tán. lìng rén shǎo zǐ. shí zhī bào féi. yǐ qí fēng xū gù yě. nüè bìng jīn chuāng wù shí. bù kě tóng niú ròu shí. shēng cùn bái chóng. tóng qiáo mài shí. huàn rè fēng. tuō xū méi. tún luǎn. wèi gān. wēn. wú dú. zhǔ jìng xián diān jí. guǐ zhù gǔ dú. chú hán rè bēn tún. wǔ lóng xié qì luán suō. xuán tí. zhǔ wǔ zhì. fú rè zài cháng. cháng yōng nèi shí. sì zú. zhǔ shāng tà zhū bài chuāng. xià rǔ zhī. xīn. zhǔ jìng xié yōu huì. xuě bù zú. bǔ xū liè. duō shí hào xīn qì. bù kě tóng zhū yú shí. dù. wēi wēn. bǔ zhōng yì qì. zhǐ kě lì. zhǔ gǔ zhēng rè láo. shā láo chóng. bǔ léi. zhù xuě mài. zhǐ lì. sì jì yí shí. fèi. wēi hán. néng bǔ fèi. bù kě tóng bái huá cài shí. lìng zhì qì. fā huò. gān. wēn. zhǔ jiǎo qì. lěng xiè chì bái zàng xū. bù kě tóng yú zǐ shí. shèn. lěng. hé lǐ shèn qì. tōng lì páng guāng. bǔ xū láo. xiāo jī zhì. dōng bù kě shí. sǔn zhēn qì. fā xū yōng. pí. zhǔ pí wèi xū rè. shé. jiàn pí. bǔ bù zú. lìng rén néng shí. tóu. bǔ xū fá. qù jìng xián wǔ zhì. zhǔ jí shú shí zhī. nǎo. bù kě shí. qí zhī. zhǔ shēng fà. zhī gāo. zhǔ è chuāng. lì xuě mài. jiě fēng rè. pí fū fēng. rùn fèi. jiě bān māo. yuán qīng dú. là yuè zhě. shā chóng. jì shí wū méi. pí. wèi gān. hán. zhū. shuǐ chù. qí qì xiān rù shèn. jiě shào yīn kè rè. jiā bái mì shí. rùn zào chú fán. jiā mǐ fěn. yì qì duàn lì. cháng zàng. zhǔ xià jiāo xū jiē. dà xiǎo cháng fēng rè . yí shí zhī.

Pork. Flavor: bitter. [Thermoquality:] slightly cold. It masters closed blood-vessels and weak sinews and bones. It stimulates [the production of] phlegm, and decreases human fertility. [Regular] consumption [of pork] as food lets one become fat within a short period of time because [pork brings] wind [into the body, and] loosens [one's flesh]. Anybody suffering from malaria or from wounds resulting from metal [weapons] should not eat [pork]. It must not be consumed together with beef, [lest] tape-worms emerge. If one eats [pork] together with buckwheat, one will suffer from heat and wind, and his eyebrows will fall out.
Piglet testicles: Flavor: sweet. [Thermoquality:] warm. No toxicity. They master convulsions due to fright, the falling sickness, demonic possession, and the *gu*-poison. They eliminate cold and heat, the running piglet [syndrome],[1] the five protuberance ills, evil qi, and cramps.
Suspended toes: They master the five [types of] piles, deep-lying heat in the intestines, and intestinal abscesses slowly devouring [the body] internally.
The four legs: they master injuries caused by flogging, and all badly [healing] wounds. They drive down the milk-sap.
The heart: It masters fright-evil, mourning and rage, and insufficient blood; it supplements depletions and strengthens [in cases of] weakness. If one consumes large amounts of [hogs' hearts], this will diminish the qi of one's [own]

heart. It must not be eaten together with *zhuyu*.

[Hog] stomach: [Thermoquality:] slightly warm. It supplements the center and supports one's qi. It quenches thirst and ends dysentery. It masters wasting resulting from bone-steaming and heat. It kills the worms [causing] wasting. It supplements emaciation, supports the blood-vessels, and stops dysentery. One may eat it during all four seasons.

[Hog] lung: [Thermoquality:] slightly cold. It is able to supplement lung [qi]. It must not be eaten together with *baihuacai*. That would cause qi stagnation, and would stimulate [intestinal] disturbance.

[Hog] liver: [Thermoquality:] warm. It masters [evil] qi [that have moved down into the] legs, cold leakage [of urine], red and white [colored stools], and depletion in one's depots. It must not be consumed together with fish-roe.

[Hog] kidneys: [Thermoquality:] cold. They harmonize and regulate one's kidney qi, and they open the passage through the bladder. They supplement depletions and taxations, and they disperse accumulations and stagnations. [Hog kidneys] must not be eaten during winter; they would injure one's true qi, and stimulate obstructions coupled with depletion.

[Hog] spleen: It masters depletion and heat in one's spleen and stomach.

[Hog] tongue: It fortifies the spleen, and supplements insufficiencies. It gives man [hunger so that] he can eat.

[Hog] head: It supplements depletions and deficiencies, and eliminates convulsions resulting from fright, as well as the five [types of] piles. One should boil [a hog's head] until it is well done before eating it. [Hog] brain cannot be consumed.

[Hog] fat from a [hog's] mane masters the growth of hair.

Lard paste: It masters bad sores, and opens the passage through the blood-vessels. It dissolves wind-heat, as well as wind in the skin, and it moistens the lung. It dissolves the poison of cantharides and of the *yuanqing* [beetle]. During the twelfth month it kills worms. It must not be consumed [together with] black plums.

[Hog] skin: Flavor: sweet; [thermoquality:] cold. Hog is a domestic animal [associated with the agent] water. Its qi first enter the kidneys, and they dissolve heat that has settled in the minor-yin [conduits]. If one consumes it with white honey added to it, it will moisten dryness and it will eliminate uneasiness. If one adds rice-flour to it, it nourishes one's qi, and interrupts dysentery.

[Hog] intestines: They master depletion and exhaustion in the lower [section of the triple] burner. In case of heat caused by wind in the large and small intestines it is appropriate to consume them.

Notes

[1] The term "running piglet" refers to one of the "five accumulations". It is an accumulation that forms in the kidneys and gives rise to the *bēn tún* ("running piglet") qi, causing a sensation of upward shooting movement in the thorax, heart, and throat. *Bēn tún* qi is often abbreviated as *bēn tún*.

[2] The associations between the five domesticated animals serving as nourishment and the five agents are as follows: chicken/fowls – wood; sheep/goats – fire; oxes – soil; dogs – metal; pigs – water.

9.c *Chóng xiū zhèng hé jīng shǐ zhèng lèi bèi yòng běn cǎo* 15
重修政和經史證類備用本草
(Rén bù 人部)
Rén rǔ zhī 人乳汁
Human Milk-Sap

人乳汁。主補五藏。令人肥白悅澤。陶隱居云。張蒼常服人乳。故年百歲餘。肥白如瓠。唐本注云。別錄云。首生男乳。療目赤痛多泪。解獨肝牛肉毒。合豉濃汁服之。神效。又取和雀屎。去目赤努肉。**臣禹錫等謹按蜀本**云。人乳。味甘。平。無毒。日華子云。人乳。冷。益氣。治瘦悴。悅皮膚。潤毛髮。點眼止泪。并療赤目。使之明潤也。【聖惠方】治卒中風不語。舌根强硬。陳醬五合。三年者妙。人乳汁五合。二件相和研。以生布絞取汁。不計時候。少少與服。良久當語。千金方。治月經不通。飲人乳汁三合。金匱方。噉蛇牛肉殺人。何以知之。噉蛇者。毛髮向後順者是也。食之欲死。飲人乳汁一升立愈。衍義曰。人乳汁治目之功多。何也。人心生血。肝藏血。肝受血則能視。蓋水入於經。則其血乃成。又曰。上則爲乳汁。下則爲月水。故知乳汁則血也。用以點眼。豈有不相宜者。血爲陰。故其性冷。藏寒人。如乳餅酪之類。不可多食。雖曰牛羊乳。然亦不出乎陰陽造化爾。西戎更以駝馬乳爲酥酪。老人患口瘡不能食。飲人熱乳良。

澤	zé	smooth; slippery
陶隱居	táo yǐn jū	Tao Yinju, sobriquet of Táo Hóngjǐng 陶弘景 (412-536), Daoist and author of a materia medica
張蒼	zhāng cāng	Zhang Cang, statesman of the Qin-Han era; lived 256-152
瓠	hù	a gourd
唐本	táng běn	*Tang ben*, short title of *Táng xīn xiū běn cǎo* 唐新修本草, the "Newly Revised Edition of the *Materia Medica* of the Tang Dynasty", published in 659
別錄	bié lù	*Bie lu*, short title of *Míng yī bié lù* 名醫別錄, the "Additional Notes of Renowned Physicians", a book (or individual notes) added by Táo Hóngjǐng to the *Shen nong ben cao* in CE 500
首	shǒu	first
淚	lèi	tears
豉	chǐ	salted beans
神	shén	spirit(-like); miraculous
雀	què	small birds
屎	shǐ	excrement
努肉	nǔ ròu	flesh(-like) growths (in one's eyes). Also written: 胬肉
臣	chén	civil servant; imperial subject
禹錫	yǔ xī	Yuxi, personal name of Zhǎng Yǔxī 掌禹錫 (992-1068), civil servant and commentator of the *Shu materia medica*
蜀本	shǔ běn	*Shu ben*, short title of *Shǔ chóng guǎng yīng gōng běn cǎo* 蜀重廣英公本草, the "Shu Materia Medica" compiled between 934 and 965
平	píng	balanced (thermo-qualities of pharmaceutical drugs)

日華子	rì huá zǐ	Rihuazi, according to Li Shizhen the sobriquet of a man called Da Ming 大明, Tang dynasty author of the *Rìhuázǐ běn cǎo*日華子本草
悴	cuì	sad; distressed
點	diǎn	eye-drops; to drop (a liquid into the eyes)
聖惠方	shèng huì fāng	*Sheng hui fang*, short title of *Tài píng shèng huì fāng* 太平聖惠方, the "Prescriptions of the Grand Peace [Reign Period Compiled] under Imperial Auspices", a prescription collection of 992 CE
陳醬	chén jiàng	old bean sauce
合	gé	one tenth of a Chinese pint
件	jiàn	item; thing
研	yán	to rub; to grind (in a mortar)
布	bù	a piece of cloth
絞	jiǎo	to twist; to squeeze
良久	liáng jiǔ	quite a long time
千金方	qiān jīn fāng	*Qian jin fang*, short title of *Bèi jí qiān jīn fāng* 備急千金要方, the "Important Prescriptions Worth Thousands in Gold, Prepared for Use in Urgent Need" by Sūn Sīmiǎo 孫思邈 (581-682?)
月經	yuè jīng	a (woman's) monthly period
金匱方	jīnguì fāng	*Jin gui fang*, short title of *Jīn guì yù hán yào luè fāng lùn* 金匱玉函要略方論, the "Concise Discussion of Important Prescriptions from the Golden Coffer and Jade Sheath", by Zhāng Jī 張機 (142-220?)
噉	dàn	to eat; to bite
蛇	shé	snake
升	shēng	one Chinese pint (a measurement of changing quantities in the course of the dynasties)
立	lì	immediately

衍義	yán yì	*Yan yi*, short title of *Běn cǎo yán yì* 本草衍義, the "Expanded Interpretation of *Materia Medica*" by Kǒu Zōng-shì 寇宗 奭 of 1116
餅酪	bǐng lào	cheese
西戎	xī róng	the Xirong, Western tribes
駝	tuó	camel
酥酪	sū lào	curd

Rén rǔ zhī. zhǔ bǔ wǔ zàng. lìng rén féi bái yuè zé. táo yǐn jū yún. Zhāng cāng cháng fú rén rǔ. gù nián bǎi suì yú. féi bái rú hù. táng běn zhù yún. bié lù yún. shǒu shēng nán rǔ. liáo mù chì tòng duō lèi. jiě dú gān niú ròu dú. hé chǐ nóng zhī fú zhī. shén xiào. yòu qǔ hé què shǐ. qù mù chì nǔ ròu. **chén yǔ xī děng jǐn àn shǔ běn** yún. rén rǔ. wèi gān. píng. wú dú. rì huá zǐ yún. rén rǔ. lěng. yì qì. zhì shòu cuì. yuè pí fū. rùn máo fà. diǎn yǎn zhǐ lèi. bìng liáo chì mù. shǐ zhī míng rùn yě. 【shèng huì fāng】 zhì cù zhòng fēng bù yǔ. shé gēn qiáng yìng. chén jiàng wǔ hé. sān nián zhě miào. rén rǔ zhī wǔ hé. Èr jiàn xiāng hé yán. yī shēng bù jiǎo qǔ zhī. bù jì shí hòu. shǎo shǎo yǔ fú. liáng jiǔ dāng yǔ. qiān jīn fāng. zhì yuè jīng bù tōng. yǐn rén rǔ zhī sān hé. jīn kuì fāng. dàn shé niú ròu shā rén. hé yǐ zhī zhī. dàn shé zhě. máo fà xiàng hòu shùn zhě shī yě. shí zhī yù sǐ. yǐn rén rǔ zhī yì shēng lì yù. · yán yì yuē. rén rǔ zhī zhì mù zhī gōng duō. hé yě. rén xīn shēng xuě. gān zàng xuě. gān shòu xuě zé néng shì. gài shuǐ rù yú jīng. zé qí xuě nǎi chéng. yòu yuē. shàng zé wéi rǔ zhī. xià zé wéi yuè shuǐ. gù zhī rǔ zhī zé xuě yě. yòng yǐ diǎn yǎn. qǐ yǒu bù xiāng yí zhě. xuě wéi yīn. gù qí xìng lěng. zàng hán rén. rú rǔ bǐng lào zhī lèi. bù kě duō shí. suī yuē niú yáng rǔ. rán yì bù chū hū yīn yáng zào huà ěr. xī róng gèng yǐ tuó mǎ rǔ wéi sū lào. lǎo rén huàn kǒu chuāng bù néng shí. yǐn rén rè rǔ liáng.

Human milk-sap masters the supplementation of the five depots. It lets man become fat, and [causes his skin to turn] white, pleasant, and smooth. Tao Yinju has stated: Zhang Cang regularly consumed human milk. Hence, at the age of more than one hundred years he was still fat and [his skin still] white like a gourd. The commentary to the Tang edition [of the *Ben cao*] stated: In the *Bie lu* it was stated: Milk [generated] when a first male [child] is born cures red eyes and pain [in one's eyes], as well as frequent tears. It dissolves the poison in isolated liver and beef. If taken together with thick juice [pressed from] salted beans, the effects are miraculous. Also, if taken together with the excrements of small birds, it eliminates red eyes, and flesh[-like] growths [in one's eyes]. The imperial subject Yuxi and others, carefully commenting on the Shu edition [of the *Ben cao*] stated: Human milk, flavor: sweet; [thermoquality:] balanced, no toxicity. Rihuazi stated: Human milk, [thermoquality:] cold. Supports one's qi, cures emaciation and distress, makes the skin look pleasant, moistens one's body hair and the hair on the head. If one drops it into the eyes, it stops tears. Furthermore, it heals red eyes and causes them to be clear and moist. The *Sheng hui fang* [stated]: It cures inability to speak and a hardening of the base of one's tongue if one was suddenly struck by wind. [Take] old bean sauce – five ge; three years old is best – and human milk sap – five ge – and grind the two into a mixture. Then take a fresh piece of cloth and squeeze [the mixture through it]. Take the sap [produced this way] and give [the patient] little by little to eat from it without specifying a particular time of the day [for regular intake]. After quite a long time, [the patient] will speak again. The *Qian jin fang* [stated]: To treat a blocking of the monthly period, one drinks three ge human milk sap. The *Jin kui fang* [stated]: How can one know that beef [is from a cow that] has been bitten by a snake and will kill the person [that eats from it]? [If a cow or an ox] has been bitten by a snake, its hair is turned backwards along [the body of the animal]. If one eats from it and is about to die, one should drink one pint of human milk-sap, and one will be cured immediately. The *Yan yi* [stated]: Human milk-sap has many therapeutic effects on the eyes. How is that? The human heart produces blood; the liver stores blood. As long as the liver receives blood, one can see. That is, when water enters into the conduit [of the heart], blood will be generated. It said also: When it moves upward, it turns into milk-sap; when it moves downward, it turns into monthly fluid. Hence, one knows that milk-sap is nothing but blood. If one takes it to drop it into one's eyes, how could that not be appropriate? Blood is [categorized as] yin. Thus, its nature is cold. People harboring cold should not eat much of things like milk and cheese. Although it has been stated that the milk of cows and sheep [can be consumed], they too, though, do not stand apart from the yin-yang [schema of] creation. The Western tribes also use the milk of camels and horses to produce curd. Old people who suffer from sores in their mouth, and cannot eat, drink hot human milk with good [results].

9.d *Běn cǎo gāng mù* 38 本草綱目 (Fú qì bù 服器部) Sǐ rén zhěn xí 死人枕席 A Dead Person's Head-Rest or Mat

---

死人枕席 拾遺 【主治】尸疰。石蛔。又治疣目。以枕及席拭之二七遍令爛。去疣。藏器。療自汗盜汗。死人席縁燒灰。煮汁浴身。自愈。時珍。聖惠方。【發明】藏器曰。有嫗人患冷滯。積年不瘥。宋徐嗣伯診之。曰。此尸疰也。當以死人枕煮服之。乃愈。于是往古冢中取枕。枕已一邊腐缺。嫗服之。即瘥。張景聲十五歲。患腹脹面黃。衆藥不能治。以問嗣伯。嗣伯曰。此石蛔爾。極難療。當取死人枕煮服之。得大蛔蟲。頭堅如石者五六升。病即瘥。沈僧翼患眼痛。又多見鬼物。嗣伯曰。邪氣入肝。可覓死人枕煮服之。竟可埋枕於故處。如其言。又愈。王晏問曰。三病不同。皆用死人枕而俱瘥。何也。答曰。尸疰者。鬼氣也。伏而未起。故令人沉滯。得死人枕治之。魂氣飛越。不復附體。故尸疰自瘥。石蛔者。醫療既僻。蛔蟲轉堅。世間藥不能遣。須以鬼物驅之。然後乃散。故用死人枕煮服之。邪氣入肝。則使人眼痛而見魍魎。須邪物以鉤之。故用死人枕之氣。因不去之。故令埋於故處也。時珍曰。按謝士泰刪繁方。治尸疰。或見尸。或聞哭聲者。取死人席。斬棺內餘。棄路上者。一虎口。長三寸。水三升。煮一升服。立效。此即用死人枕之意也。故附之。

枕	zhěn	a head-rest; a pillow
席	xí	a mat
拾遺	shī yí	*Shi yi*, short title of *Běn cǎo shī yí*本草拾遺, "Additions to the *Materia Medica*" by Chén Càngqì陳藏器 (early 8th century)
尸疰	shī zhù	corpse possession, i.e. possession by the *hun*-soul of an alien corpse
石蛔	shí huí	stone(-like) roundworms
疣	yóu	swelling
拭	shì	to wipe (the eyes)
遍	biàn	a time; a turn
爛	làn	brightness (of eyes)
藏器	càng qì	Cangqi, personal name of Chén Càngqì 陳藏器, *materia medica* author
盜汗	dào hàn	robber sweat; night sweat
緣	yuán	a hem
燒	shāo	to burn
灰	huī	ashes
時珍	shí zhēn	Shizhen, personal name of Lǐ Shízhēn 李時珍 (1518-1593), author of the *Běn cǎo gāng mù*本草綱目
發明	fā míng	explanation
嫗	yù	an old woman
積年	jī nián	many years
瘥	chài	to recover; to get well
徐嗣伯	xú sì bó	Xu Sibo, physician and author of prescription works of the 5th century
煮	zhǔ	to boil; to decoct
於是	yú shī	thereupon; then
冢	zhǒng	tomb
邊	biān	a side
張景聲	zhāng jǐng shēng	Zhang Jingsheng, name of an otherwise unknown patient

沈僧翼	shěn sēng yì	Shen Sengyi, name of an otherwise unknown patient
覓	mì	to search for
埋	mái	to bury
王晏	Wáng Yàn	name of an otherwise unknown person
沉	chén	deep
附	fù	to attach
僻	pì	secluded; remote
遣	qiǎn	to banish; to send away
魍魎	wǎng liǎng	sprites
鉤	gōu	hook; sickle; to take on a hook; to pull
謝士泰	xiè shì tài	Xie Shitai, a 6th/7th century author of medical works
刪繁方	shān fán fāng	*Shan fan fang*, prescription collection written by Xie Shitai
斬	zhǎn	to cut in two
棺	guān	a coffin
棄	qì	to discard; to abandon

Sǐ rén zhěn xí shī yí【zhǔ zhì】shī zhù. shí huí. yòu zhì yóu mù. yǐ zhěn jí xí shì zhī èr qī biàn lìng làn. qù yóu. zàng qì. liáo zì hàn dào hàn. sǐ rén xí yuán shāo huī. zhǔ zhī yù shēn. zì yù. shí zhēn. shèng huì fāng.【fā míng】zàng qì yuē. yǒu yù rén huàn lěng zhì. jī nián bù cuó. sòng Xú sì bó zhěn zhī. yuē. cǐ shī zhù yě. dāng yǐ sǐ rén zhěn zhǔ fú zhī. nǎi yù. yú shī wǎng gǔ zhǒng zhōng qǔ zhěn. zhěn yǐ yì biān fǔ quē. yù fú zhī. jí cuò. Zhāng jǐng shēng shí wǔ suì. huàn fù zhàng miàn huáng. zhòng yào bù néng zhì. yǐ wèn sì bó. sì bó yuē. cǐ shí huí ěr. jí nán liáo. dāng qǔ sǐ rén zhěn zhǔ fú zhī. dé dà huí chóng. tóu jiān rú shí zhě wǔ liù shēng. bìng jí cuò. chén sēng yì huàn yǎn tòng. yòu duō jiàn guǐ wù. sì bó yuē. xié qì rù gān. kě mì sǐ rén zhěn zhǔ fú zhī. jìng kě mái zhěn yú gù chù. rú qí yán. yòu yù. wáng yàn wèn yuē. sān bìng bù tóng. jiē yòng sǐ rén zhěn ér jù cuò. hé yě. dá yuē. shī zhù zhě. guǐ qì yě. fú ér wèi qǐ. gù lìng rén chén zhì. dé sǐ rén zhěn zhì zhī. hún qì fēi yuè. bù fù fù tǐ. gù shī zhù zì cuò. shí huí zhě. yī liáo jì pì. huí chóng zhuǎn jiān. shì jiān yào bù néng qiǎn. xū yǐ guǐ wù qū zhī. rán hòu nǎi sàn. gù yòng sǐ rén zhěn zhǔ fú zhī. xié qì rù gān. zé shǐ rén yǎn tòng ér jiàn wǎng liǎng. xū xié wù yǐ gōu zhī. gù yòng sǐ rén zhěn zhī qì. yīn bù qù zhī. gù lìng mái yú gù chù yě. [shí zhēn yuē]. àn xiè shì tài shān fán fāng. zhì shī zhù. huò jiàn shī. huò wén kū shēng zhě. qǔ sǐ rén xí. zhǎn guān nèi yú. qì lù shàng zhě. yì hǔ kǒu. cháng sān cùn. shuǐ sān shēng. zhǔ yì shēng fú. lì xiào. cǐ jí yòng sǐ rén zhěn zhī yì yě. gù fù zhī.

A dead person's head-rest or mat: [Introduced into materia medica by the Ben cao] shi yi. **Masters Therapies of**: Corpse possession;[1] stone[-like] roundworms. [This item] also cures swollen eyes. If one wipes [swollen eyes] with a [dead person's] head-rest or mat twice seven times, [the eyes] will turn bright and the swelling will go away. [These indications were given by] Cangqi. [This item] cures sweating without external cause, and night-sweating. One takes the hem of a mat of a dead person, burns it to ashes, boils these [ashes with water], and washes the body with the [resulting] sap. That brings the cure. [These indications were given by Li] Shizhen and by the Sheng hui fang. **Explanations**: Cangqi said: There was an old woman who suffered from blockages of cold; for many years she did not recover. Xu Sibo of the Song dynasty examined her and said: This is [a case of] corpse possession. You should get a dead person's head-rest, boil it [in water], and take it [as drug]. Then you will be healed. Thereupon [the old woman] went into an old tomb and took a [dead-person's] head-rest from it. This head-rest had already rotted on one side. The woman took it and she recovered. [Later,] fifteen-year-old Zhang Jingsheng [suffered from] abdominal swelling and a yellow face. No medication was able to heal [his illness]. Hence, he consulted Sibo. Sibo said: This is [a case of] stone[-like] roundworms. It is extremely difficult to cure! You should take a dead person's head-rest and take it as a decoction. He produced 5 to 6 pints of large roundworms with heads as hard as a stone. As a result, he recovered from his illness. [Later,] Shen Sengyi suffered from pain in his eyes; in addition, he often saw demonic beings. Sibo said: Evil qi have entered your liver; you may search for a dead person's head-rest, boil it [in water], and take [the resulting decoction as a drug]. Finally, you may bury the head-rest at its old place again. [The patient] followed the words [of Sibo] and he, too, was cured. Wang Yan asked him: These three illnesses were all different, and yet they were all cured with a dead person's head-rest. How is that? [Sibo] answered: In case of corpse possession, demonic qi lie hidden [in the patient's body] and have not arisen yet. Hence, they cause obstructions deep in that person. If one finds a dead person's head-rest and [uses] it to treat [patients], the [alien corpse's] hun-qi will fly off, unable to attach themselves to the [patient's] body again. Hence, his corpse possession will get better. Stone[-like] roundworms: under medical treatment, they hide in a remote section [of the human body], and harden. No drug in this world would be able to eliminate them. One must make use of something demonic to drive them out; only then will they disperse. Hence, [I let the person suffering from roundworms] boil a dead person's head-rest [in water and] ingest it. If evil qi enter the liver and cause pain in one's eyes, as well as visions of sprites, one must resort to something evil in order to get them on the hook. Hence, one makes use of the qi of a dead person's head-rest. The [patient's qi] follow and do not leave the [head-rest qi.] Hence, one lets it be buried in its [original] place. [Li] Shizhen says: Xie Shitai, in his Shan fan fang, [has stated]: "If one wishes to treat corpse possession, corpse visions, or [cases where someone] hears wailing sounds, one takes [a piece of the width of] a tiger mouth, [that is, a piece of] three inches length, from a dead persons's mat, i.e. one of those surplus [pieces] discarded on the street once [the mat] has been cut to [fit] into the coffin, and boils it in three pints of water until [the water has been] reduced to one pint. The intake [of such a decoction] produces immediate results." The rationale behind this [prescription is the same as] that behind the use of a dead person's head-rest. Hence, I have added this [prescription here].

Note

[1] A living person is supposed to harbor two souls or spirits, i.e. a *hun*-soul and a *po*-soul. While the latter ceases to exist at the time of death, the former roams around and may take possession of some other human being. The resulting situation is called "corpse possession"

9.e *Běn cǎo qiú zhēn* 3 本草求真
Chái hú 柴胡
[The Drug] Chaihu

柴胡。耑入膽。味苦微辛。氣平微寒。據書載治傷寒熱傳足少陽膽。緣膽爲清淨之府。無出無入。邪入是經。正在表裏之界。汗吐與下當禁。惟宜和解。故仲景之治傷寒邪入少陽。而見寒熱往來。脇痛耳聾 ..。婦人熱入血室。用之以泄其邪 ..。胎前產後。小兒痘疹。五疳羸熱諸瘧。先寒後熱謂寒瘧。先熱後寒謂溫瘧。但熱不寒謂癉瘧。亦謂溫瘧。寒多熱少謂牡瘧。幷癧疽瘡瘍。咸宜用之 ..。若病在太陽。用之太早。猶引賊入門。病在陰經。用之則重傷其表。必得邪至少陽而藥始可用矣 ..。至云能治五癆。必其諸臟諸腑。其癆挾有實熱者。暫可用此解散。實熱是外邪內鬱而實。真虛而挾實熱。亦當酌其所宜。雖引清陽之氣左旋上行。然升中有散。若無歸耆同投。其散滋甚。虛熱不可寒。血衰火毒者不可燥。豈容誤哉 ..。兼之性滑善通。凡溏泄大便者。當善用之。熱結不通者。當佐當歸黃芩以投。差無誤耳。是以陰虛火炎。骨蒸勞熱。腎虛泄瀉。書載不應服。解散宜北柴胡。虛熱宜海陽軟柴胡爲良。酒炒用。半夏爲使。惡皂莢。畏女

菀。藜蘆。時珍曰。行手足少陽。以黃芩爲佐。行手足厥陰。以黃連爲佐。

據	jù	according to
書載	shū zài	recorded in the literature
緣	yuán	because
正	zhèng	exactly
界	jiè	a boundary; a border
禁	jìn	to prohibit
仲景	zhòng jǐng	Zhongjing, style-name of Zhāng Jī 張機, 142-220 (?), author of the prescription work *Shāng hán zá bìng lùn* 傷寒雜病論, "On Harm Caused by Cold and Various [Other] Diseases"
寒熱往來	hán rè wǎng lái	alternative fits of cold and heat
血室	xuě shì	the blood-chamber (of women; i.e. the womb)
胎前	tāi qián	pregnancy
五疳	wǔ gān	the five types of *gan*-illness
癉瘧	dǎn nüè	the solitary (heat-)*nüe*, i.e. solitary (heat-)malaria
牡	mǔ	male
癰疽	yōng jū	welling and deep-seated abscesses
瘡瘍	chuāng yáng	open sores
咸	xián	all; in all cases
賊	zèi	robber
至	zhì	as for; as far as
五癆	wǔ láo	the five types of consumption
歸	guī	short for *danggui*, a drug prepared from Angelica sinensis (Oliv.) Diels
旋	xuán	to come back; to move in a circle
滋	zī	more; very
容	róng	to allow; to tolerate
溏泄	táng xiè	turbid diarrhea
當歸	dāng guī	*danggui*; a drug prepared from Angelica sinensis (Oliv.) Diels

黃芩	huáng qín	*huangqing*, a drug prepared from Scutellaria baicalensis Georgi
差無誤	chā wú wù	not the slightest mistake
炎	yán	a flame; to flame
海陽	Hǎiyáng	Haiyang, a place name in today's Guangzhou
炒	chǎo	to stir-fry
半夏	bàn xià	*banxia*, a drug prepared from Pinellia ternata (Thumb.) Breit.
皂莢	zào jiá	*zaojia*, a drug prepared from Gleditsia sinensis Lam.
女菀	nǚ wǎn	*nüwan*, a drug prepared from Aster fastigiatus Fisch.
厥陰	jué yīn	the ceasing-yin (conduits)
黃連	huáng lián	*huanglian*, a drug prepared from Coptis chinensis Franch. (and other Coptis plants)

Chái hú. zhuān rù dǎn. wèi kǔ wēi xīn. qì píng wēi hán. jù shū zài zhì shāng hán rè chuán zú shào yáng dǎn. yuán dǎn wéi qīng jìng zhī fǔ. wú chū wú rù. xié rù shī jīng. zhèng zài biǎo lǐ zhī jiè. hàn tù yǔ xià dāng jìn. wéi yí hé jiě. gù zhòng jǐng zhī zhì shāng hán xié rù shào yáng. ér jiàn hán rè wǎng lái. xié tòng ěr lōng. fù rén rè rù xuě shì. yòng zhī yǐ xiè qí xié. tāi qián chǎn hòu. xiǎo ér dòu zhěn. wǔ gān léi rè zhū nüè. xiān hán hòu rè wèi hán nüè. xiān rè hòu hán wèi wēn nüè. dàn rè bù hán wèi dǎn nüè. yì wèi wēn nüè. hán duō rè shǎo wèi mǔ nüè. bìng yōng jū chuāng yáng. xián yí yòng zhī. ruò bìng zài tài yáng. yòng zhī tài zǎo. yóu yǐn zèi rù mén. bìng zài yīn jīng. yòng zhī zé zhòng shāng qí biǎo. bì dé xié zhì shào yáng ér yào shǐ kě yòng yǐ. zhì yún néng zhì wǔ láo. bì qí zhū zàng zhū fǔ. qí láo xié yǒu shí rè zhě. zàn kě yòng cǐ jiě sàn. shí rè shī wài xié nèi yù ér shí. zhēn xū ér xié shí rè. yì dāng zhuó qí suǒ yí. suī yǐn qīng yáng zhī qì zuǒ xuán shàng xíng. rán shēng zhōng yǒu sàn. ruò wú guī qí tóng tóu. qí sàn zī shèn. xū rè bù kě hán. xuě shuāi huǒ dú zhě bù kě zào. qǐ róng wù zāi. jiān zhī xìng huá shàn tōng. fán táng xiè dà biàn zhě. dāng shàn yòng zhī. rè jié bù tōng zhě. dāng zuǒ dāng guī huáng qín yǐ tóu. chā wú wù ěr. shī yǐ yīn xū huǒ yán. gǔ zhēng láo rè. shèn xū xiè xiè. shū zài bù yīng fú. jiě sàn yí běi chái hú. xū rè yí hǎi yáng ruǎn chái hú wéi liáng. jiǔ chǎo yòng. bàn xià wéi shǐ. wù zào jiá. wèi nǚ wǎn. lí lú. shí zhēn yuē. xíng shǒu zú shào yáng. yǐ huáng qín wéi zuǒ. xíng shǒu zú jué yīn. yǐ huáng lián wéi zuǒ.

Chaihu: Enters only the gallbladder. Flavor: bitter; slightly acrid. Qi: balanced; slightly cold. According to the literature, it cures harm caused by cold when heat has been transmitted into the foot-minor-yang [conduit of the] gallbladder. Because the gallbladder is the palace of cleanliness and purity, it has no [opening for anything dirty to] leave it and no [opening for anything dirty to] enter it. If evil [qi] enter the conduit [associated with the gallbladder], they remain exactly at the border between its outside and inside.[1] Sweating, vomiting, and purging must be avoided [as treatments here]; the only [therapy] appropriate is to harmonize and to resolve[2]. Hence, [Zhang] Zhongjing, in treating harm caused by cold with evil [qi] having entered the minor-yang [conduit] and the appearance of fits of cold and heat, of pain in one's ribs, of deafness, ... and of heat entering a woman's blood chamber, used [*chaihu*] in order to drain these evil [qi]. ... During pregnancy, after delivery, in cases of pox pustules of small children, in case of the five *gan*-diseases, emaciation and heat, all kinds of *nüe*[3], if one feels cold first and develops heat afterwards, that is called cold-nüe. If one develops heat first and feels cold afterwards, that is called warmth-nüe. If one develops only heat and does not feel cold, that is called solitary [heat-]nüe; it is also called warmth-nüe. If one feels cold a lot and develops only a little heat, that is called male nüe, as well as welling and deep-seated abscesses and open sores, in all these cases it is appropriate to use it. ... If one uses [*chaihu*] while the disease is still in the major-yang [conduit], that would be too early, and [such a therapy would be] comparable to an invitation to a robber to enter one's door. If one uses [*chaihu*] wile the disease is in one of the yin conduits, that would severely harm the exterior. Only when the evil [qi] have reached the minor-yang [conduit] should drugs be applied. ... When it is stated [in the literature that *chaihu*] cures the five types of consumption that is true only when all the depots and all the palaces [have been affected]. In cases of consumption coupled with repletion-heat, one may use this [drug] temporarily in order to dissolve and disperse [heat and repletion]. A repletion-heat is present when external evil [qi penetrate the body's] interior causing obstructions there and, hence, repletion. In cases of a depletion of one's true [qi] coupled with a repletion-heat, one should [carefully] consider whether an application [of *chaihu*] is appropriate indeed. Although [this drug] guides clear-yang qi, on the left, to move upward, [one should be aware of the fact that] its ascending [function] includes also a dispersing [function]. If [*chaihu*] is not given together with *gui* or *qi*, its dispersing [effects] will be even stronger! In cases of depletion [coupled with] heat, it is impossible to [give] cooling [drugs], and in cases of weakened blood or toxic fire it is impossible to [prescribe drugs with a] drying [effect]. How could one allow for a mistake here?! ... In addition to [the effects listed so far, *chaihu*] has a lubricating nature; it is an excellent [drug to stimulate the] passage [of qi]. In all cases of turbid diarrhea it is fine to use this [drug]. In cases of heat conglomeration and blocked passage, it should be assisted by *danggui* and *huangqin*. That would certainly not be wrong. Accordingly, the literature states that [*chaihu*] should not be taken in cases of depletion of yin [qi] and flaming fire, bone-steaming, taxation with heat, depletion of kidney [qi], and [clear] diarrhea. [If one wishes] to resolve and disperse, he should use *chaihu* from the north. In cases of depletion with heat, soft *chaihu* from Haiyang is appropriate. Before use, [*chaihu*] is to be stir-fried in wine. *Banxia* serves as its messenger[-drug]. It hates *zaojia*, and it fears *nüwan* and *lilu*. [Li] Shizhen has said: If [chaihu is supposed to] pass through the hand- and foot-minor-yang [conduits], it should be assisted by huangqin; if [it is supposed to] pass through the hand- and foot-ceasing-yin [conduits], it should be assisted by huanglian.

Notes

[1] "Outside" and "inside" refer here to gallbladder and liver respectively. The gallbladder is the "palace" associated with the foot-minor-yang conduit. It is categorized – like all the body's "palaces" – as "exterior". The liver is the "depot" associated with the foot-minor-yang conduit. It is categorized – like all the body's "depots" – as "interior".

[2] *Jiě* 解 is short for *jiě biǎo* 解表 here. The idea is to strengthen the guardian qi in the "skin structures", *còu lǐ* 腠理, so that evil qi will be unable to penetrate the inner body.

[3] *Nüè* 瘧 is a label for a disease known as malaria in Europe. See above, 4.d.

9.f *Běn cǎo gāng mù* 8 本草綱目
Fěn xī 粉錫
Powdered Tin

粉錫。本經下品。【釋名】解錫。本經。鉛粉。綱目。鉛華。綱目。胡粉。弘景。定粉。藥性。瓦粉。湯液。光粉。日華。白粉。湯液。水粉。綱目。官粉。〔弘景曰〕即今化鉛所作胡粉也。而謂之粉錫。似與今乖。〔時珍曰〕鉛錫一類也。古人名鉛爲黑錫。故名粉錫。釋名曰。胡者。糊也。和脂以糊面也。定瓦言其形。光白言其色 ...【正誤】〔恭曰〕鉛丹。胡粉。實用炒錫造。陶言化鉛。誤矣。〔震亨曰〕胡粉是錫粉。非鉛粉也。古人以錫爲粉。婦人用以附面者。其色類肌肉。不可入藥用。〔志曰〕..。抱朴子·內篇云。愚人不信黃丹。胡粉是化鉛所作。蘇恭以二物俱炒錫作。大誤矣。〔時珍曰〕錫炒則成黑灰。豈有白粉。蘇恭已誤。而朱震亨復踵其誤。何哉。【集解】〔時珍曰〕按墨子云。禹造粉。張華博物志云。紂燒鉛錫作粉。則粉之來亦遠矣。今金陵。杭州。韶州。辰州皆造之。而辰粉尤真。其色帶青。彼人言造法。每鉛百斤。鎔化。削成薄片。卷作筒。安木甑內。甑下。甑中各安醋一瓶。外以鹽泥固濟。紙封甑縫。風爐安火四兩。養一七。便掃入水缸內。依舊封養。次次如此。鉛盡爲度 ..。每粉一斤。入豆粉二兩。蛤粉四兩。水內攪勻。澄去清水。用細灰按成溝。紙隔數層。置粉於上。將乾。截成瓦定形。待乾收起 ..。【氣味】辛。寒。無毒。〔權曰〕甘。辛。涼。〔時珍曰〕胡粉能制硫黃。又雌黃得胡粉而失

色。胡粉得雌黃而色黑。蓋相惡也。又入酒中去酸味。收蟹不沙。

【主治】伏尸毒螫。殺三蟲。本經 ..。療惡瘡。止小便利。墮胎。別錄。治積聚不消 ..。止小兒疳痢。甄權 ..。治食復勞復。墜痰消脹。治疥癬狐臭。黑鬚髮。時珍。【發明】〔弘景曰〕胡粉金色者。療尸蟲彌良。〔藏器曰〕久痢成疳者。胡粉和水及雞子白服。以糞黑爲度。爲其殺蟲而止痢也。

粉錫	fěn xī	Powdered Tin (i.e. white lead; lead carbonate)
本經	běn jīng	the "Original Classic" (i.e. the *Shén nóng běn cǎo jīng* 神農本草經)
解錫	jiě xī	Dissolved Tin
鉛粉	qiān fěn	Lead Powder
綱目	gāng mù	abbreviated title of the *Běn cǎo gāng mù* ("Materia Medica Arranged According to Drug Descriptions and Technical Aspects") compiled by Lǐ Shí-zhēn 李時珍 (1518-1593)
鉛華	qiān huá	Lead Shine
胡粉	hú fěn	Foreign Powder
弘景	hóng jǐng	Hongjing, abbreviated name of Táo Hóngjǐng 陶弘景 (456-536), Daoist and author of a materia medica
定	dìng	ingot, used here for 錠 *dìng*
定粉	dìng fěn	"Ingot Powder"; powder pressed into an ingot shape
藥性	yào xìng	*Yao xing*, abbreviated title of the *Yào xìng běn cǎo* 藥性本草 ascribed to Zhēn Quán 甄權 of the 7th century
瓦粉	wǎ fěn	"Brick Powder"; powder pressed into a brick shape

湯液	tāng yè	*Tang ye*, abbreviated title of the *Tāng yè běn cǎo* 湯液本草 by Wáng Hàogǔ 王好古of the 13th century
光粉	guāng fěn	Radiant Powder
白粉	bái fěn	White Powder
水粉	shuǐ fěn	Water Powder
官粉	guān fěn	Superior Powder
乖	guāi	perversion; error
錫	xī	tin
釋名	shì míng	*Shi ming*, "Explanation of Names"; title of a Han dynasty book on terminology
糊	hú	paste
正	zhèng	to correct
誤	wù	mistake
恭	gōng	Gong, abbreviated taboo version of the name of Sū Jìng 蘇敬, co-author of the *Táng běn cǎo* 唐本草
鉛丹	qiān dān	Lead Balls (i.e. minium; lead tetroxide)
造	zào	to produce
震亨	zhèn hēng	Zhenheng, abbreviated name of Zhū Zhèn hēng 朱震亨 (1281-1358), scholar and medical author, best known under his sobriquet Zhū Dānxī 朱丹溪
志	zhì	Zhi, personal name of Mǎ Zhì 馬志 (fl. 975), co-author of the *Kāi bǎo běn cǎo* 開寶本草
抱朴子-內篇	bào pǔ zǐ nèi piān	*Bao pu zi nei pian*, the "Inner Section of the [Book Written by the] Master Embracing Purity"; a work by Gě Hóng 葛洪 281-341
黃丹	huáng dān	Yellow Balls (i.e. minium; lead tetroxide)
蘇恭	sū gōng	Su Gong, taboo version of the name of Sū Jìng 蘇敬 (fl. 657), co-author of the *Táng běn cǎo* 唐本草
朱震亨	zhū zhèn hēng	Zhu Zhenheng, scholar and medical author (1281-1358)

踵	zhǒng	to follow; to imitate
墨子	mò zǐ	Mozi, Master Mo; the philosopher Mò Dì 墨翟
禹	yǔ	the legendary emperor Yǔ
張華	zhāng huá	Zhang Hua, scholar and statesman of the 3rd c. CE
博物志	bó wù zhì	*Bo wu zhi*, title of a collection of essays by Zhāng Huá
紂	Zhòu	(King) Zhòu, the last ruler of the Yin dynasty, 12th c. BCE
金陵	jīn líng	Jinling, a place name
杭州	háng zhōu	Hangzhou, name of a prefecture
韶州	sháo zhōu	Shaozhou, name of a prefecture
辰州	chén zhōu	Chenzhou, name of a prefecture
真	zhēn	pure; genuine
帶	dài	belt; to carry with; connected with
斤	jīn	a catty
鎔化	róng huà	to smelt
削成	xiāo chéng	to cut into
片	piàn	a strip
卷	juǎn	to roll up
筒	tǒng	a tube
安	ān	to place
甑	zèng	a steamer
醋	cù	vinegar
瓶	píng	a jar
濟	jì	to complete
封	fēng	to seal up
縫	fèng	seam; slit
爐	lú	stove; furnace
風爐	fēng lú	a wind-stove (i.e. a stove that is fanned by the natural flow of wind/air, and that does not need a bellows)
兩	liǎng	a tael
掃	sǎo	a broom; to brush

水缸	shuǐ gāng	a large open-mouthed water jar
舊	jiù	formerly; before
次次	cì cì	time and again; continuously
爲度	wéi dù	take as measure; take as limit; until
蛤粉	gé fěn	powdered oyster shells
攪	jiào	to stir up
澄	chéng	to let settle
溝	gōu	a ditch
層	céng	a layer
置	zhì	to place; to arrange
截	jié	to cut
權	quán	Quan, abbreviated name of Zhēn Quán甄權, 7th century author of the *Yào xìng běn cǎo* 藥性本草
硫黃	liú huáng	sulphur
雌黃	cí huáng	auripigment
蟹	xiè	a crab
沙	shā	crumbly; in crumbs
螫	zhē	poison; poisonous
三蟲	sān chóng	the three worms (which inhabit the human body and may cause illness)
墮胎	duò tāi	to cause an abortion
甄權	zhēn quán	Zhen Quan, 7th century pharmaceutical author
食復	shí fù	recurrence (of an illness) due to (inappropriate) eating
勞復	láo fù	recurrence (of an illness) due to (physical) taxation
墜	zhuì	to bring down; to make fall down
疥癬	jiè xuǎn	itching skin diseases, consisting of either eruptive, scattered, small patches (*jiè* 疥), or noneruptive, large patches (*xuǎn* 癬)
狐臭	hú xiù	fox odor (from under the arm-pits)
尸蟲	shī chóng	corpse worms (i.e. the three worms inhabiting the human body)

彌	mí	very; especially
鷄子白	jī zǐ bái	egg-white
糞	fèn	feces

Fěn xī. běn jīng xià pǐn. 【shì míng】 jiě xī. běn jīng. qiān fěn. gāng mù. qiān huá. gāng mù. hú fěn. hóng jǐng. dìng fěn. yào xìng. wǎ fěn. tāng yè. guāng fěn. rì huá. bái fěn. tāng yè. shuǐ fěn. gāng mù. guān fěn. 〔hóng jǐng yuē〕 jí jīn huà qiān suǒ zuò hú fěn yě. ér wèi zhī fěn xī. sì yǔ jīn guāi. 〔shí zhēn yuē〕 qiān xī yí lèi yě. gǔ rén míng qiān wéi hēi xī. gù míng fěn xī. shì míng yuē. hú zhě. hú yě. hé zhī yǐ hú miàn yě. dìng wǎ yán qí xíng. guāng bái yán qí sè. 【zhèng wù】 〔gōng yuē〕 qiān dān. hú fěn. shí yòng chǎo xī zào. táo yán huà qiān. wù yǐ. 〔zhèn hēng yuē〕 hú fěn shī xī fěn. fēi qiān fěn yě. gǔ rén yǐ xī wéi fěn. fù rén yòng yǐ fù miàn zhě. qí sè lèi jī ròu. bù kě rù yào. 〔zhì yuē〕 bào pǔ zǐ· nèi piān yún. yú rén bù xìn huáng dān. hú fěn shì huà qiān suǒ zuò. sū gōng yǐ èr wù jù chǎo xī zuò. dà wù yǐ. 〔shí zhēn yuē〕 xī chǎo zé chéng hēi huī. qǐ yǒu bái fěn. sū gōng yǐ wù. ér zhū zhèn hēng fù zhǒng qí wù. hé zāi. 【jí jiě】 〔shí zhēn yuē〕 àn mò zǐ yún. yǔ zào fěn. Zhāng huá bó wù zhì yún. Zhòu shāo qiān xī zuò fěn. zé fěn zhī lái yì yuǎn yǐ. jīn jīn líng. háng zhōu. sháo zhōu. chén zhōu jiē zào zhī. ér chén fěn yóu zhēn. qí sè dài qīng. bǐ rén yán zào fǎ. měi qiān bǎi jīn. róng huà. xiāo chéng bó piàn. juǎn zuò tǒng. ān mù zèng nèi. zèng xià. zèng zhōng gè ān cù yì píng. wài yǐ yán ní gù jì. zhǐ fēng zèng fèng. fēng lú ān huǒ sì liǎng. yǎng yī qī. biàn sǎo rù shuǐ gāng nèi. yī jiù fēng yǎng. cì cì rú cǐ. qiān jìn wéi dù. měi fěn yì jīn. rù dòu fěn èr liǎng. gé fěn sì liǎng. shuǐ nèi jiào yún. chéng qù qīng shuǐ. yòng xì huī àn chéng gōu. zhǐ gé shù céng. zhì fěn yú shàng. jiāng gān. jié chéng wǎ dìng xíng. dái gān shōu qǐ. 【qì wèi】 xīn. hán. wú dú. 〔quán yuē〕 gān. xīn. liáng. 〔shí zhēn yuē〕 hú fěn néng zhì liú huáng. yòu cí huáng dé hú fěn ér shī sè. hú fěn dé cí huáng ér sè hēi. gài xiāng wù yě. yòu rù jiǔ zhōng qù suān wèi. shōu xiè bù shā. 【zhǔ zhì】 fú shī dú zhē. shā sān chóng. běn jīng. liáo è chuāng. zhǐ xiǎo biàn lì. duò tāi. bié lù. zhì jī jù bù xiāo. zhǐ xiǎo ér gān lì. zhēn quán. zhì shí fù láo fù. zhuì tán xiāo zhàng. zhì jiè xuǎn hú xiù. hēi xū fà. shí zhēn. 【fā míng】 〔hóng jǐng yuē〕 hú fěn jīn sè zhě. liáo shī chóng mí liáng. 〔càng qì yuē〕 jiǔ lì chéng gān zhě. hú fěn hé shuǐ jí jī zǐ bái fú. yǐ fèn hēi wéi dù. wéi qí shā chóng ér zhǐ lì yě.

Powdered Tin. [Listed among the] lower class [of drugs] in the original classic [of Shennong].

Elucidation of Names: Dissolved Tin. [A name mentioned in the] original classic.

Lead Powder. [A name introduced by the Ben cao] gang mu. Lead Shine. [A name introduced by the *Ben cao*] *gang mu*. Foreign Powder. [A name introduced by Tao] Hongjing. Ingot Powder. [A name introduced by the] *Yao xing* [*ben cao*]. Brick Powder. [A name introduced by the] *Tang ye* [*ben cao*]. Radiant Powder. [A name introduced by] Rihua [zi]. White Powder. [A name introduced by the] *Tang ye* [*ben cao*]. Water Powder. [A name introduced by the *Ben cao*] *gang mu*. Superior Powder. [Tao] Hongjing has said: This is today's Foreign Powder. It is made through a transformation of lead. To call it Powdered Tin may be a recent mistake. [Li] Shizhen says: Lead and tin are of one kind. In ancient times the people called lead the "black tin". Hence, [the present substance] was called Powdered Tin. [The book] "Explanation of Names" says: Hu ("Foreign") stands for hu ("paste"). [This substance is] mixed with fat and used to paste the face. "Ingot" and "Brick" refer to the shape [of this product on the market]. "Radiance" and "White" refer to its color...

Correction of Mistakes: [Su] Gong has said: Lead balls and Foreign Powder are, in fact, produced by roasting tin. When Tao [Hongjing] states that it is [the result of] a transformation of lead, that is a mistake. [Zhu] Zhenheng has said: Foreign Powder is Tin Powder. It is not Lead Powder. In ancient times, the people made a powder from tin, and the women used it to apply it to their face because its color is that of flesh. It cannot be used as drug. Zhi has said: ... Baopu zi, in his Nei bian, has stated: "Ignorant people do not believe that Yellow Balls and Foreign Powder are produced through a transformation of lead." When Su Gong held that both substances are made by roasting tin, that was a great mistake. [Li] Shizhen says: When tin is roasted, black ashes result. How could White Powder [be produced this way]? Su Gong [had written down this] error already, and then Zhu Zhenheng followed him and made the same mistake. How could that happen?

Collected Explanations: [Li] Shizhen says: Mozi has stated: "Yu produced powder." Zhang Hua, in his Bo wu zhi, has stated: "[King] Zhou burned lead and tin and produced the powder." That shows, the origin of this powder already lies in the distant [past]. Today it is produced in Jinling, Hangzhou, Shaozhou, and Chenzhou, and the powder from Chen[zhou] is the purest. Its color carries some greenish-blue [elements]. The people there relate the process of production [as follows]. For each [production process] one hundred catties of lead are smelted, cut into thin stripes, and rolled to form tubes. Then one [takes a first portion of these tubes and] places them [into the upper section of] a wooden steamer. A jar filled with vinegar is placed into the lower and central [sections of the] steamer. [Now] the steamer is covered entirely, from outside, with brine-paste, and all its slits are closed with paper. [After these preparations, the steamer] is placed on a wind-stove [heated by] a fire from four taels [of coal. The fire is] nourished for one [period of] seven [days], after which [the lead powder] is brushed [from the top section of the steamer] into a larger water container. Just as before, [the steamer is filled again with further lead tubes], sealed, and [the fire is] nourished [again]. This is continued in the same manner until all the lead is used up. ... For each catty of the [resulting] powder, two taels of bean powder and four taels of powdered oyster-shells are added [The mixture] is stirred in water until [all ingredients are] evenly [distributed]. One allows [the powder] to settle, and discards the clear water [above it]. Now one takes finely ground ashes and presses ditches into them. One uses paper to separate different levels. Then the powder is brought on top of this in order to dry. [Then] they are formed into bricks and ingots. These are taken off [the paper] once they are dried. ...

Qi and Flavor: Acric, cold. No toxicity. [Chen] Quan has said: Sweet, acrid, cool. [Li] Shizhen says: Foreign Powder is able to check sulphur. Also, if auripigment gets in contact with Foreign Powder, it loses its color, and if Foreign Powder gets in contact with auripigment, its color turns black. That is to say, they hate each other. If brought into wine, it eliminates [the latter's] sour [flavor. It may be used to] conserve crabs. It keeps [their meat] from becoming crumbly.

Masters Therapies of: hidden corpse poison. Kills the three worms.[1] [These indications were given in the] original classic. ... Heals malign sores. Stops incessant urination. Causes abortion. [These indications were given in the Ming yi] bie lu. Cures accumulations [resulting from a] failure to digest. ... Stops *gan*-disease with dysentery in small children. [These indications were given by] Chen Quan. ... Cures recurrence [of an illness] due to one's [physical] taxation. It causes phlegm to sink down [in the body], decreases swellings, and cures itching skin-diseases, as well as fox odor [from under one's armpits. Furthermore,] it blackens one's hair. [These indications were added by Li] Shizhen.

Explanations: [Tao] Hongjing has said: Foreign Powder of golden color is particularly good for curing [patients suffering from] corpse worms. [Chen] Cangqi has said: If a chronic dysentery turns into a gan-disease, one takes Foreign Powder with water and egg-white until one's stools turn black. It stops dysentery because it kills the worms [causing it].

Note

[1] The concept of the "three worms" is outlined in *juan* 18 of Chao Yuanfang's 巢元方 etiological treatise *Zhu bing yuan hou lun* 諸病源候論 of the 7th century. Accordingly, as a result of depletion-heat in the stomach and the intestines, further depletion is caused in the five depots. The three worms inhabiting the body take advantage of this situation, seize the depleted regions, and eat away the five depots

Lesson Ten

Needle Treatment

Needle treatment was mentioned first by the historian Sima Qian 司馬遷 in his *Shiji* 史記 of 90 BCE. No earlier evidence, neither written nor archaeological, is available to trace the origins of this therapeutic method, and one may assume that the technique of piercing the skin with fine needles of various sizes was developed in China from unknown antecedents during the second century BCE. Acupuncture as a type of needle treatment based on the concepts of qi flow in the human body's conduits and legitimated by the doctrines of systematic correspondence became the mainstay of the medicine of correspondence, and has been, erroneously, identified with Chinese traditional health care per se in Western literature of the past two or three decades. Historical evidence suggests that therapeutic intervention by means of needling appears to have remained secondary to pharmaceutics in China throughout the past two millennia. Like the development of Chinese materia medica, acupuncture reached its peak in the sixteenth century, but unlike pharmaceutics which continued to be practiced at the level reached, acupuncture declined and fell almost into oblivion, a status from which it was rescued, for pragmatic and political reasons, only about three decades ago. Acupuncture was never a unified, stringently conceptualized system of therapy. New "holes" to be pierced and techniques continued to be discovered through experience or were deduced theoretically, and were propagated by different schools. While the restriction of pulse diagnosis to the wrists, advocated by the *Nan jing* 難經, presumably as a consequence of the assumption of a circulatory flow of qi through the organism, was accepted subsequently, and replaced the palpation of the individual conduits themselves, a second restriction suggested by the *Nan jing*, possibly as a consequence of the same assumption, did not fall on fertile grounds. The *Nan jing* no longer recommended the piercing of the individual conduits at locations spread all over the body, but emphasized the piercing of theoretically deduced "holes" in the four distal extremities only. One of the ideas underlying the piercing of well-defined insertion points in the extremities all over the body was to allow qi to enter (in cases of depletion) or to leave (in cases of repletion) the organism through these holes. Another idea was to stimulate, through the insertion of needles into specific points or conduits associated with specific functional units, an increase or decrease of the functions of these units, or to free the passage through the conduits from blockages of various sorts. Although the classic sources document a considerable practice of blood-letting, this application appears to have been particularly prominent on the level of folk acupuncture in later centuries.

Key Terms Introduced in Lesson Ten

腧	shū	transport (acupuncture insertion point)
鑱鍼	chán zhēn	the chisel needle
員鍼	yuán zhēn	the round needle
鍉鍼	dī zhēn	the arrowhead needle
鋒鍼	fēng zhēn	the lance-point needle
鈹鍼	pī zhēn	the sword needle
員利鍼	yuán lì zhēn	the round-sharp needle
毫鍼	háo zhēn	the hair needle
長鍼	cháng zhēn	the long needle
大鍼	dà zhēn	the large needle
分間	fēn jiān	the region of the partings [of the flesh]
分氣	fēn qì	the qi in the partings [of the flesh]
痼	gù	chronic illness
機關	jī guān	the (sections where the bones) move and have their joints
井	jǐng	a well (generic name for all first insertion points on the twelve conduit-streams in the extremities)
滎	yíng	a brook (generic name for all second insertion points on the twelve conduit-streams in the extremities)
輸	shū	a transporter (generic name for all third insertion points on the twelve conduit-streams in the extremities)
經	jīng	a stream (generic name for all fourth insertion points on the twelve conduit-streams in the extremities)
合	hé	a confluence (generic name for all final insertion points on the conduit-streams in the extremities)

轉	zhuǎn	to twirl [a needle after insertion]
痏	wěi	the wound [where a needle was inserted]
納	nà	to insert [a needle]
七竅	qī qiào	the seven orifices
腰痛	yāo tòng	lumbar pain
血絡	xuě luò	the blood [vessel] network
輸刺	shū cì	piercing of transport [holes]; i.e. piercing of the five insertion points "well" through "confluence" in the distal extremities[1]
遠道刺	yuǎn dào cì	piercing from a distance; i.e. piercing at a point far away from the affected area
經刺	jīng cì	piercing of conduits; i.e. piercing of the conduit primarily affected by a disease
絡刺	luò cì	piercing of network [vessels]; i.e. piercing of small vessels in the region directly below the skin to drain blood
分刺	fēn cì	piercing of the partings [of the flesh]
大寫刺	dà xiè cì	piercing to induce drainage of large [quantities of pus or blood]
毛刺	máo cì	piercing [of the skin as cautiously as if with a] hair
巨刺	jù cì	grand piercing; i.e. piercing a site on the right side of the patient if the illness is located on the left, and vice versa
焠刺	cuì cì	cauterization piercing [with a heated needle]
偶刺	ǒu cì	paired piercing; i.e. piercing of two sites of pain on the back and front of a patient
報刺	bào cì	retaliation piercing; i.e. method to treat pain changing its location. A needle is inserted at a site of pain. The physician locates with his hand a second site of pain, withdraws the needle from the first and inserts it at the second site
恢刺	huī cì	broad piercing; i.e. piercing next to a cramped or painful sinew. The needle is moved back and forth to widen the opening at the insertion point

齊刺	qí cì	combination piercing; i.e. the insertion of one needle each to the left and right of a needle inserted directly into an affected area
揚刺	yáng cì	scattered piercing; i.e. the insertion of four needles around a first needle
直針刺	zhí zhēn cì	direct piercing; i.e. piercing into a lifted skin-fold without damaging the flesh
輸刺	shū cì	transport piercing; i.e. fast and deep insertion and withdrawal of a needle
短刺	duǎn cì	short piercing; i.e. deep insertion of a needle until it comes close to a bone
浮刺	fú cì	surface piercing; i.e. a slanted superficial insertion
陰刺	yīn cì	yin piercing; i.e. piercing of the foot-minor-yin conduit on both its right and left course
傍刺	páng cì	side-wise piercing; i.e. piercing to the side of a needle already inserted
贊刺	zàn cì	supportive piercing; i.e. shallow piercing to drain blood and support the dispersion of pain and swellings
焠鍼	cuì zhēn	cauterizing needle
艾	ài	moxa; common mugwort
火鍼	huǒ zhēn	the fire needle
灼	zhuó	to cauterize
仆	pū	to fall to the ground; to collapse
發針	fā zhēn	to withdraw the needle
蒼蒼	cāng cāng	green
痹	bì	closure; blockage
姙孕	rèn yùn	pregnant
符水	fú shuǐ	amulet [dissolved in] water
吟	yín	to moan
恙	yàng	illness; indisposition
痕	hén	a scar; mark

10.a *Huáng dì nèi jīng, Líng shū* 1
黃帝內經·靈樞
Jiǔ zhēn shí èr yuán 九針十二原
The Nine Needles and the Twelve Origins

凡用鍼者。虛則實之。滿則泄之。宛陳則除之。邪勝則虛之。大要曰。徐而疾則實。疾而徐則虛。言實與虛。若有若無。察後與先。若存若亡。爲虛爲實。若得若失。虛實之要。九鍼最妙。補瀉之時。以鍼爲之。瀉曰必持內之。放而出之。排陽得鍼。邪氣得泄。按而引鍼。是謂內溫。血不得散。氣不得出也。補曰隨之。隨之意。若妄之。若行若按。如蚊虻止。如留如還。去如弦絕。令左屬右。其氣故止。外門已閉。中氣乃實。必無留血。急取誅之。持鍼之道。堅者爲寶。正指直刺。無鍼左右。神在秋毫。屬意病者。審視血脈者。刺之無殆。方刺之時。必在懸陽。及與兩衛。神屬勿去。知病存亡。血脈者。在腧橫居。視之獨澄。切之獨堅。九鍼之名。各不同形。一曰鑱鍼。長一寸六分。二曰員鍼。長一寸六分。三曰鍉鍼。長三寸半。四曰鋒鍼。長一寸六分。五曰鈹鍼。長四寸。廣二分半。六曰

員利鍼。長一寸六分。七曰毫鍼。長三寸六分。八曰長鍼。長七寸。九曰大鍼。長四寸。鑱鍼者。頭大末銳。去瀉陽氣。員鍼者。鍼如卵形。揩摩分間。不得傷肌肉。以瀉分氣。鍉鍼者。鋒如黍粟之銳。主按脈勿陷。以致其氣。鋒鍼者。刃三隅以發痼疾。鈹鍼者。末如劍鋒。以取大膿。員利鍼者。大如氂。且員且銳。中身微大。以取暴氣。毫鍼者。尖如蚊虻喙。靜以徐往。微以久留之而養。以取痛痺。長鍼者。鋒利身薄。可以取遠痺。大鍼者。尖如梃。其鋒微員。以瀉機關之水也。

宛陳	yù chén	long-term accumulation
大要	dà yào	*Da yao*, "Great Essential", an antique text, now lost
放	fàng	to loosen; to let go
排	pái	to open up
溫	wēn	used for 蘊 *yùn*: to accumulate; to collect
妄	wàng	used for 忘 *wàng*: to forget
蚊虻	wén méng	mosquito
弦	xián	a string
屬	shǔ	to go to
誅	zhū	to eradicate; to eliminate
寶	bǎo	valuable; best
直	zhí	straight
秋毫	qiū háo	autumn down
屬意	zhǔ yì	to focus one's attention on
殆	dài	dangerous
腧	shū	transport (acupuncture insertion point)

澄	chéng	clear
鑱鍼	chán zhēn	the chisel needle
員鍼	yuán zhēn	the round needle
鍉鍼	dī zhēn	the arrowhead needle
鋒鍼	fēng zhēn	the lance-point needle
鈹鍼	pī zhēn	the sword needle
員利鍼	yuán lì zhēn	the round-sharp needle
毫鍼	háo zhēn	the hair needle
長鍼	cháng zhēn	the long needle
大鍼	dà zhēn	the large needle
卵	luǎn	egg
揩摩	kāi mó	to rub
分間	fēn jiān	the region of the partings [of the flesh]
分氣	fēn qì	the qi in the partings [of the flesh]
陷	xiàn	to penetrate into; to insert
刃	rèn	a sword
隅	yú	an angle; an edge
發	fā	to send out; to eliminate; to emit
痼	gù	chronic illness
劍	jiàn	a double-edged sword
氂	máo	a yak's tail
喙	huì	a beak; a snout
靜	jìng	quiet
挺	tǐng	a stick
機關	jī guān	the (sections where the bones) move and have their joints

Fán yòng zhēn zhě. xū zé shí zhī. mǎn zé xiè zhī. yù chén zé chú zhī. xié shèng zé xū zhī. dà yào yuē. xú ér jí zé shí. jí ér xú zé xū. yán shí yǔ xū. ruò yǒu ruò wú. chá hòu yǔ xiān. ruò cún ruò wáng. wéi xū wéi shí. ruò dé ruò shī. xū shí zhī yào. jiǔ zhēn zuì miào. bǔ xiè zhī shí. yǐ zhēn wéi zhī. xiè yuē bì chí nèi zhī. Fàng ér chū zhī. pái yáng dé zhēn. xié qì dé xiè. àn ér yǐn zhēn. shī wèi nèi wēn. xuě bù dé sàn. qì bù dé chū yě. bǔ yuē suí zhī. suí zhī yì. ruò wàng zhī. ruò xíng ruò àn. rú wén méng zhǐ. rú liú rú huán. qù rú xián jué. lìng zuǒ shǔ yòu. qí qì gù zhǐ. wài mén yǐ bì. zhōng qì nǎi shí. bì wú liú xuě. jí qǔ zhū zhī. chí zhēn zhī dào. jiān zhě wéi bǎo. zhèng zhǐ zhí cì. wú zhēn zuǒ yòu. shén zài qiū háo. zhǔ yì bìng zhě. shěn shì xuě mài zhě. cì zhī wú dài. fāng cì zhī shí. bì zài xuán yáng. jí yǔ liǎng wèi. shén shǔ wù qù. zhī bìng cún wáng. xuě mài zhě. zài shū héng jū. shì zhī dú chéng. qiè zhī dú jiān. jiǔ zhēn zhī míng. gè bù tóng xíng. yī yuē chán zhēn. cháng yí cùn liù fēn. èr yuē yuán zhēn. cháng yí cùn liù fēn. sān yuē dī zhēn. cháng sān cùn bàn. sì yuē fēng zhēn. cháng yí cùn liù fēn. wǔ yuē pī zhēn. cháng sì cùn. guǎng èr fēn bàn. liù yuē yuán lì zhēn. cháng yí cùn liù fēn. qī yuē háo zhēn. cháng sān cùn liù fēn. bā yuē cháng zhēn. cháng qī cùn. jiǔ yuē dà zhēn. cháng sì cùn. chán zhēn zhě. tóu dà mò ruì. qù xiè yáng qì. yuán zhēn zhě. zhēn rú luǎn xíng. kāi mó fēn jiān. bù dé shāng jī ròu. yǐ xiè fēn qì. dī zhēn zhě. fēng rú shǔ sù zhī ruì. zhǔ àn mài wù xiàn. yǐ zhì qí qì. fēng zhēn zhě. rèn sān yú yǐ fā gù jí. pī zhēn zhě. mò rú jiàn fēng. yǐ qǔ dà nóng. yuán lì zhēn zhě. dà rú máo. qiě yuán qiě ruì. zhōng shēn wēi dà. yǐ qǔ bào qì. háo zhēn zhě. jiān rú wén méng huì. jìng yǐ xú wǎng. wēi yǐ jiǔ liú zhī ér yǎng. yǐ qǔ tòng bì. cháng zhēn zhě. fēng lì shēn bó. kě yǐ qǔ yuǎn bì. dà zhēn zhě. jiān rú tǐng. qí fēng wēi yuán. yǐ xiè jī guān zhī shuǐ yě.

All [therapeutic] applications of needles [are meant to achieve the following results]. If [the patient suffers from] depletion, this is to be replenished. If [the patient suffers from] fullness, this is to be discharged. If [the patient suffers from] long-term accumulations, these are to be eliminated. If evil [qi] have gained dominance, they are to be depleted. The *Da yao* states: "[If one inserts the needle] slowly and [withdraws it] quickly, that has a replenishing [effect; if one inserts the needle] quickly and [withdraws it] slowly, that has a depleting [effect]."[1] That is to say: repletion and depletion are like having and not having.[2] To examine whether it is a belated or earlier [arrival of qi] is like [examining whether it] is present or has been lost.[3] If one deals with depletion and repletion, that is as if one were to treat a gain or a loss [respectively.][4] When it comes to the essential [knowledge in the treatment of] depletion and repletion, the [application of the] nine needles is the most subtle. Whenever one supplements [a depletion] or drains [a repletion], this is to be done with needles. To drain means that one must hold [the needle] firmly and insert it [into the skin. Then] one loosens one's grip and withdraws the [needle. This way,] one opens the yang [region beneath the skin, and allows the qi there to] contact the needle. [With the withdrawal of the needle] the evil qi can flow out.[5] If one were to press [a finger on the insertion point] while pulling out the needle, that would mean [to cause] internal accumulations. The blood would not be able to disperse, and the qi would not be able to leave [the body].[6] To supplement means to follow the [direction of the movement in the vessels when inserting the needle]. While following the [direction of the movement in the vessels when inserting the needle] one's sentiments are as if one had forgotten it.[7] In moving [the needle] and in pressing [the place of insertion], one must not go [in strength] beyond the sting of a mosquito. [The needle is allowed to] rest [in the skin until the qi have arrived], and is then withdrawn again, and it should leave [the skin as fast as] a [tense] string that has been cut. One lets the left [hand] move to where the right [hand has just removed the needle, and presses the insertion point with one's fingers]. This way, the qi will be halted [and cannot flow out]. After the gate to the outside has been closed, the qi inside are replenished. No blood should remain. [If blood appears there] it must quickly be eliminated.[8] The best way to hold the needle is [to grasp it] firmly. [The needle should] point exactly [downward] and it should pierce straight [into the skin]. One should not [allow] the needle [to move diagonally to] the left or right. One's spirit must focus on [details as fine as] autumn down; one's attention must be entirely with the patient. One examines the blood vessels [with sufficient care] so that needling them will cause no danger. At the moment one inserts the needle, it is essential to lift the [patient's] yang, and to [pay attention to] his two guardians. [One beholds whether the patient's] spirit stays with him or has left already, and hence knows whether the patient will survive or die.[9] Where the blood-vessels cross over a transport [point where the needles are to be inserted], they can be discerned most clearly, and they can be felt in all their firmness.

The names of the nine needles refer to their different shapes. The first is called the chisel needle. It is one inch and six tenths [of an inch] long. The second is called the round needle. It is one inch and six [tenths of an inch] long. The third is called the arrowhead needle; it is three and a half inches long. The fourth is called the lance point needle; it is one inch and six tenths [of an inch] long. The fifth is called the sword needle. It is four inches long, and two and a half tenths [of an inch] broad. The sixth is called the roundsharp needle. It is one inch and six tenths [of an inch] long. The seventh is called the hair needle. It is three inches and six tenths [of an inch] long. The eighth is called the long needle. It is seven inches long. The ninth is called the large needle. It is four inches long. The chisel needle: it has a large head and a pointed tip. [It serves] to drain yang qi. The round needle: this needle is shaped like an egg. It [is used to] rub in the region of the partings [of the flesh]. It cannot injure the muscles and the flesh. It [serves to] drain qi from the partings [of the flesh]. The arrowhead needle: its head is pointed like a grain of millet. It is used to press the vessels, but should not be deeply inserted. It serves to cause [regular] qi to arrive. The lance-point needle: it is a three-edged sword. It serves to drive out chonic diseases. The sword needle: its end resembles the head of a sword. It serves to eliminate large amounts of pus. The round-sharp needle: its size resembles the [long and thin but at the same time strong hairs in the] tail of a yak. It has a round [shaft] and a pointed [tip]. Its central piece is rather large. It serves to eliminate violent qi. The hair needle: it is pointed like the snout of a mosquito. [One may let it] rest quietly [in the skin] until [the qi] slowly moves on. [Its body is] delicate, and it remains [in the skin] for a long time to nourish [the regular qi]. It serves to eliminate pain and/or blockages. The long needle: its head is sharp, and its body is thin. It serves to eliminate blockages in distant regions. The large needle: it is pointed like a stick. Its head is slightly rounded. It serves to drain water from the joints [where the bones] move.

Notes

[1] The *Huang Di nei jing ling shu yi shi* 黄帝内经灵枢译释 (referred to as HDNLSYS below), 1986, p. 5, interprets this passage as follows: "The pattern to slowly insert and quickly withdraw the needle, and to press the opening with one's finger immediately after the withdrawal of the needle, that is a pattern of supplementation. To quickly insert and slowly withdraw the needle, and not to close the insertion point after the withdrawal of the needle, that is a pattern of draining." The basis of this interpretation is in *Ling shu* treatise 3: Xiao zhen jie 小鍼解.

[2] Zhang Jiebin (Jingyue) (fl. 1624), the author of the *Lei jing*, commented on this statement: "Repletion and depletion refer to the presence and absence of qi. The qi by itself has no material shape. Hence it is 'like existing and like not existing.' Those who are able to investigate this, their mind will enter the boderline of existence and non-existence (有無之間 *yǒu wú zhī jiàn*)."

[3] The Xiao zhen jie states: "That is to say, if one is going to fill or drain a depletion or repletion of qi earlier or later [in the course of a treatment], one should examine [first of all] whether the [evil] qi have retreated already, or are still present." The HDNJLSSY, p. 5, interprets 察後與先 *chá hòu yǔ xiān* as: "Examine whether a disease moves slowly or quickly, and then decide the order of where to treat [the organism] first, and where to treat it later." And it interprets 若存若亡 *ruò cún ruò wáng* as "in accordance with the presence of depletion or repletion, decide wether to let the needle remain [in the skin] or not, and [if you decide] it should remain [in the skin, you must decide] for how long."

[4] Some editions have 爲虛與實 *wèi xū yǔ shí* instead of 爲虛爲實 *wèi xū wèi shí.*

[5] The HDNJLSSY, pp. 5-6, interprets this passage as follows: "Whenever one applies a [therapeutic] pattern of draining, one must hold the needle firmly and insert it quickly. After one has gained contact with the qi, the needle is slowly withdrawn again. It is moved around to create a large hole and to open up the external, [i.e.] the yang [region underneath the skin] so as to allow the qi to flow out freely." 放 *Fàng* is interpreted here not as "to loosen [one's grip]", but as 搖 *yáo*, "to move wildly".

[6] HDNJLSSY, p. 6: "To supplement by mistake in a situation where one has to drain [would be the following procedure]. One first presses the insertion point [with one's finger], and then slowly inserts the needle. This way one causes the blood and the qi to accumulate internally but not to disperse to the outside, and hence the evil qi cannot leave [the body] either." 引 *Yǐn* is interpreted here as "to insert". Other commentators have interpreted 引 *yǐn* as equivalent to 出鍼 *chū zhēn*, "to withdraw the needle".

[7] Some commentators have interpreted 妄 *wàng* as "casual", "aimless": "One inserts the needle in the direction of the movement in the vessels, acting like a person with no particular goal in mind."

[8] Some commentators have interpreted the technique of this "elimination" as insertion of a needle to drain the blood to the outside

[9] The meaning of 懸陽 *xuán yáng* and 兩衛 *liǎng wèi* is by no means clear. Chinese commentators have suggested different interpretations, none of which is entirely satisfying. Zhang Jiebin in his 類經 *Lei jing* interprets 懸 *xuán* as 舉 *jǔ* "to lift", "to support", and 兩衛 *liǎng wèi* as, first, the guardian qi flowing in the external regions of the body, and, second, the qi of the spleen since the spleen is the protector of the well-being of all the other functional units of the organism. (The function of the spleen, in this view, is to supplement all the other functional units with the products of digestion). Both these kinds of qi must not be harmed. Hence, a practitioner should pay attention to their condition. The 靈樞經校釋 *Ling shu jing jiao shi* of the Hebei Medical College 1982, pp. 15-16, interprets 懸陽 *xuán yáng* as "the eyes", and 衛 *wèi* as 衡 *héng*, "the space between the eyebrows": "While needling [the patient], one must watch his eyes and the space between his eyebrows."

10.b *Xú líng tāi xiān sheng yī shū quán jí* 1
徐靈胎先生醫書全集
(Yī xué yuán liú lùn 醫學源流論)
Zhēn jiǔ shī chuán lùn
針灸失傳論
On the Loss of Tradition in Needling and Cauterization (I)

靈素兩經。其詳論臟腑經穴疾病等說。為針法言者。十之七八。為方藥言者。十之二三。上古之重針法如此。然針道難而方藥易。病者亦樂于服藥。而苦于針。所以後世方藥盛行。而針法不講。今之為針者。其顯然之失有十。而精微尚不與焉。兩經所言。十二經之出入起止。淺深左右。交錯不齊。其穴隨經上下。亦參差無定。今人祗執同身寸。依左右一直豎量。幷不依經曲折。則經非經而穴非穴。此一失也。兩經治病。云某病取某穴者固多。其餘則指經而不指穴。如靈 ..。厥病篇云 ..。耳聾取手陽明。嗌乾取足少陰。皆不言其穴 ..。今則每病指定幾穴。此二失也。兩經論治。井。滎。輸。經。合最重 ..。凡只言某經。而不言某穴者。大都皆指井滎五者為言。今則皆不講矣。此三失也。補瀉之法。內

經云。吸則內針。無令氣忤。靜以久留。無令邪布。吸則轉針。以得氣爲故。候呼引針。呼盡乃去。大氣皆出爲瀉。呼盡內針。靜以久留。以氣至爲故。候吸引針。氣不得出。各在其處。推闔其門。令神氣存。大氣留止爲補。又必迎其經氣。疾內而徐出。不按其痏爲瀉。隨其經氣。徐內而疾出。即按其痏爲補。其法多端。今則轉針之時。以大指推出爲瀉。搓入爲補。此四失也。納針之後。必候其氣。刺實者。陰氣隆至乃去針。刺虛者。陽氣隆至乃出針。氣不至。無問其數。氣至即去之。勿復針 ..。今則時時轉動。俟針下寬轉。而後出針。不問氣之至與不至。此五失也。

靈	líng	abbreviated title of the *Líng shū* 靈樞, one of the books constituting the *Huang Di nei jing* 黃帝內經 corpus
素	sù	abbreviated title of the *Sù wèn* 素問, one of the books constituting the *Huang Di nei jing* corpus
上古	shàng gǔ	high antiquity
重	zhòng	to value
失	shī	loss
交錯	jiāo cuò	interlocking; intertwined
齊	qí	regular; uniform
參差	cēn cī	irregular; not uniform
同身寸	tóng shēn cùn	[individually] standardized body inch
一直	yì zhí	in straight lines
竪	shù	to set up; to establish

量	liáng	to measure
幷	bìng	a particle adding emphasis if placed before a negative
曲	qū	a bend; a curve
折	zhé	broken; a curve
取	qǔ	to select [a hole for piercing]
厥病篇	jué bìng piān	the treatise Jue bing ("Recession Diseases") of the *Líng shū* 靈樞
井	jǐng	a well (generic name for all first insertion points on the twelve conduit-streams in the extremities)
滎	xíng	a brook (generic name for all second insertion points on the twelve conduit-streams in the extremities)
輸	shū	transporter (generic name for all third insertion points on the twelve conduit-streams in the extremities)
經	jīng	a stream (generic name for all fourth insertion points on the twelve conduit-streams in the extremities)
合	hé	a confluence (generic name for all final insertion points on the conduit-streams in the extremities)
只	zhǐ	only
忤	wǔ	to irritate
轉	zhuǎn	to twirl [a needle after insertion]
候	hòu	to wait
推	tuī	to push
闔	hé	to close
迎	yíng	to move against
痏	wěi	the wound [where a needle was inserted]
搓	cuō	to rub between the hands
納	nà	to insert [a needle]
隆	lóng	abundant

俟	sì	as soon as
寬	kuān	broad; extensive

Líng sù liăng jīng. qí xiáng lùn zàng fŭ jīng xuè jí bìng dĕng shuō. wéi zhēn fă yán zhĕ. shí zhī qī bā. wéi fāng yào yán zhĕ. shí zhī èr sān. shàng gŭ zhī zhòng zhēn fă rú cĭ. rán zhēn dào nán ér fāng yào yì. bìng zhĕ yì lè yú fú yào. ér kŭ yú zhēn. suŏ yĭ hòu shì fāng yào shèng xíng. ér zhēn fă bù jiăng. jīn zhī wéi zhēn zhĕ. qí xiăn rán zhī shī yŏu shí. ér jīng wēi shàng bù yŭ yān. liăng jīng suŏ yán. shí èr jīng zhī chū rù qĭ zhĭ. qiăn shēn zuŏ yòu. jiāo cuò bù qí. qí xuè suí jīng shàng xià. yì cēn cī wú dìng. jīn rén zhĭ zhí tóng shēn cùn. yī zuŏ yòu yì zhí shù liáng. bìng bù yī jīng qū zhé. zé jīng fēi jīng ér xuè fēi xuè. cĭ yì shī yĕ. liăng jīng zhì bìng. yún mŏu bìng qŭ mŏu xuè zhĕ gù duō. qí yú zé zhĭ jīng ér bù zhĭ xuè. rú líng jué bìng piān yún. ĕr lōng qŭ shŏu yáng míng. yì gān qŭ zú shào yīn. jiē bù yán qí xuè. jīn zé mĕi bìng zhĭ dìng jĭ xuè. cĭ èr shī yĕ. liăng jīng lùn zhì. jĭng. xíng. shū. jīng. hé zuì zhòng. dōng cì jĭng. fán zhĭ yán mŏu jīng. ér bù yán mŏu xuè zhĕ. dà dū jiē zhĭ jĭng xíng wŭ zhĕ wéi yán. jīn zé jiē bù jiăng yĭ. cĭ sān shī yĕ. bŭ xiè zhī fă. nèi-jīng yún. xī zé nèi zhēn. wú lìng qì wŭ. jìng yĭ jiŭ liú. wú lìng xié bù. xī zé zhuăn zhēn. yĭ dé qì wéi gù. hòu hū yĭn zhēn. hū jìn năi qù. dà qì jiē chū wéi xiè. hū jìn nèi zhēn. jìng yĭ jiŭ liú. yĭ qì zhì wéi gù. hòu xī yĭn zhēn. qì bù dé chū. gè zài qí chù. tuī hé qí mén. lìng shén qì cún. dà qì liú zhĭ wéi bŭ. yòu bì yíng qí jīng qì. jí nèi ér xú chū. bù àn qí wĕi wéi xiè. suí qí jīng qì. xú nèi ér jí chū. jí àn qí wĕi wéi bŭ. qí fă duō duān. jīn zé zhuăn zhēn zhī shí. yĭ dà zhĭ tuī chū wéi xiè. cuō rù wéi bŭ. cĭ sì shī yĕ. nà zhēn zhī hòu. bì hòu qí qì. cì shí zhĕ. yīn qì lóng zhì năi qù zhēn. cì xū zhĕ. yáng qì lóng zhì năi chū zhēn. qì bù zhì. wú wèn qí shù. qì zhì jí qù zhī. wù fù zhēn. jīn zé shí shí zhuăn dòng. sì zhēn xià kuān zhuăn. ér hòu chū zhēn. bù wèn qì zhī zhì yŭ bù zhì. cĭ wŭ shī yĕ.

In their detailed discussions of the depots and palaces, of the conduits and their holes, and of the illnesses, the two classics *Ling[shu]* and the *Su[wen]* refer to the patterns of needling seven or eight times out of ten, while they refer to prescriptions and drugs only two or three times out of ten. That shows how much [the people] in high antiquity valued the method of needling. However, the "Way of the Needle" is difficult, while it is easy [to use] prescriptions and drugs. Also, the patients enjoy the intake of drugs, but they suffer from the needles. Hence, in later times the [use of] prescriptions and drugs flourished widely while nobody talked about the patterns of needling [anymore]. Nowadays, the application of the needles is marked by ten obvious losses, and that does not even include all the subtleties [that have been forgotten in the meantime]. When the two classics outline the origins and the ends of the twelve conduits, where they appear and where they stop, where they lie near the surface or in the depth, to the left or to the right, [all this shows that these vessels] are intertwined and have no uniform [courses]. Similarly, the holes [for inserting the needles are] located irregularly without any fixed order, following the upward and downward [courses] of the conduits. Nowadays, the people only grasp the [individually] standardized body inch,[1] and set up their measurements in straight [lines from] left or right. Never do they follow the curves and bends [in the courses] of the conduits. Thus, the conduits [they identify] are not the conduits [specified in the classics], and the holes [they identify] are not the holes [specified in the classics]. That is the first loss. When the two classics [refer to] the treatment of diseases, they do, of course, state quite often "in cases of such-and-such a disease, select such-and-such a hole". In all other cases, though, they refer to the conduits and not to the holes. As it is stated, for instance, ... in the chapter Juebing of the *Ling[shu]*: "... In cases of deafness, select the hand-yang-brilliance [conduit for treatment]", "in cases of a dry throat select the foot-minor-yin [conduit for treatment]." In all these [and many other] instances, [the classics] do not specify any particular hole. ... Nowadays, for each disease a number of holes are specified. That is the second loss. The two classics discuss the well, brook, transporter, stream, and confluence [insertion points located on the lower segments of the four extremities] with greatest emphasis. ... Whenever they speak of but a particular conduit, and do not mention a particular hole, they refer, for the most part, to one of the five [generic holes] such as well, brook, [etc.] Nowadays, these [holes] are not mentioned any longer at all. That is the third loss. On the methods of supplementing and draining, the *Nei jing* states: When [the patient] inhales, insert the needle. Do not allow the qi to be irritated [by confronting them during an exhalation]. Let [the needle] remain quietly in its position for a while. Do not allow evil qi to spread. [When the patient] inhales [again], twirl the needle because this way it collects qi [around itself]. Wait until [the patient] exhales and pull the needle [out of his skin]. With the completion of that exhalation, the needle should be removed. Large [quantities of] qi will leave [with the needle through the site of insertion]. That is drainage. [In order to supplement], one inserts the needle at the moment an exhalation ends. Let [the needle] remain in its position quietly for a while to let the qi arrive. Wait until an inhalation and withdraw the needle [because during an inhalation] the qi cannot leave, and they stay where they are. [Once the needle is removed, one uses one's fingers] to close the gate [that was opened by the needle] with some pressure, and cause the spirit qi to stay [inside]. Large [quantities of] qi [that were inserted together with the needle] will remain [inside too]. That is supplementation. [In the classics it is stated] further that if [one points the needle, upon its insertion], contrary to the [movement of the] qi in the vessels, inserts quickly and withdraws slowly without closing the wound [afterwards], that is draining. If [one inserts the needle] following the [direction of the movement of the] qi in the conduits, inserts slowly and withdraws quickly, and then presses the wound [in order to close it], that is supplementation. The methods [of draining and supplementing] follow many principles, but nowadays while [people] twirl the needle they use their thumbs to push [qi] out [of the vessels], and that is their draining. Or, they rub [the qi, while twirling the needle] into [the hole], and that is their supplementing. That is the fourth loss. After the needle has been inserted, one must wait until the qi [have arrived]. If one needles a repletion, yin qi must arrive in large quantities, and only then is the needle to be removed. If one needles a depletion, yang qi must arrive in large amounts before one may withdraw the needle. If no qi arrive [immediately, the needle is inserted] many times again and again, and it is withdrawn only – and not inserted again – when the qi have [finally] arrived. ... Nowadays, [the people] constantly twirl and move [the needle and do not let it remain quietly for a while]. As soon as the needle is lowered into [the flesh], it is twirled extensively, and then it is withdrawn again. Nobody asks whether the qi have arrived or not. That is the fifth loss.

Note

[1] As a person may be tall or short, corpulent or thin, a method was devised in ancient China to locate the insertion points for piercing in relation to the body size of an individual. It was assumed that the middle joint of the index finger, which is about one inch long, varies in its length in direct proportions with the size of the body. Hence, the length of this joint was defined as "individually standardized body inch".

10.c *Xú líng tāi xiān sheng yī shū quán jí* 1
徐靈胎先生醫書全集
(Yī xué yuán liú lùn 醫學源流論)
Zhēn jiǔ shī chuán lùn 針灸失傳論
On the Loss of the Tradition in Needling and Cauterization (II)

凡針之深淺。隨時不同。春氣在毛。夏氣在皮膚。秋氣在肌肉。冬氣在筋骨。故春夏刺淺。秋冬刺深。反此有害。今則不論四時。分寸各有定數。此六失也。古之用針。凡瘧疾。傷寒。寒熱咳嗽。一切臟腑七竅等病。無所不治。今則止治經脉形體痿痹屈伸等病而已。此七失也。古人刺法。取血甚多。靈樞血絡論言之最詳。而頭痛腰痛。尤必大瀉其血。凡血絡有邪者。必盡去之。若血射出而黑。必令變色。見赤血而止。否則病不除而反有害。今人則偶爾見血。病者醫者。已惶恐失據。病何由除。此八失也。內經刺法。有九變十二節。九變者。輸刺。遠道刺。經刺。絡刺。分刺。大寫刺。毛刺。巨刺。焠刺。十二節者。偶刺。報刺。恢刺。齊刺。揚刺。直針刺。輸刺。短刺。浮刺。陰刺。傍刺。贊刺。以上二十一法。視病所宜。不可更易。一法不備。則一

病不愈。今則祇直刺一法。此九失也。古之針制有九。鑱針。員針。鍉針。鋒針。鈹針。員利針。毫針。長針。大針。亦隨病所宜而用。一失其制。則病不應。今則大者如員針。小者如毫針而已。豈能治痼疾暴氣。此十失也。

七竅	qī qiào	the seven orifices
腰痛	yāo tòng	lumbar pain
血絡	xuě luò	the blood [vessel] network
射	shè	to shoot; to spurt
惶恐	huáng kǒng	to fear; to be frightened
失據	shī jù	to lose one's orientation (for instance, due to fright)
九變^	jiǔ biàn	the nine variations (in the method of piercing)
十二節	shí èr jié	the twelve sections (of the method of piercing)
輸刺	shū cì	piercing of transport [holes]; i.e. piercing of the five insertion points "well" through "confluence" in the distal extremities[1]
遠道刺	yuǎn dào cì	piercing from a distance; i.e. piercing at a point far away from the affected area
經刺	jīng cì	piercing of conduits; i.e. piercing of the conduit primarily affected by a disease
絡刺	luò cì	piercing of network [vessels]; i.e. piercing of small vessels in the region directly below the skin to drain blood
分刺	fēn cì	piercing of the partings [of the flesh]
大寫刺	dà xiè cì	piercing to induce drainage of large [quantities of pus or blood]
毛刺	máo cì	piercing [of the skin as cautiously as if with a] hair

巨刺	jù cì	grand piercing; i.e. piercing a site on the right side of the patient if the illness is located on the left, and vice versa
焠刺	cuì cì	cauterization piercing [with a heated needle]
偶刺	ǒu cì	paired piercing; i.e. piercing of two sites of pain on the back and front of a patient
報刺	bào cì	retaliation piercing; i.e. method to treat pain changing its location. A needle is inserted at a site of pain. The physician locates with his hand a second site of pain, withdraws the needle from the first and inserts it at the second site
恢刺	huī cì	broad piercing; i.e. piercing next to a cramped or painful sinew. The needle is moved back and forth to widen the opening at the insertion point
齊刺	qí cì	combination piercing; i.e. the insertion of one needle each to the left and right of a needle inserted directly into an affected area
揚刺	yáng cì	scattered piercing; i.e. the insertion of four needles around a first needle
直針刺	zhí zhēn cì	direct piercing; i.e. piercing into a lifted skinfold without damaging the flesh
輸刺	shū cì	transport piercing; i.e. fast and deep insertion and withdrawal of a needle
短刺	duǎn cì	short piercing; i.e. deep insertion of a needle until it comes close to a bone
浮刺	fú cì	surface piercing; i.e. a slanted superficial insertion
陰刺	yīn cì	yin piercing; i.e. piercing of the foot-minor-yin conduit on both its right and left course
傍刺	páng cì	side-wise piercing; i.e. piercing to the side of a needle already inserted
贊刺	zàn cì	supportive piercing; i.e. shallow piercing to drain blood and support the dispersion of pain and swelling

備	bèi	to master completely
制	zhì	design [of the needles]

Fán zhēn zhī shēn qiǎn. suí shí bù tóng. chūn qì zài máo. xià qì zài pí fū. qiū qì zài jī ròu. dōng qì zài jīn gǔ. gù chūn xià cì qiǎn. qiū dōng cì shēn. fǎn cǐ yǒu hài. jīn zé bù lùn sì shí. fēn cùn gè yǒu dìng shù. cǐ liù shī yě. gǔ zhī yòng zhēn. fán nüè jí. shāng hán. hán rè ké sòu. yí qiè zàng fǔ qī qiào děng bìng. wú suǒ bù zhì. jīn zé zhǐ zhì jīng mài xíng tǐ wěi bì qū shēn děng bìng ér yǐ. cǐ qī shī yě. gǔ rén cì fǎ. qǔ xuě shèn duō. líng shū xuě luò lùn yán zhī zuì xiáng. ér tóu tòng yāo tòng. yóu bì dà xiè qí xuě. fán xuě luò yǒu xié zhě. bì jìn qù zhī. ruò xuě shè chū ér hēi. bì lìng biàn sè. jiàn chì xuě ér zhǐ. foǔ zé bìng bù chú ér fǎn yǒu hài. jīn rén zé ǒu ěr jiàn xuě. bìng zhě yī zhě. yǐ huáng kǒng shī jù. bìng hé yóu chú. cǐ bā shī yě. nèi-jīng cì fǎ. yǒu jiǔ biàn shí èr jié. jiǔ biàn zhě. shū cì. yuǎn dào cì. jīng cì. luò cì. fēn cì. dà xiè cì. máo cì. jù cì. cuì cì. shí èr jié zhě. ǒu cì. bào cì. huī cì. qí cì. yáng cì. zhí zhēn cì. shū cì. duǎn cì. fú cì. yīn cì. páng cì. zàn cì. yǐ shàng èr shí yī fǎ. shì bìng suǒ yí. bù kě gèng yì. yì fǎ bù bèi. zé yí bìng bù yù. jīn zé zhǐ zhí cì yì fǎ. cǐ jiǔ shī yě. gǔ zhī zhēn zhì yǒu jiǔ. chán zhēn. yuán zhēn. dī zhēn. fēng zhēn. pī zhēn. yuán lì zhēn. háo zhēn. cháng zhēn. dà zhēn. yì suí bìng suǒ yí ér yòng. yì shī qí zhì. zé bìng bù yìng. jīn zé dà zhě rú yuán zhēn. xiǎo zhě rú háo zhēn ér yǐ. qǐ néng zhì gù jí bào qì. cǐ shí shī yě.

Whether [one inserts] a needle deeply or not depends on the different [requirements of the four] seasons. In spring, the qi are in the body hair. In summer, the qi are in the skin. In autumn, the qi are in the flesh. In winter, the qi are in the sinews and bones. Hence, piercing is shallow in spring and summer, while one pierces into the depth in autumn and winter. If one acts contrary to these [patterns], harm will result. Nowadays, [people] do not consider the four seasons. The number of tenths and inches [by which the needles are inserted] is always fixed [to be the same]. That is the sixth loss. In ancient times, the needles were used to treat all cases of *nüe*-disease, harm caused by cold, [fits of] cold and heat, cough, as well as all diseases affecting the depots, palaces, and the seven orifices. Nowadays, [the needles are used] only to treat the conduit-vessels and the physical body if they are affected by such diseases as limpness and blockage, [or those affecting one's ability] to bend and stretch [one's body]. That is the seventh loss. The piercing methods [employed] by the people in ancient times very often [included] bloodletting. That is outlined in great detail in the *Ling shu* in its discussion of the blood[-vessel] network.

In particular, in cases of headache and lumbar pain, one must drain blood in large quantities. Whenever some evil [qi] are located in the blood[-vessel] network, they must be eliminated completely. When the blood spurts out black [in color], one must let [it spurt] until the color has changed. When red blood appears one must stop [the flow]. If the [blood] is not [let in these quantities], the disease will not be removed, and, on the contrary, more harm will result. Nowadays, if people happen to see some blood, both patients and physicians are frightened and lose all orientation. How, then, can a disease be eliminated [under these circumstances]? That is the eighth loss. According to the *Nei jing*, the methods of piercing may undergo nine variations and may be divided into twelve sections. The nine variations include piercing transport [holes only], piercing from a distance, piercing conduits, piercing network [vessels], piercing the partings [of the flesh], piercing to induce drainage of large [amounts of pus or blood], piercing [the skin as cautiously as if with a] hair, grand piercing, and cauterization piercing. The twelve sections include paired piercing, retaliation piercing, broad piercing, combination piercing, scattered piercing, direct piercing, piercing transport [holes], short piercing, surface piercing, yin piercing, side-wise piercing, and supportive piercing. These twenty-one methods mentioned above [should be used] in accordance with the requirements of the diseases [to be treated]. One cannot exchange [one method] for another. If one fails to master one of these methods, even a single illness cannot be cured. Nowadays, [the people] cling to the one method of direct piercing. That is the ninth loss. In ancient times, the needles were shaped in nine [different ways, including] the chisel needle, the round needle, the arrowhead needle, the lance-point needle, the sword needle, the round-sharp needle, the hair needle, the long needle, and the large needle. They, too, were employed in accordance with the requirements of the diseases [to be treated]. Every time one misses the [correct] shape [of the needle to be used in a specific therapy], the disease will fail to respond [to the treatment]. Nowadays, [the people use] large [needles] like round needles, and small ones like hair needles. How could they treat chronic diseases or violent qi [successfully]? That is the tenth loss.

Note

[1] The following definitions of technical terms are based on the *Huang di nei jing*, *Ling shu*, treatise Guan zhen. It should be noted that different interpretations were developed for some of these terms in later times.

10.d *Gǔ jīn yī tǒng dà quán* 7
古今醫統大全
Huǒ zhēn 火鍼
Fire Needle

經曰。焠鍼者。以痳油滿盞。燈草令多如大指許叢。其燈火燒鍼頭。頻以痳油蘸其鍼。燒令通紅。用方有功。若不紅者。反損於人。不能去病。燒時令鍼頭低下。恐油熱傷手。先令他人燒鍼。醫者臨時用之。以免致手熱。纔覺鍼紅。醫則取鍼。先以鍼安穴上。自然乾。鍼之亦佳。凡行鍼點艾。相似以墨記之。使鍼時無差穴。道差則無功。火鍼甚難。須有臨陣之將心。方可行鍼。先以左手按定其穴。然後鍼之。切忌太深。深則反傷經絡。不可太淺。淺則治病無功。但消息取中也。凡大醉之後。不可用鍼。不適淺深。有害無利。凡行火鍼。必先安慰病人。令勿驚動。較之火鍼及灸。灸則直受艾灼燒。過痛則久也。火鍼雖則畏人。其鍼下疾。一鍼便去。不久也。凡下火鍼。一鍼之後。疾速換去。不可久留。尋即以左手速按鍼孔上。則疼止。不按則疼甚。火鍼不宜鍼脚氣。反加腫痛。不能行履。火鍼者。宜破癰疽發背。潰膿在內。外皮無頭者。

但按毒上軟處以潰膿。闊大者。按頭尾及中。以點記。宜下三鍼。决破出膿。一鍼腫上。不可按之。即以指從兩旁捺之。令膿隨手而出。或腫大膿多。鍼時須側身廻避。恐膿射出污身。

焠鍼	cuì zhēn	cauterizing needle
麻油	má yóu	hemp oil
盞	zhǎn	small bowl; numerical for lamps
燈草	dēng cǎo	reed used for lamp wicks
許	xǔ	about
叢	cóng	crowded; clump of herbs
燈火	dēng huǒ	the flame of a lamp
燒	shāo	to heat
鍼頭	zhēn tóu	the point of a needle
頻	pín	repeatedly
蘸	zhàn	to dip into
紅	hóng	red
低	dī	to hang down
臨時	lín shí	when the time has come
纔	cái	only when
鍼	zhēn	needle; to insert a needle
自然	zì rán	naturally; by itself
佳	jiā	excellent; good
點	diǎn	to light
艾	ài	moxa; common mugwort
墨	mò	ink
記	jì	to record; to mark
差	chā	to differ; to miss
陣	zhèn	battle order
將	jiāng	a general
切	qiè	particle used to add emphasis before a negative

消息	xiāo xí	ebb and flow; to act within the limits of one's assessment
火鍼	huǒ zhēn	the fire needle
安慰	ān wèi	to comfort
較	jiào	to compare
灼	zhuó	to cauterize
下	xià	to lower
一	yì	as soon as
換	huàn	to remove
尋	xún	subsequently
孔	kǒng	hole
發背	fā bèi	to develop on one's back (as a sore)
潰	kuì	to scatter; to disperse
闊大	kuò dà	capacious
捺	nà	to press heavily downwards
側身	cè shēn	to turn to the side; to turn half way round
廻避	huí bì	to turn away

Jīng yuē. cuì zhēn zhě. yǐ má yóu mǎn zhǎn. dēng cǎo lìng duō rú dà zhǐ xǔ cóng . qí dēng huǒ shāo zhēn tóu. pín yǐ má yóu zhàn qí zhēn. shāo lìng tōng hóng . yòng fāng yǒu gōng. ruò bù hóng zhě. fǎn sǔn yú rén. bù néng qù bìng. shāo shí lìng zhēn tóu dī xià. kǒng yóu rè shāng shǒu. xiān lìng tā rén shāo zhēn. yī zhě lín shí yòng zhī. yǐ miǎn zhì shǒu rè. cái jué zhēn hóng. yī zé qǔ zhēn. xiān yǐ zhēn ān xuè shàng. zì rán gān. zhēn zhī yì jiā. fán xíng zhēn diǎn ài. xiāng sì yǐ mò jì zhī. shǐ zhēn shí wú chā xuè. dào chā zé wú gōng. huǒ zhēn shèn nán. xū yǒu lín zhèn zhī jiāng xīn. fāng kě xíng zhēn. xiān yǐ zuǒ shǒu àn dìng qí xuè. rán hòu zhēn zhī. qiè jì tài shēn. shēn zé fǎn shāng jīng luò. bù kě tài qiǎn. qiǎn zé zhì bìng wú gōng. dàn xiāo xí qǔ zhōng yě. fán dà zuì zhī hòu. bù kě yòng zhēn. bù shì qiǎn shēn. yǒu hài wú lì. fán xíng huǒ zhēn. bì xiān ān wèi bìng rén. lìng wù jìng dòng. jiào zhī huǒ zhēn jí jiǔ. jiǔ zé zhí shòu ài zhuó shāo. guò tòng zé jiǔ yě. huǒ zhēn suī zé wèi rén. qí zhēn xià jí. yì zhēn biàn qù. bù jiǔ yě. fán xià huǒ zhēn. yì zhēn zhī hòu. jí sù huàn qù. bù kě jiǔ liú. xún jí yǐ zuǒ shǒu sù àn zhēn kǒng shàng. zé téng zhǐ. bù àn zé téng shèn. huǒ zhēn bù yí zhēn jiǎo qì. fǎn jiā zhǒng tòng. bù néng xíng lǚ. huǒ zhēn zhě. yí pò yōng jū fā bèi. kuì nóng zài nèi. wài pí wú tóu zhě. dàn àn dú shàng ruǎn chù yǐ kuì nóng. kuò dà zhě. àn tóu wěi jí zhōng. yǐ diǎn jì. yí xià sān zhēn. jué pò chū nóng. yì zhēn zhǒng shàng. bù kě àn zhī. jí yǐ zhǐ cóng liǎng páng nà zhī. lìng nóng suí shǒu ér chū. huò zhǒng dà nóng duō. zhēn shí xū cè shēn huí bì. kǒng nóng shè chū wū shēn.

The Classic states: [To prepare] a cauterizing needle, [the following procedure is to be carried out]. A small bowl is filled with hemp-oil and with a clump of lamp [wick] reed of about the size of a thumb. While the point of the needle is heated in the flame of the lamp, it is dipped repeatedly into the hemp oil. The needle is heated until it is red through and through. If used right in this moment, it will show its [desired] effect. If it is not red [through and through], it will – contrary [to one's intentions] – cause harm to the person [treated], and will not be able to eliminate the illness. During the heating, the point of the needle is directed downwards, so that the heat of the oil may not harm the hand [holding the needle]. Prior [to the treatment], one asks someone else to heat the needle. The physician takes it [only] at the moment of [his applying it], thereby avoiding that his hand becomes hot. Only when he realizes that the needle is red, the physician takes it. He first places the needle above the hole [to be pierced], and it is best to wait until the [oil on the needle] has dried out by itself before one [inserts the] needle. Whenever one is about to apply the [fire] needle, one should light some moxa [on the location to be pierced]. That [allows for an identification of the insertion point to be pierced] as if one had marked it with ink, and one will not miss this hole at the moment the needle is to be inserted. If the [correct] path is missed, [the treatment will have] no effect. The [application of the] fire needle is very difficult. One should have the mind of a general facing a battle order: only then can the needle be set in action. One begins by pressing one's left hand on the hole, thereby fixing it, and then needles it. One must not [insert] too deeply; a deep [insertion] will – contrary [to one's intentions] – harm conduits and network [vessels. Also,] one must not [leave the needle] too close to the surface. If it remains near the surface, the treatment of the illness will show no effect. Within the limits of one's assessment, one takes a central [position between too deep and too shallow]. One must never use the needle after [one has drunk enough wine to be] highly intoxicated. If the requirements of shallow and deep [needling] are not met, [a treatment] will cause harm, but no benefits. Before a fire-needle is applied, one should always comfort the patient, so that he does not move out of fear. One should compare for him the fire-needle with [moxa] cauterization. [In cases of moxa] cauterization, [the patient] receives the moxa burning directly [on his skin]. After the application of the heat one has to endure the pain for a long time. The fire-needle may appear dreadful to some, but the needle is inserted quickly, and so soon as the needling occurs, [the needle] is removed again. It does not stay for long. Whenever the fire-needle is lowered [into the skin], after the needling has occurred, the [needle] is quickly removed again, and must not remain [in the skin for] long. Immediately [after it has been removed], one quickly presses one's left hand on the needling hole, and the pain stops. If one fails to apply this pressure, the pain will be tremendous. A fire-needle is inappropriate to needle qi [that have accumulated in the] legs. On the contrary, it would increase the swelling and the pain, and [the person treated this way] would be unable to walk. The fire-needle is suitable in breaking welling and deep-seated abscesses developing on one's back, and in eliminating the pus inside [the body. In cases of abscesses where the pus below] the skin has not formed a head yet on the outside, one simply puts pressure on the soft spot above the poison in order to have the pus disperse [internally. Abscesses covering an] extensive area are pressed where [the pus forms] a head, also at their ends and at their center in order to mark [the spots to be pierced]. Then three needles are inserted to break [such abscesses] open and have the pus come out. When a swelling is needled from above [its top], it should not be pressed there. [In this case] one must press this [location] heavily with one's fingers from both sides and let the pus come out following [the movement of] one's hands. In some cases, when the swelling is large, with much pus, one should, at the moment of needling, turn half around and away [from the patient] so that one's body is not soiled when the pus spurts out.

10.e *Huáng dì nèi jīng, Líng shū* 39
黃帝內經·靈樞
Xuě luò lùn 血絡論
On Network [Vessels Filled With] Blood.

黃帝曰。願聞其奇邪而不在經者。岐伯曰。血絡是也。黃帝曰。刺血絡而仆者何也。血出而射者何也。血少。黑而濁者何也。血出清而半爲汁者何也。發鍼而腫者何也。血出若多若少。而面色蒼蒼者何也。發鍼而面色不變。而煩悗者何也。多出血而不動搖者何也。願聞其故。岐伯曰。脈氣盛而血虛者。刺之則脫氣。脫氣則仆。血氣俱盛。而陰氣多者其血滑。刺之則射。陽氣畜積。久留而不寫者。其血黑以濁。故不能射。新飲而液滲于絡。而未合和于血也。故血出而汁別焉。其不新飲者。身中有水。久則爲腫。陰氣積于陽。其氣因于絡。故刺之血未出而氣先行。故腫。陰陽之氣。其新相得而未和合。因而寫之。則陰陽俱脫。表裏相離。故脫色而蒼蒼然。刺之血出多。色不變而煩悗者。刺絡而虛經。虛經之屬于陰者。陰脫故煩悗。陰陽相得而合爲痹者。此爲內溢于經。外注于絡。如是者。陰陽俱

有餘。雖多出血。而弗能虛也。黃帝曰。相之奈何。岐伯曰。血脈者。盛堅橫以赤。上下無常處。小者如鍼。大者如筯。則而寫之萬全也。故無失數矣。失數而反。各如其度。黃帝曰。鍼入而肉著何也。岐伯曰。熱氣因于鍼。則鍼熱。熱則肉著于鍼。故堅焉。

奇邪	qí xié	irregular qi
仆	pū	to fall to the ground; to collapse
濁	zhuó	thick
發針	fā zhēn	to withdraw the needle
蒼蒼	cāng cāng	ashen
悗	mèn	frightened
寫	xiè	used here for 瀉 *xiè*, to drain
因	yīn	used here for 由 *yóu*, "originating from"
痹	bì	closure; blockage
相	xiàng	to examine with one's eyes
橫	héng	bulging
筯	zhù	chopstick
數	shù	short for 度數 *dù shù*: a pattern
度	dù	rule
著	zhù	to stick to; to adhere

Huáng-dì yuē. yuàn wén qí qí xié ér bù zài jīng zhě. qí bó yuē. xuě luò shī yě. huáng-dì yuē. cì xuě luò ér pū zhě hé yě. xuě chū ér shè zhě hé yě. xuě shǎo. hēi ér zhuó zhě hé yě. xuě chū qīng ér bàn wéi zhī zhě hé yě. fā zhēn ér zhǒng zhě hé yě. xuě chū ruò duō ruò shǎo. ér miàn sè cāng cāng zhě hé yě. fā zhēn ér miàn sè bù biàn. ér fán mèn zhě hé yě. duō chū xuě ér bù dòng yáo zhě hé yě. yuàn wén qí gù. qí bó yuē. mài qì shèng ér xuě xū zhě. cì zhī zé tuō qì. tuō qì zé pū. xuě qì jù shèng. ér yīn qì duō zhě qí xuě huá. cì zhī zé shè. yáng qì xù jī. jiǔ liú ér bù xiè zhě. qí xuě hēi yǐ zhuó. gù bù néng shè. xīn yǐn ér yè shèn yú luò. ér wèi hé hé yú xuě yě. gù xuě chū ér zhī bié yān. qí bù xīn yǐn zhě. shēn zhōng yǒu shuǐ. jiǔ zé wéi zhǒng. yīn qì jī yú yáng. qí qì yīn yú luò. gù cì zhī xuě wèi chū ér qì xiān xíng. gù zhǒng. yīn yáng zhī qì. qí xīn xiāng dé ér wèi hé hé. yīn ér xiè zhī. zé yīn yáng jù tuō. biǎo lǐ xiāng lí. gù tuō sè ér cāng cāng rán. cì zhī xuě chū duō. sè bù biàn ér fán mèn zhě. cì luò ér xū jīng. xū jīng zhī shǔ yú yīn zhě. yīn tuō gù fán mèn. yīn yáng xiāng dé ér hé wéi bì zhě. cǐ wéi nèi yì yú jīng. wài zhù yú luò. rú shī zhě. yīn yáng jù yǒu yú. suī duō chū xiě. ér fú néng xū yě. huáng-dì yuē. xiàng zhī nài hé. qí bó yuē. xuě mài zhě. shèng jiān héng yǐ chì. shàng xià wú cháng chù. xiǎo zhě rú zhēn. dà zhě rú jīn. zé ér xiè zhī wàn quán yě. gù wú shī shù yǐ. shī shù ér fǎn. gè rú qí dù. huáng-dì yuē. zhēn rù ér ròu zhù hé yě. qí bó yuē. rè qì yīn yú zhēn. zé zhēn rè. rè zé ròu zhù yú zhēn. gù jiān yān.

Huang Di: I should like to hear about those irregular evil [qi] that do not settle in the conduits.
Qi Bo: They are in the network [vessels that contain] blood.[1]
Huang Di: If one pierces a network [vessel containing] blood, and [the patient] collapses, why is that? If the blood spurts out [of such a vessel when pierced], why is that? If the blood comes out in small amounts [only, but is] black and thick, why is that? If the blood comes out [such that half of it is] pure [blood] while the other half is another liquid, why is that? If a swelling occurs after one has withdrawn the needle, why is that? If blood leaves [the patient's vessels] varying in larger or smaller quantities, and if the color of his face turns ashen, why is that? If at the moment one withdraws the needle, the [patient's] complexion does not change, but he feels distressed and frightened, why is that? If the blood is allowed to leave in large quantities, but [the patient remains completely] unmoved, why is that? I should like to inquire about the causes [of all these possibilities].
Qi Bo: If someone's vessels hold very [large quantities of] qi, while his blood is depleted, he will lose his qi as soon as [his vessels] are pierced. Once he has lost his qi, he will collapse. If both blood and qi are present in abundance, and if the yin qi [are present in particularly] large amounts, the [flow of the] blood is smooth, and it will spurt out as soon as [the vessels] are pierced.[2] If yang qi accumulate and remain [at one and the same place] for a long time, without being drained, the blood will turn black and thick, and, hence, cannot spurt out.[3] If [the patient] has drunk [some liquid] only a short while ago, and if this liquid has already flown into his network [vessels], but has not mixed with [the patient's] blood yet, these liquids will still separate from the blood when [the latter] leaves [the vessels]. If [the patient] has not drunk [any liquid] recently, and yet he retains water in his body for a long time, this will lead to swelling.

When yin qi gather in the yang [section], then these qi [leave the body] from the network [vessels]. Hence, if these [network vessels] are pierced, the [yin] qi will move [to the hole opened through the piercing] before the blood leaves [the body], and swelling will occur.[4] When the draining occurs at a moment where yin and yang qi have just contacted each other without forming a union yet, then [the patient] will lose both yin and yang [qi]. The [qi of the] exterior and interior [sections of the body] will separate from each other again, and as a result, [the patient] loses his complexion and turns ashen.[5] If one's piercing causes large quantities of blood to leave [the vessels], with the patient feeling distressed and frightened even though his complexion does not change, [in that case] one has pierced the network [vessels] but has caused a depletion in the conduits. Because the conduits that were depleted [this way] belong to the yin, yin [qi] are lost, and [the patient] feels distressed and frightened.[6] If [evil qi from the] yin and yang [regions] mix with each other, and cause a blockage, this causes them to flow into the conduits internally, and pour into the network [vessels] externally. As a result, both the yin and the yang [sections suffer from] superabundance [of evil qi], and this [superabundance] cannot be depleted even if large amounts of blood [are drained to] leave [the body].

Huang Di: What about a visual examination of the [network vessels containing blood]?

Qi Bo: When the blood vessels are filled [with evil qi], they are firm, bulging, and red. They turn upward and downward, without holding any regular place. If the smallest are like needles, and the largest are like chopsticks, then draining them will always have positive results. That is to say, [when piercing network vessels containing blood], one must never deviate from the correct pattern. If one loses the correct pattern, and acts contrary to it, all kinds [of negative consequences result] in accordance with the rules [outlined above].

Huang Di: When the flesh sticks to a needle inserted into it, why is that?

Qi Bo: That is because hot qi have followed the needle, and the needle has become hot as a result. When a needle is hot, the flesh will stick to it. Hence, the needle will [get stuck] firmly [in the flesh, and it will be difficult to twirl it].

Notes

[1] *Huang Di nei jing*, *Su wen* treatise 62, Miu ci lun 繆刺論, states: "When evil [qi] reside in the hair of the skin, they enter [the body] and settle in the secondary network [vessels].There they stay, and do not leave. They cause obstructions blocking all passage. They cannot enter the conduts and flow into the major network [vessels] where they cause irregular diseases." Zhang Jingyue 張景岳 explained in his *Lei jing* 類經: "The network [vessels containing] blood are the network vessels (*luò mài*) and secondary network [vessels, *sūn luò*] that can be seen in the skin."

[2] "That is to say, both the innerbody and the outerbody conduits and vessels are all filled with blood

and qi, but the yin qi in the vessels are especially abundant. Hence, the flow of the blood is smooth and unobstructed, and it will spurt out as soon as a vessel is opened." Chen Biliu 陳壁琉 and Zheng Zhuoren 鄭桌人: *Ling shu jing bai hua jie* 靈樞經白話解, Hongkong, n.d., p. 302.

[3] Zhang Jingyue: "If yang qi remain [at one and the same place] for a long time, and are not drained, yang evil will be increasingly abundant day by day, while the yin blood will dry up at the same time. Hence, the blood turns black and thick. It will leave [- if a vessel is pierced -] in small amounts only and cannot spurt."

[4] Zhang Yin'an 張隱庵 (1610-1674?) stated in his *Ling shu ji zhu* 靈樞集注 of 1672: "The depots, the palaces, the conduits, and the vessels are yin. The skin, the flesh, and the striations are yang. If the yin qi of the depots and palaces accumulate in the yang section of the skin, and if these qi leave [the body] from the major and secondary network [vessels], that is, if the qi move first before the blood leaves [the body], then this is a situation where the qi of the depots and palaces move first and the blood leaves [the body] following the qi."

[5] "If a draining of the vessels is performed at the moment when the camp qi and the guardian qi, as well as the blood and the [regular] qi, are about to merge but have not formed a complete union yet, then the blood, the guardian [qi], and the camp qi all separate and disperse." Chen Biliu and Zheng Zhuoren, Hongkong, n.d., 30.

[6] Zhang Jingyue: "If one wishes to drain blood, one pierces [the patient's] network [vessels]. If too much blood [is allowed] to leave [the body], this will cause a depletion in the conduits. The conduits are yin, and they govern the depots. A depletion in the depots signals a loss of yin [qi]. Hence, [the patient] is distressed and frightened."

[7] Early editions of this text have 筋 *jīn*, "sinew". More recent commentaries read this character as 筯 *zhù*, "chopstick".

10.f *Yī shuō* 2 醫說 Mén fù zhēn ér 捫腹鍼兒 Touching the Abdomen and Needling a Child

朱新仲祖居桐城。時親戚間有一婦人。娠孕將產。七日而子不下。藥餌符水無不用。待死而已。名醫李幾道偶在朱公舍。朱引至婦人家視之。李曰。此百藥無所施。惟有鍼法。吾藝未至此。不敢措手爾。遂還。而幾道之師龐安常。適過門。遂同謁朱。朱告之故。曰。其家不敢屈公。然人命至重。公能不惜一行救之否。安常許諾。相與同往。才見孕者。即連呼曰不死。令其家人以湯溫其腰腹間。安常以手上下拊摩之。孕者覺腸胃微痛。呻吟間生一男子。母子皆無恙。其家驚喜拜謝。敬之如神。而不知其所以然。安常曰。兒已出胞。而一手誤執母腸胃。不復能脫。故雖投藥而無益。適吾隔腸捫兒手所在。鍼其虎口。兒既痛。即縮手。所以遽生。無他術也。試令取兒視之。右手虎口有鍼痕。其妙如此。

朱新仲	zhū xīn zhòng	Zhu Xinzhong, style-name of Zhū Yi 朱翌 (1097-1167), a Song era official and literatus

祖	zǔ	ancestor; grandfather
桐城	tóng chéng	the city of Tong in Anhui province
親戚	qīn qì	relatives
妊孕	rèn yùn	pregnant
餌	ěr	cake
符水	fú shuǐ	amulet [dissolved in] water
李幾道	Lǐ Jǐdào	name of an otherwise unknown physician
公	gōng	a gentleman; Sir; Mr.
藝	yì	skill
措手	cuò shǒu	to set the hand to
還	huán	to return
龐安常	páng ān cháng	Pang Anchang, style-name of Páng Ānshi龐安時
謁	yè	to visit
故	gù	fact
屈	qū	to bother
惜	xī	to pity
許諾	xǔ nuò	to promise
相與	xiāng yǔ	together
才	cái	then; just then
連	lián	at once
拊摩	fǔ mó	to pat
吟	yín	to moan
恙	yàng	illness; indisposition
拜謝	bài xiè	to thank
敬	jìng	to revere
隔	gé	to push aside
縮	suō	to draw in
遽	jù	suddenly; immediately
試	shì	to examine
痕	hén	a scar; mark

Zhū xīn zhòng zǔ jū tóng chéng. shí qīn qì jiān yǒu yí fù rén. rèn yùn jiāng chǎn. qī rì ér zǐ bù xià. yào ěr fú shuǐ wú bù yòng. dái sǐ ér yǐ. míng yī lǐ jǐ dào ǒu zài zhū gōng shě. zhū yǐn zhì fù rén jiā shì zhī. lǐ yuē. cǐ bǎi yào wú suǒ shī. wéi yǒu zhēn fǎ. wū yì wèi zhì cǐ. bù gǎn cuò shǒu ěr. suí huán. ér jǐ dào zhī shī páng ān cháng. shì guò mén. suí tóng yè zhū. zhū gào zhī gù. yuē. qí ji ā bù gǎn qū gōng. rán rén mìng zhì zhòng. gōng néng bù xī yì xíng jiù zhī foǔ. ān cháng xǔ nuò. xiāng yǔ tóng wǎng. cái jiàn yùn zhě. jí lián hū yuē bù sǐ. lìng qí jiā rén yǐ tāng wēn qí yāo fù jiān. ān cháng yǐ shǒu shàng xià fǔ mó zhī. yùn zhě jué cháng wèi wēi tòng. shēn yín jiān shēng yì nán zǐ. mǔ zǐ jiē wú yàng. qí jiā jìng xǐ bài xiè. jìng zhī rú shén. ér bù zhī qí suǒ yǐ rán. ān cháng yuē. ér yǐ chū bāo. ér yì shǒu wù zhí mǔ cháng wèi. bù fù néng tuō. gù suī tóu yào ér wú yì. shì wū gé cháng mén ér shǒu suǒ zài. zhēn qí hǔ kǒu. ér jì tòng. jí suō shǒu. suǒ yǐ jù shēng. wú tā shù yě. shì lìng qǔ ér shì zhī. yòu shǒu hǔ kǒu yǒu zhēn hén. qí miào rú cǐ.

Zhu Xinzhong's grandfather lived in the city of Tong. At one time, a pregnant woman among his relatives was about to deliver. After seven days the child had still not come down. Cakes filled with drugs, amulets dissolved in water, everything was used on her. Finally, she awaited only her death. Coincidentally, the renowned physician Li Jidao resided at Mr. Zhu's [home], and Zhu took him to the home of that woman to take a look at her. Li said: "No drug could be of use here, only needling [may bring help]. My own skills have not yet reached [the level needed] in this case; I do not dare to set my hand to her." Hence, he went back again, and it happened that [Li] Jidao's teacher, Pang Anchang, just passed by the gate, and [Li and Pang] together went to see Zhu. Zhu informed [Pang] of what had happened, and said [to him]: "Her family would never dare to bother you, Sir! Still, human life is most important. Sir, could not you feel pity with her, and proceed to her immediately to save her?" [Pang] Anchang promised [to do so], and joined the others to proceed [to the patient]. As soon as he saw the pregnant [woman] he exclaimed: "She need not die!" Then [Pang] Anchang asked one of the family to warm the [patient's] waist and abdomen with hot water, and he patted her upper and lower [waist and abdomen] with his hands. The pregnant [woman] felt a slight pain around her intestines and stomach, and amidst her moaning and groaning she gave birth to a male child. Mother and child were both well. Her family was both startled and happy, and they expressed their gratitude. They revered [Pang] as if he were a spirit, but nobody knew how he had done this. [Pang] Anchang said: "The child had left the womb already when one of its hands inadvertently grasped the mother's intestines and stomach. Hence, it could not separate itself. Consequently, even though she was given drugs, this was of no use. Just now, I pushed her intestines aside and felt for the child's hand. Then I needled its tiger mouth, whereupon the child felt some pain and drew its hand in, and was born immediately. There was no other technique involved." To test [his words] he asked the child to be brought, and examined its right hand. The tiger mouth [location] had a mark resulting from a needle. [Pang Anchang's skills] were as miraculous as this.

Appendix

Special Research Aids

A. General Survey

I. Dictionaries – Glossaries

I.1. General

Ying Han Han Ying Zhong Yi Ci Dian
英漢漢英中醫詞典

Zhong Guo Yi Xue Da Ci Dian
中國醫學大辭典

Zhong Yi Da Ci Dian
中醫大辭典

Zhong Guo Yi Xue Bai Ke Quan Shu
中國醫學百科全書

Zhong Guo Yi Xue Bai Ke Quan Shu
中國醫學百科全書

Zhong Guo Da Bai Ke Quan Shu·Zhong Guo Chuan Tong Yi Xue
中國大百科全書·中國傳統醫學

Zhong Guo Da Bai Ke Quan Shu·Zhong Yi
中國大百科全書·中醫

Jian Ming Zhong Yi Ci Dian
簡明中醫辭典

I.2. Pharmaceutical

Zhong Hua Ben Cao
中華本草

Zhong Hua Ben Cao Jing Xuan Ben
中華本草·精選本

Xian Dai Zhong Yao Xue Da Ci Dian
現代中藥學大辭典

Zhong Yao Da Ci Dian
中藥大辭典

Zhong Guo Yao Xue Da Ci Dian
中國藥學大辭典

Jian Ming Zhong Yao Yao Ming Ci Dian
簡明中藥藥名詞典

Zhong Yao Yao Li Da Ci Dian
中藥藥理大辭典

Zhong Yi Fang Ji Da Ci Dian
中醫方劑大辭典

I.3. Further Selected Topics

Zhong Guo Qi Gong Ci Dian
中國氣功詞典

Zhong Yi Ming Ci Shu Yu Xuan Shi
中醫名詞術語選釋

Gu Dai Ji Bing Ming Hou Shu Yi
古代疾病名候疏義

Zhong Xi Bing Ming Dui Zhao Biao
中西病名對照表

Zu Guo Yi Xue Yu Xian Dai Yi Xue Bing Zheng Ming Cheng Dui Zhao
祖國醫學與現代醫學病症名稱對照

Gu Dai Er Ke Ji Bing Xin Lun
古代兒科疾病新論

Zhong Yi Ming Ci Ci Dian
中醫名詞辭典

Historisch-Terminologisches Wörterbuch der Yüan-Zeit: Medizinwesen

Les Caractères Médicaux Dans L'Écriture Chinoises

Schriftzeichenanalysen medizinischer Termini technici in der chinesischen Sprache

Zhong Yi Ming Yan Ci Dian
中醫名言辭典

Huang Di Nei Jing Ci Dian "Dictionary of the Huang Di Nei Jing
黄帝內經辭典

Nei Jing Ci Dian "Dictionary of the Nei Jing"
內經辭典

Zhong Guo Yi Ji Zi Dian
中國醫籍字典

Yi Yong Gu Han Yu Zi Dian
醫用古漢語字典

Zhong Yi Nan Zi Zi Dian
中醫難字字典

I.4. Chinese-English

Han Ying Chang Yong Zhong Yi Yao Da Ci Hui
漢英常用中醫藥詞滙

Han Ying Chang Yong Yi Xue Ci Hui
漢英常用醫學詞滙

Han Ying Shuang Jie Chang Yong Zhong Yi Ming Ci Shu Yu
漢英雙解常用中醫名詞術語

II. Bibliographies

II.1. General

Zhong Guo Yi Ji Kao
中國醫籍考

Chugoku Isho Honzō -ko
中國醫書本草考

Zhong Guo Yi Xue Shu Mu
中國醫學書目

Xu Zhong Guo Yi Xue Shu Mu
續中國醫學書目

Zhong Yi Tu Shu Lian He Mu Lu
中醫圖書聯合目錄

Quan Guo Zhong Yi Tu Shu Lian He Mu Lu
全國中醫圖書聯合目錄

Zhong Guo Yi Ji Ti Yao
中國醫籍提要

Zhong Yi Gu Ji Zhen Ben Ti Yao
中醫古籍珍本提要

中國分省醫籍考
Zhong Guo Fen Sheng Yi Ji Kao

II.2. Pharmaceutical

Xian Cun Ben Cao Shu Lu
現存本草書錄

Medicine in China. A History of Pharmaceutics

Li Dai Zhong Yao Wen Xian Jing Hua
歷代中藥文獻精華

II.3. Further Selected Areas/Periods

Song Yi Qian Yi Ji Kao
宋以前醫籍考

San Bai Zhong Yi Ji Lu
三百種醫籍錄

Hebei Yi Ji Kao
河北醫籍考

Zhong Yi Wai Ke Yi Ji Cun Yi Kao
中醫外科醫籍存佚考

II.4. Secondary Sources

Yi Xue Shi Lun Wen Zi Liao Suo Yin (1903-1978)
醫學史論文資料索引

Zhong Guo Yi Shi Wai Wen Wen Xian Suo Yin
中國醫史外文文獻索引

Zhong Guo Yi Xue Wai Wen Zhu Shu Shu Mu
中國醫學外文著述書目

III. Biographies

III.1. General

Zhong Guo Li Dai Yi Jia Zhuan Lu
中國歷代醫家傳錄

Zhong Yi Ren Ming Ci Dian
中醫人名辭典

Zhong Yi Ren Wu Ci Dian
中醫人物詞典

Zhong Guo Yi Xue Ren Ming Zhi
中國醫學人名誌

Zhong Guo Li Dai Ming Yi Lu
中國歷代名醫錄

Zhong Guo Li Dai Ming Yi Zhuan
中國歷代名醫傳

III.2. Selected Groups

Sichuan Yi Lin Ren Wu
四川醫林人物

IV. Miscellaneous

Zhong Guo Li Dai Yi Shi
中國歷代醫史

Zhong Guo Yi Shi Nian Biao
中國醫史年表

Zhong Yi Chang Yong Gong Ju Shu Shou Ce
中醫常用工具書手

B. Detailed Survey

I. Dictionaries – Glossaries

I.1. General

Ying Han Han Ying Zhong Yi Ci Dian 英漢漢英中醫詞典 "English-Chinese Chinese-English Dictionary of Chinese Medicine" by Nigel Wiseman. Publisher: Hunan Science and Technology Press 湖南科學技術出版社. Forewords by Chen Keji 陳可冀 and Paul Unschuld. Author's preface dated February 1995. First edition: 1995. 1 vol. 105 + 805 pp. 2 indexes: Pinyin Index, Stroke Index.

This dictionary offers a comprehensive listing (pp. 1-387) of English terms associated with Chinese medicine and their original Chinese equivalents, and of Chinese medical terms and their English equivalents (pp. 391-770). Soon after its publication, this dictionary became a standard tool for translators seeking meaningful and standardized English equivalents for Chinese medical terms and concepts. Based on his familiarity with several European languages and with classic and contemporary Chinese, and on his comprehensive knowledge of both the theoretical foundations and the clinical reality of Chinese medicine, Wiseman has compiled a work of unprecendeted standards. It includes more than 10,000 Chinese terms and the names of 2,000 formulas and 1,700 drugs, as well as of 1,500 needle insertion points. In the Chinese-English section, Chinese terms are ordered according to pinyin alphabet. For each term, Chinese characters are followed by pinyin pronunciation and English equivalent. Wiseman has chosen a pragmatic approach, mostly adopting literal translations, rarely offering interpretative renderings (as in "common cold" for *gǎn mào*). In his search for suitable English equivalents, he has occasionally brought historical English terms, obsolete in Western medicine for centuries, back to usage. Where Chinese terms are based on ancient metaphors which may no longer be recognized as such by today's Chinese readers, he offers modern interpretations in addition to a literal rendering (as in "viscus", "treasury", "storehouse" for zàng). Following recent trends, Latin identifications of Chinese herbs are given without their authors. A unique feature of this dictionary is its most detailed reflection, in a lenghty "Introduction", on "The Translation of Chinese Medical Terminology" (Chinese: pp. 1-35; English: pp. 37-80), with the following paragraphs: "Opposing Trends" (p.37), "Objects, Concepts, and Terms" (p. 40), "Chinese Medical Concepts" (p. 43), "Language and Terms" (p. 49), "Methods for translating terms" (p. 55), "Conclusion" (p. 78), and its list of "Commonly Used Characters of Chinese Medicine" (pp. 81-104). On these pages, Wiseman demonstrates his unparalleled competence as a Chinese medical linguist.

Zhong Guo Yi Xue Da Ci Dian 中國醫學大辭典 "Comprehensive Dictionary of Chinese Medicine" by Xie Guan 謝觀. Current publisher: Commercial Press Taiwan 臺灣商務印書館. Author's preface dated 1 January 1921. 4 vols., 4690 pp. + 127 pp. Supplement. Two indexes: stroke-number; four corners.
This is still the most comprehensive Chinese-Chinese dictionary of Chinese medicine. No Western language terms were employed to explain Chinese technical terms or identify drugs. Entries on herbal and animal drugs are accompanied by drawings of the original herbs and animals. A few anatomical features are illustrated by drawings as well. The dictionary includes biographical and bibliographical data. One of the features distinguishing this dictionary from all others is its detailed guide to the sources, indications, ingredients, and modes of preparation of a vast number of standard prescriptions. Explanations of technical terms are preceded by a reference to the source of their oldest known usage. The total number of entries exceeds seventy thousand.

Zhong Yi Da Ci Dian 中醫大辭典"Comprehensive Dictionary of Chinese Medicine" by Li Yongchun 李永春 et al. Publisher: People's Hygiene Press 人民衛生出版社, Beijing. First edition: see individual volumes. 8 vols. No. of pages: see individual volumes.
Vol. 1: "Theoretical Foundations" 基礎理論分冊. First edition: January 1982. 355 pp. Contains 5778 entries from areas such as functional units of the organism, conduits, pathology, diagnosis, treatment, and basic theory.
Vol. 2: "Internal Medicine" 內科分冊

Vol. 3: "Gynecology and Pediatrics" 婦科兒科分冊. First edition: July 1981. 215 pp. Contains 3917 entries from gynecology and pediatrics.
Vol. 4: "Standard Prescriptions" 方劑分冊. First edition: May 1983. 612 pp. Contains detailed descriptions of 7500 prescriptions from Chinese traditional medical literature. Each entry includes the name of a preparation, its original literary source, ingredients, pharmaceutical preparation, and therapeutic indications. An appendix offers a comparative survey of measures of length, measures of capacity, and weights from the Zhou dynasty to 1911.
Vol. 5: "Medical History and Literature" 醫史文獻分冊. First edition: October 1981. 276 pp. Contains 2589 entries on historical personalities in Chinese medicine, 2258 entries on Chinese traditional medical literature, and 234 entries on historical institutions and administration in Chinese medicine.
Vol. 6: "External Medicine. Bonesetting. Nose-Eyes-Mouth-Tongue-Ears" 外科骨科五官科分冊. First edition: April 1987. 295 pp. Contains 4218 entries on external medicine, traumatology, and otorhinolaryngology. Historical texts named here as references are given with time of compilation and author only if these data are not included in vol. 5 "Medical History and Literature". The same applies to historical recipes. If they are mentioned in vol. 4, "Standard Prescriptions", they are repeated here only with their names. If not, their composition is listed in full.
Vol. 7: "Chinese Drugs" 中藥分冊. First edition: October 1982. 437 pp. Contains 6995 entries on primary and secondary names of drugs, and their botanical, zoological, and mineralogical identification. Latin names are given for original herbs, animals, and specific drug ingredients.
Vol. 8: "Acupuncture/Moxibustion. Massage. Chinese Traditional Gymnastics. Maintenance of Life" 針灸推拿氣功養生分冊. First edition: March 1986. 222 pp. Contains 2660 entries from the realms of acumoxatherapy (including the conduits, insertion points, piercing and moxa patterns, and relevant human body parts), massage and other manual therapies, as well as qigong and maintenance-of-life techniques. Where appropriate, the entries offer explanations on the history and meaning of concepts and practices, and define both traditional and contemporary technical terminology employed in the context of these practices.
All volumes have an alphabetical pinyin list of characters at the end, and a stroke-number index to Chinese characters, as well as a stroke-number index to terms consisting of combined characters, at their beginning. Vol. 7 has an appendix with two additional indexes: a stroke-number index to names of original herbs and animals used to prepare drugs, and a stroke-number index to the names of drugs referred to within the entries on other drugs.

Zhong Guo Yi Xue Bai Ke Quan Shu 中國醫學百科全書 "Chinese Encyclopedia of Medicine" by a committee with Qian Xinzhong 錢信忠 as Editor-in-Chief. Publisher: Shanghai Science and Technology Press上海科學技術出版社. 17 *juan* in 17 volumes on Chinese Medicine published beginning with 1983. This is a comprehensive project undertaken to offer a broad spectrum of data on Chinese Medicine, Basic Medical Science, Clinical Medicine, Preventive Medicine, and some special medical issues. It covers all medical sub-disciplines and was compiled with a focus on the prevention and clinical treatment of illness. The total layout comprises 20 000 articles in 93 *juan*. The first 17 *juan* of the encyclopedia were planned to cover Chinese Medicine. The themes of the individual volumes were defined as follows. Those volumes that have been published are given here with their year of publication; the remaining were never written.

Historiography of Medicine   1987
Basic Theory of Chinese Medicine   1988
Chinese Pharmaceutical Sciences   1988
Prescriptions in Chinese Medicine   1988
Internal Medicine   1988
Gynecology   1983
Pediatrics   1983
External Medicine   1985
Bone-setting and Traumatology
Ophthalmology   1985
Otorhinolaryngology   1984
Acupuncture   1988
Qigong   1988
Tuina Push-and-Pull Massage   1987
Mongolian Medicine
Tibetan Medicine
Uighur Medicine

Zhong Guo Yi Xue Bai Ke Quan Shu 中國醫學百科全書 · 中醫學 "Chinese Encyclopedia of Medicine, Chinese Medicine" by "Chinese Medicine" Compilation Committee 《中醫學》編輯委員會, Editor-in-Chief: Shi Dianbang 施奠邦. Publisher: Shanghai Science and Technology Press上海科學技術出版社. First edition: 1997. 3 vol. 2371 pp. Two appendixes: Table of events in the history of Chinese Medicine and Prescriptions of all clinical disciplines. One stroke index to all entries.

Starting from the Chinese Encyclopedia of Medicine but leaving behind its division into single *juan* volumes, the present book offers a comprehensively rearranged and thoroughly revised version of the section on Chinese Medicine. The division into medical subdisciplines was discarded, some data were omitted, others have been added. The book is now divided into the following ten sections: general discourse, history of Chinese Medicine, basic theory, therapeutic principles and methods, Chinese materia medica, prescriptions, acupuncture, tuina push-and-pull-massage, qigong, clinical medicine. The number of entries amounts to less than in the original single-*juan* volumes edition, with some of the retained entries having been written anew.

Zhong Guo Da Bai Ke Quan Shu · Zhong Guo Chuan Tong Yi Xue 中國大百科全書·中國傳統醫學 "Encyclopedia of China. Chinese Traditional Medicine" by Shi Dianbang 施奠邦 (Ed.-in-Chief). Publisher: Encyclopedia of China Press 中國大百科出版社. First edition: 1992. 1 vol. 754 pp. Two appendixes: Table of major events in the history of Chinese traditional medicine and Comparative list of unabbreviated and abbreviated Chinese characters. 3 indexes: stroke index to the first Chinese character of each entry, index of articles (Englisch), and pinyin index to contents.
This is the first attempt in China to present the contents of Chinese Medicine in the form of a one volume encyclopedia. The sequence of entries in the main text follows the pinyin alphabetical order of first characters. Also, there are 1082 entries in accordance with the system of Chinese Medicine. All entries are accompanied by a corresponding English term. Some entries have a detailed illustration. Important entries are followed by a listing of references. The contents are categorized according to the following themes: Chinese traditional medicine, Chinese medical history, basic theory, diagnostic methods, differentiation of patho-conditions, therapeutic principles and methods, Chinese materia medica, acupuncture, tuina push-and-pull-massage, nourishment of life, illness patho-conditions. Each entry is accompanied by a precise description.

Zhong Guo Da Bai Ke Quan Shu · Zhong Yi 中國大百科全書 · 中醫 "Encyclopedia of China. Chinese Medicine" by Fu Shiyuan 傅世垣 (Ed.-in-Chief). Publisher: Encyclopedia of China Press 中國大百科全書出版社. First edition: 2000. 1 vol., 713 pp. Three appendixes: Table of major events in the history of Chinese Medicine, List of Major Medical Personalities in History; List of Major Writings from the History of Chinese Medicine. Three indexes: Stroke Index to Entries; Index of Articles in Foreign Languages, and Pinyin Index of Contents .

This is a revised edition of the "Encyclopedia of China. Chinese traditional medicine" *Zhong Guo Da Bai Ke Quan Shu Zhong Guo Chuan Tong Yi Xue* 中國大百科全書·中國傳統醫學 listed above. It has added 213 new entries to the 609 entries of the former version, offering a total of 822 entries. Some of the illustrations have been corrected, others have been added. Two sections of the main text are new: "List of frequently used Chinese drugs" 常用中藥表, and "List of frequently used recipes" 常用方劑表. The contents are even more concise and accurate than in the old edition.

Jian Ming Zhong Yi Ci Dian 簡明中醫辭典 "Concise Dictionary of Chinese Medicine" by Guangzhou Chinese Medical College 廣州中醫學院, Chinese Medical Academy 中國中醫研究院. Publisher: Joint Publishing Co., Hong Kong Branch 三聯書店香港分店. First edition: September 1979. 1 vol., 1005 pp. One index: stroke-number.
This dictionary contains 12,176 entries from areas such as theoretical foundations, clinical application, acupuncture/moxibustion, Chinese pharmaceutics, prescriptions, personalities, and literature. Herbal and animal drugs are identified, in Latin, with the botanical and zoological names of the original herbs and animals respectively. Mineral drugs are identified with modern Chinese chemical terminology (no Latin formulas added). Sources of first known literary usage are given for most substances, standard prescriptions, and technical terms. An appendix includes three comparative lists of weights and measures of capacity, and a chronological table of Chinese dynasties.

I.2. Pharmaceutical

Zhong Hua Ben Cao 中華本草, "Chinese Materia Medica", by Administration of Chinese Medicine and Pharmaceutics Committee for the Compilation of a Materia Medica of China 國家中醫藥管理局中華本草編委會. Publisher: Shanghai Science and Technology Press 上海科學技術出版社. First edition: 1999. 30 *juan*, 10 vols. Eight indexes: index to Chinese names, index to scientific names of pharmaceutically used herbal, animal, and mineral substances, comparative table of Chinese and English names of chemical components, comparative table of English and Chinese names of chemical components, constitution diagrams of chemical components, index to pharmacological functions, index to pharmaceutical effects, index to pharmaceutical indications.
This book surveys the entire knowledge gathered in Chinese materia medica over the past 2000 years, in particular it reflects the advancements of phar-

maceutical science in the 20th century and constitutes the most comprehensive reference book on Chinese materia medica compiled on the Chinese mainland since 1949. The book is divided into the four parts: General Introduction, Pharmaceutical Substances, Appendixes, and Indexes. The General Introduction comprises 1 *juan* and is divided into 14 sections: history of materia medica, natural resources of Chinese materia medica, cultivation of Chinese materia medica, collection of Chinese materia medica, storage of Chinese materia medica, categories of Chinese materia medica, varieties of Chinese materia medica, identification of Chinese materia medica, chemistry of Chinese materia medica, pharmacology of Chinese materia medica, pharmaceutical preparation of Chinese materia medica, preparations of Chinese materia medica, composition of Chinese materia medica, properties of Chinese materia medica. The section on Pharmaceutical Substances comprises 26 *juan* and distinguishes between the three groups of mineral substances, herbal substances, and animal substances. The mineral substances are ordered in the sequence of their actions, plants and animals in accordance with their natural classes. The total number of substances listed is 8980, with 8534 illustrations, based on more than 10,000 literary sources. Each drug monograph addresses the following 23 parameters: proper name, secondary name(s), explanation of name(s), literary research on varieties, geographic origin, original plant/ animal/ mineral, essentials of cultivation, collection and processing, production and marketing of drug material, differentiation of drug material, chemical components, pharmacology, pharmaceutical preparation, drug qualities, effects and indications, application and composition [in recipes with other drugs], usage and dosage, advise for usage, recipes, fixed medications, current clinical research, historical discourses, various explanations by earlier authors. The appendix comprises 1 *juan* and is divided into 4 parts: Drugs of unknown identity, various prefaces/prolegomena to historical *ben cao* 本草 works, remarks on major works on materia medica in history, bibliography of historical materia medica works. The eight indexes are provided in the final two *juan*.

Zhong Hua Ben Cao Jing Xuan Ben 中華本草·精選本 "Materia Medica of China. A Volume on Carefully Selected Samples". By State Administration of Chinese Medicine and Pharmaceutics Committee for the Compilation of a Materia Medica of China 國家中醫藥管理局中華本草編委會. Publisher: Shanghai Science and Technology Press 上海科學技術出版社. First edition: 1998. 2 vols. 2630 pp. 3 indexes: index to Chinese names of materia medica, index to scientific names of plants, animals, and minerals used for Chinese materia medica, and index to classified effects of Chinese materia medica.

This book was compiled on the basis of the Materia Medica of China, *Zhong Hua Ben Cao* 中華本草. It focusses on a selection of only the most important data, and is divided into three parts: General discourse, materia medica, and indexes. In comparison with the *Zhong Hua Ben Cao* 中華本草, the "general discourse" of the present book comprises only ten themes, it has omitted the sections on gathering and storing, the chemistry, and the pharmacology of Chinese materia medica. The total number of pharmaceutical drugs selected is 535. The number of indexes was limited to three. The classification and the structure of drug monographs is identical with that in the *Zhong Hua Ben Cao* 中華本草.

Xian Dai Zhong Yao Xue Da Ci Dian 現代中藥學大辭典 "Comprehensive Dictionary of Modern Chinese Pharmaceutics" by Song Liren 宋立人et al. Publisher: People's Hygiene Press 人民衛生出版社. First edition: 2001. 2 vols. with ca. 4,400 pp. 3 indexes: Stroke-number table of contents; stroke-number index of drug names; alphabetical index of Latin identifications of Chinese pharmaceutical substances.
This dictionary combines 2254 entries of substances used in Chinese traditional materia medica, 969 entries of technical terms used in Chinese traditional pharmaceutics, 264 entries of major pharmaceutical works of the past, as well as 103 entries of persons associated with the development of Chinese traditional pharmaceutics. The two volumes include 1117 illustrations. Each entry of pharmaceutical substances includes (1) the proper name, secondary names, and general description in traditional terms; (2) original plant, animal, or mineral; (3) proper cultivation; (4) pharmaceutical processing of raw drugs; (5) pharmaceutical preparation of processed drugs; (6) description and names of pharmaceutical end product; (7) traditional modes of preparation; (8) modern findings of effective constituents; (9) pharmacology; (10) traditional description of properties; different effects resulting from different processing; internal and external dosages and amounts to be ingested by adults; (11) modern and historical notes on contraindications, synergism, prohibitions; main indications; (12) excerpts from ancient and modern literature on the nature and effects of a substance; (13) modern medications using the substance in question; (14) selected recipes; (15) clinical research. Entries of historical pharmaceutical works published prior to 1911 include title, alternative titles, author, date of publication, summary of contents, historical significance, and editions.

Zhong Yao Da Ci Dian 中藥大辭典 "Comprehensive Dictionary of Chinese Drugs" by committee, Jiangsu New Medical College. 江蘇新醫學院 Publisher:

Shanghai Science and Technology Press 上海科學技術出版社. First edition: October 1977. 3 vols. (2 vols. with together 2754 pp., containing drug monographs. 1 vol. with 764 pp., containing indexes). Six indexes:

1. stroke-number index to primary and secondary drug names
2. alphabetical indexes to the Latin scientific names of herbs and animals used in the preparation of Chinese drugs, and to the English names of minerals
3. alphabetical index to the active chemical ingredients identified in Chinese drugs
4. index to major pharmacological functions
5. index to illnesses and diseases prevented or cured by Chinese drugs listed in vols. 1 and 2

In addition, the third volume contains a comparative table of Chinese and English terms used to designate active chemical ingredients; a list of reference works used to compile the data on the active ingredients, the pharmacology, and the clinical application of the drugs listed in vols. 1 and 2, as well as a comparative table of ancient and contemporary measures.

The *Zhong Yao Da Ci Dian* is currently the most useful dictionary for data on Chinese drugs. It contains 5767 monographs with drawings illustrating original plants and animals. The individual monographs are subdivided into paragraphs relating both (selected) traditional and modern knowledge. The drugs are listed under the name given in the earliest Chinese pharmaceutical work mentioning them. Secondary names from medical and non-medical sources are quoted in addition. Further paragraphs include (where applicable) description of the drug, active ingredients, pharmacology; modes of preparation, flavor/thermo-quality (*wei/qi*)/toxicity, preferred conduit, major therapeutic effects, mode of application and dosage, contraindications, selected prescriptions from classical sources, reports on contemporary clinical successes, and miscellaneous notes from earlier authors.

Zhong Guo Yao Xue Da Ci Dian 中國藥學大辭典 "Comprehensive Dictionary of Chinese Pharmaceutics" by Chen Cunren 陳存仁. Current Publisher: Cyclone Press 旋風出版社, Taibei. 2 vols. 1981 pp. One index: stroke-number.

This dictionary is an early attempt to combine traditional Chinese knowledge with current Western knowledge. The author intended to write a work succeeding the *Ben Cao Gang Mu* as a standard work of Chinese traditional materia medica. He compiled an unspecified number of drug monographs with the goal of providing Chinese traditional materia medica with a foundation in modern science. Chen Cunren discarded as untimely all references to the ancient theories of the five agents. The drug monographs follow the structure of the *Ben Cao Gang Mu* in that they are subdivided into paragraphs discussing specific topics, including earliest known name of a drug, etymology of drug names, foreign scientific names, appearance, time of collecting original substances, modes of preparation, traditional qualities (flavor, thermo-quality, toxicity), herbal or animal or mineral origin, historical accounts, secondary names used in ancient literature, and (where applicable) active ingredients identified through chemical analysis. Much of the information provided may be outdated today. This dictionary is still useful, though, for its information on secondary names, and on the etymology of drug names, as well as many historical data referred to in the monographs. An extensive preface relates the introduction of Chinese traditional materia medica to Germany, England, Japan, and the USA. Appendixes include the following data: 1. Reports on chemical ingredients found in Chinese drugs by Japanese researchers. 2. A list of drugs grown in Sichuan and Zhejiang, their preferable geographic origins, and a survey of the quantities of drugs grown in these two provinces. 3. An explanation of technical terms employed in this dictionary. 4. An investigation of measures employed in ancient prescriptions. 5. A comparative list of ancient and current weights and measures of capacity. 6. A list of abbreviations employed in this dictionary. 7. Sources used in the compilation of this dictionary, in chronological order, from the *Shen Nong Ben Cao Jing* to publications of the 1920s and 1930s.

Jian Ming Zhong Yao Yao Ming Ci Dian 簡明中藥藥名詞典 "Concise Dictionary of Drug Names From Chinese Pharmacy" by Kuang Haixue 匡海學 and Sang Shurong 桑樹榮. Publisher: Heilongjiang Science and Technology Press 黑龍江科學技術出版社. First edition: 1988. 1 vol. 15 + 592 pp. 2 indexes: Stroke-number index (table of contents) of drug names referring to main entries. Stroke number index (appendix) of drug names referring to all substances named.
This is a survey of 861 frequently used pharmaceutical substances in Chinese traditional materia medica. Where applicable, the proper name of a substance is followed by data on its first appearance in a literary context, its origin in the animal, herbal, or mineral arena (with Latin identification of sources), its traditional assessment in terms of "nature", "qi", and effects, secondary names, and its designation in prescriptions as a processed drug. Regional and botanical/zoological variants, as well as processing variants are described too, bringing the total number of substances treated to 10,467.

Zhong Yao Yao Li Da Ci Dian 中藥藥理大辭典 "Comprehensive Dictionary of Chinese Pharmacy and Pharmacology" by Lu Kuisheng 陸奎生. Publisher: Eastern Book Co. 東方圖書公司. First edition: 1962. 1 vol. 280 pp. One index: stroke-number index to primary and secondary drug names.
An unspecified number of monographs includes information on the scientific name of the original substances, a description of the original substances, their places of origin, flavor/thermo-quality/toxicity, results of scientific analysis, major therapeutic indications, and dosage. Many of these data may have become outdated in the meantime or are listed comprehensively in the Zhong Yao Da Ci Dian. Still, this little book is of continuing value for its extensive introduction of 17 pages, with details on Chinese pharmaceutical technology, and the etymology of names, providing data that are hard to find elsewhere.

Zhong Yi Fang Ji Da Ci Dian 中醫方劑大辭典 "Comprehensive Dictionary of Chinese Recipes" by Peng Huairen 彭懷仁 et al. Publisher: People's Hygiene Press人民衛生出版社. First edition 1993. 11. volumes. Table of contents. 1 vol. of indexes.
Fixed recipes constitute one of the mainstays of Chinese pharmaceutics. This dictionary lists, in ten volumes, ca. 100,000 such recipes selected from ca. 1,800 works of two millennia of Chinese prescription literature. The oldest sources date from the Qin and Han dynasties; the most recent text excerpted was published in 1986. The 11th volume has the following indexes: index to all names of prescriptions; index to all names of patho-conditions; index to all source texts. Vol. 11 ends with a comparative table of ancient and modern units of measurement. Each entry offers data, where applicable, on the following issues: earliest textual source; alternative names; composition; preparation of ingredients; general indication; main indications; contraindications; additions and omissions vis-a-vis individual patho-conditions; selected explanations of composition, synergisms, differentiation of patho-conditions, etc.; selected clinical case histories; modern research results; additional information.

I.3. Further Selected Topics

Zhong Guo Qi Gong Ci Dian 中國氣功詞典 "Dictionary of Chinese Qigong" by Lü Guangrong 呂光榮 et al. Publisher: People's Hygiene Press 人民衛生出版社. First edition: 1988. 1 vol. 66 + 529 pp. 3 indexes: Stroke number index to table of contents. Stroke number index as table of contents. General index (appendix) with sections (1) Basic Theory, (2) Human body, conduits, holes, external locations, (3) Technical terms, (4) Qigong techniques, (5) Discourses

and literary sources, (6) Famous phrases, (7) Patho-conditions suitable for Qigong treatment, (8) Persons, (9) Books.
This dictionary has close to 6,000 entries with detailed explanations. The terms, phrases, titles, and designations included are characterized by the nine sections of the general index listed above.

Zhong Yi Ming Ci Shu Yu Xuan Shi 中醫名詞術語選釋 "An Explanation of Selected Phrases and Technical Terms from Chinese Medicine" by Guangdong Chinese Medical College 廣東中醫學院, Academy of Traditional Chinese Medicine 中醫研究院. Publisher: Knowledge Press 知識出版社, Hong Kong. First edition: not specified. 1 vol., 585 pp. One index: stroke-number.
This Chinese-Chinese dictionary contains 4285 entries. It is subdivided into twelve chapters devoted to the following topics:

1. Yinyang and the five agents
2. Structural Units of the Organism, and their Functions
3. Conduits and Categories of Acupuncture Points
4. Etiology and Pathology
5. Diagnostic Techniques
6. Rules of Treatment; Pharmacy; Prescriptions
7. Acupuncture and Moxibustion
8. Pediatrics
9. Gynecology
10. Injuries and External Medicine
11. Ear, Nose, Throat, and Eye Diseases
12. Medical History

This dictionary does not include references to historical personalities, names of drugs, names of prescriptions, and names of individual acupuncture points. An appendix contains 1. a list of explanations of eighty single-character terms commonly used in Chinese medicine; 2. a bibliography of traditional Chinese medical literature; 3. drawings of major parts of the body and the skeleton, with Chinese names of body parts, locations, bones, etc. shown in situ; and 4. comparative lists of ancient and contemporary weights and measures.

Gu Dai Ji Bing Ming Hou Shu Yi 古代疾病名候疏義 "Commentaries to the Names and Symptoms of Illnesses/Diseases in Ancient Times" by Yu Yan 余巖. Current publisher: Taiwan Free Publ. Co. 臺灣自由出版社, Taibei. Author's preface dated 1949. 1 vol. 369 pp. + 13 pp. Supplement + 73 pp. Index. 1 index: stroke-number index to the names of illnesses/diseases.
From 1937 through1947, the author has analysed the classic (non-medical) texts of ancient China to prepare a list of all illnesses/diseases mentioned, and

to explain (a) what the respective terms and phrases were meant to designate in their historical context, and (b) what pathological conditions in terms of modern medical science they may have stood for. The author attempted to avoid simplistic parallels, and to refrain from forced interpretations. The altogether 675 terms and phrases are grouped under six major headings, in accordance with the texts they were taken from: 1. *Er Ya* 爾雅(9); 2. *Fang Yan*方言 (15); 3. *Shuo Wen Jie Zi* 說文解字(354); 4. *Shi Ming* 釋名(55); 5. *Guang Ya* 廣雅 (49); 6. The Thirteen Classics: *Yi Jing* 易經 (13), *Shu Jing* 書經 (12), *Shi Jing* 詩經(42), *Zhou Li*周禮 (6), *Gu Liang Zhuan* 穀梁傳(4), *Xiao Jing*孝經, *Lun Yu*論語 and *Meng Zi*孟子 (together 8). The entire book was written in classic Chinese. German, English, and/or Latin terms are added to the explanations where applicable.

Zhong Xi Bing Ming Dui Zhao Biao 中西病名對照表 "Comparative Tables of Chinese and Western Names of Illnesses" by Ye Juquan 葉橘泉. Publisher: Arts and Book Co. 藝美圖書公司. First edition: April 1972. 1 vol. 75 pp. No index. General table of contents.
This book is devided into eleven sections: 1. Illnesses of the respiratory organs (30 entries). 2. Illnesses of the digestive organs (66 entries). 3. Illnesses of the urinary and reproductive organs (26 entries). 4. Illnesses of the circulatory organs, and of the blood (15 entries). 5. Illnesses affecting the nervous system (51 entries). 6. Metabolic illnesses (11 entries). 7. Polyarthritic, dermatological, and lymphatic illnesses (60 entries). 8. Illnesses affecting the ears (4 entries). 9. Illnesses affecting the eyes (14 entries). 10. Gynecological illnesses (27 entries). 11. Pediatric illnesses (17 entries). Each page is divided into an upper section listing traditional illness terms, a middle section quoting definitions of these terms from classic medical literature, and a lower section offering explanations in modern terms (no English equivalents given).

Zu Guo Yi Xue Yu Xian Dai Yi Xue Bing Zheng Ming Cheng Dui Zhao 祖國醫學與現代醫學病症名稱對照 "A Comparison of Terms for Illnesses and Symptoms from Our Native Medicine and Modern Medicine" by Zhang Ruixiang 張瑞祥 and Sun Jiaji 孫家驥. Publisher: Qinghai People's Press 青海人民出版社. Xining. First edition: February 1979. 1 vol. 45 pp. No index.
A listing of terms from Chinese traditional medicine with their supposed equivalents in modern scientific Chinese, English, and Latin terminology. The list is divided into five groups: 1. Inner Medicine and Pediatrics (109 terms and phrases). 2. External Medicine (69). 3. Obstetrics and Gynecology (30). 4. Dermatology (90). 5. Illnesses of the Five Orifices (60).

Gu Dai Er Ke Ji Bing Xin Lun 古代兒科疾病新論 “New Discussion of Illnesses/Diseases in Ancient Pediatrics” by Gao Jinglang 高鏡朗. Publisher: Shanghai Science and Technology Press 上海科學技術出版社. First edition: 1954. Second edition: July 1982. 1 vol. 145 pp. No index.
Grouped in five chapters, this little book lists 144 issues related to child health. The book is not designed as a dictionary for quick consultation on specific terms and phrases, rather it is a concise introduction to Chinese traditional pediatrics with an explanation of ancient terms and concepts, often on the basis of modern scientific interpretations. The five chapters, with their two to seven sub-paragraphs, carry the following headings:

I. “On Newborns” (1. “Management of Newborns”, 2. “The Illnesses of Newborns”)
II. “Upbringing and Nourishment” (1. “General Rules of Upbringing”, 2. “The Nourishment of Sucklings and Infaxnts”)
III. “Dietetic Illnesses (1. “Chronic Digestive Insufficiency”, 2. “Vitamin Deficiency Illnesses”)
IV. “Systems’ Illnesses” (1. “Illnesses of the Respiratory System”, 2. “Illnesses of the Throat”,3. “Illnesses of the Digestive System”, 4. “Illnesses of the Nervous System”, 5. “Illnesses of the Urinary System”, 6. “Illnesses of the Skin”, 7. “Illnesses of the Inner Secretory Glands”)
V. “Infectious Diseases” (1. “Epidemics”, 2. “Illnesses due to Bacteria”, 3. “Illnesses due to Viruses”, 4. “Illnesses du to Intestinal Parasites”, 5. “Illnesses due to Protozoons”, 6. “Illnesses due to Spirochaetas”, 7. “Illnesses due to Rickettsia”)

Zhong Yi Ming Ci Ci Dian 中醫名詞辭典 “Dictionary of Chinese Medical Terms” by Chen Xihe 陳西河. Publisher: Wuzhou Press 五洲出版社, Taibei. First edition: 1986. 1 vol. 204 pp. 1 index: stroke-number.
Chinese-Chinese dictionary of more than 2200 commonly used terms in Chinese medicine. Short entries with no attempts at Western, modern, or scientific explanations. Entirely traditional explanation of terms and concepts.

Historisch-Terminologisches Wörterbuch der Yüan-Zeit: Medizinwesen by Paul Ratchnevsky et al. Publisher: Akademie-Verlag Berlin. First edition: 1967. 1 vol. 118 pp. No index.
Alphabetical pinyin listing of more than 500 terms and phrases from Yuan dynasty sources, and their explanation in German. Also provided are explanations of titles and institutions, as well as data on eminent persons linked to medicine during the Mongol era. This *Wörterbuch* is particularly useful be-

cause the bibliographical sources underlying the information quoted in each entry are provided.

Les Caractères Médicaux Dans L'Écriture Chinoises by Docteur Lucien-Graux. Publisher : Les Éditions G. Grès & Cie, Paris. First edition : 1914. 1 vol. 276 pp. Table of contents. No index.
Following two short essays on the nature of the Chinese script in general, and on the radicals of Chinese characters in specific, the author offers etymological analyses of 270 single Chinese characters with medical, anatomical, or related meanings. Each entry starts with a transliteration of the Chinese pronunciation of the term (using the French system of romanization developed by Arnold Vissière), and a translation of the term. Where possible, the author applies Western medical terms of his time, but he also employs descriptive renderings. Next, the Chinese character is given, occasionally in addition to its standard version in an ancient form to clarify its meaning. The pictogram is followed by a text describing the general usage of the term, and relating the meaning of the pictogram to its actual pictographic message. No Chinese or Western sources are quoted. The volume contains several appendixes, including a translation (without source) of a "Chinese Opinion On Medicine", a listing of Chinese prescriptions, a listing of ten 19th century French works on Chinese medicine, and a listing of ten titles of Chinese medical classics with their authors. The volume is concluded by the table of contents.

Schriftzeichenanalysen medizinischer Termini technici in der chinesischen Sprache by Gottfried Schramm. Publisher: VEB Otto Harrassowitz, Leipzig. First edition: 1958. 1 vol. 107 pp. Table of contents, and index of German terms. No index of Chinese characters.
The author analyses 81 Chinese pictograms and combinations of pictograms with medical or related meaning. Each entry starts with the common form of the character discussed, and analyses, next, its structural elements, and the relationship of these elements with the meaning of the character. Etymological discussions of the terms from earlier Chinese and European sources are quoted, and one or more ancient pictographic predecessors of the common version of the pictograms are given where necessary. Quotes from ancient classics are added to further clarify the meaning of the terms.

Zhong Yi Ming Yan Ci Dian 中醫名言辭典 "Dictionary of Famous Statements in Chinese Medicine" by Qiu Peiran 裘沛然. Publisher: Hunan Science and Technology Press 湖南科學技術出版社. First edition: 1992. 1 vol. 924 pp. 3 indexes: Stroke-number indexes (1) to first appearance of first characters

of statements with page number, (2) to all statements (given in full text) with consecutive numerical reference to individual entries. Pinyin alphabetical index to transliteration of first appearance of first characters of statements.
This dictionary lists 2260 "famous statements" associated with Chinese medicine in the course of the past 2000 years. The statements, comprising one line to several lines of characters, are followed by a reference to their source text and a detailed explanation in Chinese. The index to all statements given in full text is particularly helpful in that it permits one not only to find phrases or statements one is aware of, but also to search for and find statements associated with a general theme one may be interested in.

Huang Di Nei Jing Ci Dian 黃帝內經辭典 "Dictionary of the Huang Di Nei Jing" by Guo Aichun 郭靄春 et al. Publisher: Tianjin Science and Technology Press 天津科學技術出版社. First edition: 1991. 1 vol. 169 + 1296 pp. With an appendix: "Index to Articles on the *Huang Di Nei Jing*, 1910 – 1988" by Wei Xiangwu.
3 indexes: (1) Stroke-number index of single characters to table of contents. (2) Pinyin index of single characters to table of contents. (3) Stroke number index (table of contents) of single characters and phrases with reference to page number of entry. Where applicable, ancient unabbreviated forms are listed together with the modern abbreviated forms of characters. Pinyin transliteration and tones are given for each character. Where a single character is used in the source texts in different meanings, these are explained separately with context examples.
This dictionary offers a comprehensive list of 2747 single characters, and of 4979 binoms and phrases of several characters from the *Huang Di Nei Jing Su Wen* and *Ling Shu*. Each entry begins with a single character (large print) and its pinyin transliteration followed by one or several explanations of its meaning with source context examples. This is followed, where applicable, by a list of binomical usages with explanations and source context examples.

Nei Jing Ci Dian 內經辭典 "Dictionary of the Nei Jing" by Zhang Dengben 張登本 and Wu Changchun 武長春. Publisher: People's Hygiene Press 人民衛生出版社. First edition, 1990. 1 vol. 5 + 591 + 19 pp. With an appendix: The headings of the Su Wen and Ling Shu treatises. 1 index: Radical index to single characters.
This dictionary lists 2286 single characters and, in addition, 5560 binoms and phrases of several characters from the *Huang Di Nei Jing Su Wen* and *Ling Shu*. Each entry begins with a single character (large print) in its unabbreviated version, a count of its appearance in the Nei Jing (Su Wen and Ling Shu),

its pinyin transliteration plus Chinese *fan qie* pronunciation, tone, and rhyme type (ancient and modern). Next is given the count of its appearance as a single character (with the character repeated, where applicable, in its abbreviated form), followed by an explanation of one or several meanings with source context examples. This is followed, where applicable, by binomical appearances, each with count and explanations.

Zhong Guo Yi Ji Zi Dian 中國醫籍字典 "Dictionary of Chinese Medical Literature" by Chinese Medical Literature Research Institute of Shanghai Chinese Medical College 上海中醫學院中醫文獻研究所. Publisher: Jiangxi Science and Technology Press 江西科學技術出版社. First edition: 1989. 59 + 530 pp. 3 indexes: Stroke-number index to radical index; radical index and stroke-number index to main body of entries.
This dictionary lists ca. 6100 single characters in their abbreviated forms, with unabbreviated forms added in brackets where applicable, and their pinyin transliteration. Ca. 1700 entries offer unusual writings and characters in their unabbreviated form with references to the respective main entries. Aside from the vocabulary found in classical Chinese medical literature, characters with medical connotations were taken from the *Er Ya, Fang Yan, Shuo Wen Jie Zi, Shi Ming, Guang Ya, Ji Yun, Shi Jing, Li Ji, Zuo Zhuan, Shan Hai Jing*, and the dynastic histories. The entries include ancient drug names, and secondary names of pharmaceutically used substances, form words frequently used in ancient medical texts, as well as some expressions associated with medicine. The explanations include source context examples.

Yi Yong Gu Han Yu Zi Dian 醫用古漢語字典 "Dictionary of Ancient Medical Chinese" by Huang Yuntai 黃雲臺. Publisher: Guangxi Science and Technology Press 廣西科學技術出版社. First edition: 1992. 28 + 283 pp. 3 indexes: Stroke-number index to radical index. Radical and pinyin alphabetical index to main body of entries.
This dictionary offers explanations of 1752 single characters selected as frequently used from ancient Chinese medical literature to help readers of classic medical texts understand terms and meanings no longer in common use in modern Chinese language. Each entry offers a character in large print followed by Chinese *fan qie* and occasional homophone, as well as pinyin explanations of pronunciation. Meanings are explained with source context examples.

Zhong Yi Nan Zi Zi Dian 中醫難字字典 "Dictionary of Difficult Characters in Chinese Medicine" by Li Rong 李榮. Publisher: Sichuan Science and

Technology Press 四川科學技術出版社. First edition: 1986. 1 vol. 191 pp. 2 indexes: Stroke-number index and pinyin index.
The author considers the wealth of Chinese medical literature inaccessible if a beginning student is familiar with only frequently used Chinese characters. In the present dictionary, he listed ca. 2000 characters he considered "difficult". These do not include characters which are extremely rarely used. Rather, the author selected characters which in their medical-pharmaceutical context have a special meaning, those which are difficult to write or to recognize from others, those which are often mispronounced, and so on. The range of sources includes Chinese traditional medical literature, recent TCM teaching primers, as well as Chinese texts on modern Western medicine and pharmacy. Thus, one encounters characters designed to represent chemical substances. The entries are listed according to subjects, beginning with sections on "Chinese basic medical theory", "Chinese pharmaceutics", and "Chinese prescriptions", all medical specialties, and ending with sections on various literary genres, such as *Nei Jing, Shang Han Lun, Jin Gui Yao Lue*, warmth diseases, and "ancient Chinese medical literature". An appendix combines a table of abbreviated and unabbreviated characters (with a rare explanation of the origins and different meanings of abbreviated and unabbreviated characters), a table of variant forms of Chinese characters, a comparative table of ancient and modern expressions of day and night times, and a list of the twelve months and their ancient equivalents.

I.4. Chinese-English

Han Ying Chang Yong Zhong Yi Yao Da Ci Hui 漢英常用中醫藥詞滙 "Common Terms of Chinese Medicine in English" by Xie Zhufan 謝竹藩 et al. Publisher: Beijing Medical College. Author's preface: December 1980. 1 vol. 540 pp. 1 index: stroke-number.
This dictionary is divided into twelve major sections (some of them being subdivided again), each of which is devoted to a specific subject area (English translation copied from the book):

1. "The Theories of Yinyang and of the Five Elements"
2. "Structure and Functions of the Human Body"
3. "Material Basis of Vital Activities of the Human Body"
4. "Causes and Mechanisms of Diseases"
5. "Method of Diagnosis"
6. "Differentiation of Symptom-Complexes"

7. “Principles and Methods of Treatment”
8. “Chinese Materia Medica”
9. “Prescriptions”
10. “Acupuncture and Moxibustion, Channels and Points”
11. “Disease and Symptoms of Various Branches of Medicine”
12. “Distinguished Physicians and Well-known Medical Works in History”

An appendix provides an alphabetical list of Latin drug names and their Chinese equivalents.

Han Ying Chang Yong Zhong Yi Ci Hui 漢英常用中醫詞滙 “Chinese-English Glossary of Common Terms in Chinese Medicine” by Ou Ming 歐明 et al. Publisher: Joint Publishing Co. Hong Kong Branch 三联 First edition: October 1982. 1 vol. 322 pp. 1 index: stroke number.
A list of terms commonly used in Chinese medicine. Wherever possible, the authors have used terms from modern Western anatomy, physiology, pathology, etc., as equivalents to the Chinese expressions listed. The appendix contains 1. a list of common Chinese drugs with English and Latin equivalents (the Latin names are incomplete, though, since no authors are given); 2. a list of acupuncture and moxibustion points with latinized pinyin transliteration and a literal translation into English; 3. a chronological table of Chinese dynasties; 4. the Heavenly Stems and Earthly Branches; 5. the twenty-four solar terms in Chinese and English translation; and 6. a conversion table of complex and simplified forms of Chinese characters.

Han Ying Chang Yong Yi Xue Ci Hui 漢英常用醫學詞滙 “Concise Chinese-English Dictionary of Medicine” by Huang Xiaokai 黃孝楷 et al. Publisher: People’s Hygiene Press, 人民衛生出版社 Beijing. First edition: 1982. 1 vol. 524 pp. 1 index: alphabetical (pinyin).
This dictionary is divided into three major sections:
1. a Chinese-English glossary of Western medical and pharmaceutical terms (pp. 1-365) 2. a Chinese-English glossary of Chinese traditional medical terms, and 3. a list of 400 Chinese drugs with their Latin and English equivalents.
An appendix contains 1. a list of the names of 400 acupoints with latinized transliteration in the pinyin and modified Wade-Giles systems, and 2. a list of Chinese names of health care institutions in contemporary China with their English translations.

Han Ying Shuang Jie Chang Yong Zhong Yi Ming Ci Shu Yu 漢英雙解常用中醫名詞術語 “Chinese-English Terminology of Chinese Medicine with Twofold Explanation” by Shuai Xuezhong 帥學忠 et al. Publisher: Hunan Science and

Technology Press 湖南科學技術出版社. First edition: January 1983. 1 vol. 765 pp. 1 index: stroke-number.

This dictionary is divided into thirteen chapters with the following headings (English translation adopted from the book):

1. "Yin and Yang, and the Five Elements"
2. "Visceral Symptoms"
3. "Channels & their Collateral Channels, and Acupuncture Points"
4. "Etiology and Pathology"
5. "Techniques and Diagnosis"
6. "The General Rules of Treatment"
7. "The Chinese Medical Formulary"
8. "Acupuncture and Moxibustion"
9. "Internal Medicine and Pediatrics"
10. "Gynecology and Obstetrics"
11. "Surgery and Traumatology"
12. "The Five Sensory Organs"
13. "The History of Traditional Chinese Medicine"

An appendix includes 1. an alphabetical pinyin list of romanized names of acupuncture points, and 2. a comparative table of pinyin and Wade-Giles romanizations. In contrast to all the other Chinese-English dictionaries/glossaries introduced here, this dictionary explains the Chinese terms and phrases first in Chinese and then in English.

II. Bibliographies

II.1. General

Zhong Guo Yi Ji Kao 中國醫籍考 "An Investigation of Chinese Medical Literature" by Tamba Mototane 丹波元胤. Current publisher: Beijing People's Hygiene Press 北京人民衛生出版社. Date of compilation: 1819. 1 vol. 1404 pp. 2 indexes: stroke-number indexes to titles and authors.

The *Zhong Guo Yi Ji Kao* includes, subdivided into eighty chapters, 2605 titles from Chinese traditional medical literature. Data provided, where applicable, are: author, title, number of *juan*, bibliographical reference, extant/unknown,quotations of entire prefaces/afterwords, excerpts from the *Si Ku Quan Shu Ti Yao* and other bibliographies, as well as sometimes lengthy notes by Tamba himself on questions of authenticity, origin, and authorship.

Chugoku Isho Honzō-ko 中國醫書本草考 "An Investigation of Chinese Medical and Materia Medica Literature" by Okanishi Tameto 岡西爲人. Publisher: Inoue Book Company 井上書店, Tokyo. First edition: 1974. 1 vol. 643 pp. + 86 pp. Appendixes. 5 indexes (Japanese alphabet): book titles, names of persons, names of drugs and plants, general index, as well as Latin drug names and Western authors.

This book includes partly reprints of previously published essays, and partly previously unpublished materials. It is divided into six chapters, with altogether sixty-one essays:

1. Explication of basic Chinese medical literature
2. On prescription works in Chinese medicine
3. The medical literature of the Jin Yuan era
4. On medical bibliographies
5. *Ben cao*-materia medica literature and Chinese drugs
6. History of Chinese acupuncture

Added to these six chapters are reproductions of the illustrations of famous historical physicians and legendary personalities from the Li Dai Ming Yi Tu Xing Shi 歷代名醫圖姓氏 section of the *Ben Cao Meng Quan* 本草蒙筌. An appendix includes, furthermore, a list of all publications of Okanishi, a short biography of Okanishi's academic life, as well as a number of obituaries on the author who died 5 May 1973.

Zhong Guo Yi Xue Shu Mu 中國醫學書目 "Bibliography of Chinese Medicine" by Kuroda Genji 黑田源次. Publisher: Ocean of Literature Press 文海出版社, Taibei. Author's preface: 1931. 1 vol. 1030 pp. 2 indexes: stroke-number indexes to book titles and authors.

This is a listing of 1273 editions of books from Chinese traditional medicine, subdivided into 31 groups. Of particular use is group 30, a listing of literary collections (*congshu* 叢書) with a guide to each individual title contained. Each edition listed is characterized by the following data, where applicable: number of *juan*, number of volumes, lines per page (horizontal and vertical), author, preface(s) with author and date, introduction with author and date, table of contents, afterword with author and date.

Xu Zhong Guo Yi Xue Shu Mu 續中國醫學書目 "Supplementary Bibliography of Chinese Medicine" by Okanishi Tameto 岡西爲人 Publisher: Ocean of Literature Press 文海出版社, Taibei. Author's preface: 1941. 1 vol. 580 pp. 2 indexes: stroke-number indexes to book titles and authors.

This supplement to Kuroda Genji's volume lists additional 1060 editions, subdivided into 29 groups. The structure of the entries is identical to that in Kuroda's volume.

Zhong Yi Tu Shu Lian He Mu Lu 中醫圖書聯合目錄 "Joint Library Catalogue on Chinese Medical Literature" by Academy of Traditional Chinese Medicine, Ministry of Health of the People's Republic of China, and Beijing Library. Publisher: Beijing Library 北京圖書館. First edition: 1961. 1 vol. 868 pp. 2 indexes: stroke-number indexes to book titles and authors.
This is an inventory of the holdings of 59 libraries in the People's Republic of China, at the end of 1959, of Chinese traditional medical literature. Besides titles in Chinese, Manchurian and Tibetan language publications are included as well. Also, foreign titles are included if they were written in Chinese originally, or have appeared in Chinese translation. The book includes a total of 7661 listings, subdivided into 16 groups with numerous subgroups. For each title are provided the following data, where applicable: title,number of *juan*, alternative or abbreviated titles, year of first printing, dynasty era, author, editions held by Chinese libraries with year and publisher and a reference to the libraries holding the respective edition.

Quan Guo Zhong Yi Tu Shu Lian He Mu Lu 全國中醫圖書聯合目錄 "Nation-Wide Joint Library Catalogue on Chinese Medical Literature" by Xie Qinglu 薛清錄. Publisher: Ancient Chinese Medical Literature Publ. Co. 中醫古籍出版社. First edition: 1991, 1 vol., 1104 pp. Four indexes added as an appendix: Stroke-number index of book titles, pinyin index of book titles, stroke index of authors, pinyin index of authors. Further appendixes: table of sixty combinations of heavenly stems and earth branches, table of historical capitals, table of tabooed characters from the names of emperors.
This is a catalogue of 12.124 books on Chinese Medicine kept at the end of 1980 in 113 libraries on the Chinese mainland. The structure of the book followed the *Zhong Yi Tu Shu Lian He Mu Lu* 中醫圖書聯合目錄 of 1961. Books are ordered along the 12 conventional subdisciplines of Chinese traditional medical literature, and their dates of appearance. Each entry is preceded by a number, which is followed by the title, the year the book was published, the dynasty, the name(s) of the author(s), editions, and one or more identification numbers of the respective libraries. In comparison with the 1961 edition, the contents have been enlarged and are easier to consult.

Zhong Guo Yi Ji Ti Yao 中國醫籍提要 "A Summary of Chinese Medical Literature" by Sun Jifen 孫繼芬 et al. Publisher: Jilin People's Press 吉林人

民出版社. 2 vols.First edition: 1984. 656 pp. One detailed table of contents. 2 indexes: stroke-number indexes to book titles and authors. List of Reference Works.

This bibliography contains rather detailed descriptions of 504 titles selected from Chinese, Japanese, and Korean traditional medical literature. The descriptions are grouped as follows:

1. Basic Theory, including the sub-groups: medical classics; diagnostics; materia medica; prescription books; on harm caused by cold; *Jin Gui* [*Yao Lue*] (and subsequent works following this tradition); thermic illnesses.
2. Clinical disciplines, including: internal medicine, gynecology, pediatrics; external medicine; five sensory organs; injuries; acupuncture/moxibustion; massage.
3. General, including: general medical books; medical case histories; medical language; reflections on medicine: complete editions of the works of specific authors, and collections according to other criteria.
4. Medical History; Forensic Medicine; Prolongation of Life.

The description of each single book provides data on the title, the year of compilation/publication, author, contents, and most recent edition. In characterizing the contents, the authors of this bibliography have emphasized innovative achievements, basic ideas, and impact on subsequent times.

Zhong Yi Gu Ji Zhen Ben Ti Yao 中醫古籍珍本提要 "A Summary of Precious Titles From Ancient Chinese Medical Literature" by Yu Ying'ao 余瀛鰲 and Fu Jinghua 傅景華. Publisher: Ancient Chinese Medical Literature Press 中醫古籍出版社. First edition: 1992. 1 vol. 40 + 609 + 36 pp. 2 indexes: stroke-number indexes of book titles and authors.

This is a concise description of 1080 pre-modern medical books kept in the library of the China Academy of Chinese Medicine in Beijing. The contents are grouped under 14 headings: (1) *Nei Jing* 內經, *Nan Jing* 難經, (2) *Shang Han* 傷寒, *Jin Gui* 金匱, (3) Warmth Diseases, (4) Diagnostics, (5) Materia Medica, (6) Prescription Works, (7) Acupuncture/Tuina Massage, (8) All Clinical Specialties, (9) Nourishment of Life, (10) General Medical Titles, (11) Case Histories/Medical Language/Medical Discourse, (12) History of Medicine, (13) Series of Books, (14) Research Tools. Each entry begins with a "short characterization of the author", followed by a "summary of the contents" of the text in question, and a list of "important editions" with date of appearance, printed/manuscript version, and a numerical reference to locations in libraries in Beijing and elsewhere. A few of the titles listed are not available in the library of the China Academy.

Zhong Guo Fen Sheng Yi Ji Kao 中國分省醫籍考 "An Investigation of Chinese Medical Literature Differentiated by Provinces" by Guo Aichun 郭靄春 et al. Publisher: Tianjin Science and Technology Press 天津科學技術出版社. Vol. 1: First edition: 1984. 1375 pp. No indexes. Vol. 2: First edition: 1987. 1409 pp.
The first volume lists a total of 4302 titles that are mentioned in local histories written prior to 1911. The overall grouping of the titles is according to their origin in one of the following six provinces: Hebei (259 titles); Henan (399); Shandong (601); Jiangsu (1441); Zhejiang (1063); and Jiangxi (539). Each of these six sections has its own preface and detailed table of contents, the latter listing the titles according to the following headings: medical classics; diagnostics; harm caused by cold; materia medica; acupuncture/moxibustion; prescriptions, with numerous sub-groups; language and case histories; nourishment of life; forensic medicine; medical history; case histories; varia. A list of all the local histories and other reference works quoted concludes each section. Each title, in the descriptive part of this bibliography, is identified by its author and dynastic era, and by characterizations quoted from local histories in full. For each quotation, the date of publication and the respective chapter of the local history, from which the quotation was taken, is provided. The second volume follows the structure of the first volume. It offers data on literature on Chinese Medicine from the following provinces: Shanxi, Anhui, Fujian, Hubei, Hunan, Guangdong, Guangxi Zhuang ethnic group Autonomous Region, Sichuan, Guizhou, Yunnan, Shaanxi, Gansu, Liaoning, Jilin, Heilongjiang, Inner Mongolia Autonomous Region, Tibet Autonomous Region, Qinghai, Ningxia Hui ethnic group Autonomous Region, Xinjiang Uighur ethnic group Autonomous Region, Taiwan, Supplement to Jiangsu, Supplement to Zhejiang. The 2nd volume concludes with an index to book titles and an index to personal names.

II.2. Pharmaceutical

Xian Cun Ben Cao Shu Lu 現存本草書錄 "A List of Materia Medica Works Extant Today" by Long Bojian 龍伯堅. Publisher: Beijing People's Hygiene Press 北京人民衛生出版社 First edition: 1957. 1 vol. 243 pp. 2 indexes: stroke-number indexes to authors and titles.
This little book lists 260 *ben cao* materia medica titles, providing, where applicable, for each book the following data: title, number of *juan*, author, all editions since first publication, as well as notes by Long Bojian on authorship, contents, categorization, prefaces.

Medicine in China. A History of Pharmaceutics by Paul U. Unschuld. Publisher: University of California Press, Los Angeles, Berkeley, London. First edition: 1985. 1 vol. 367 pp. 4 indexes: indexes to book titles, names of persons, Chinese drug names, and general index.
This book offers an analysis of approximately one hundred works from Chinese traditional pharmaceutical literature from the Han dynasty to the official pharmacopoeias of the People's Republic of China. It is divided into two major parts: *Ben cao* materia medica literature with comprehensive contents, and *ben cao* materia medica literature with specialized contents, the latter comprising works on dietetics, monographic works, works on pharmaceutical technology, rhymed works, works limited to plants, regionally specialized works, as well as lists of secondary names for drugs. A third part contains an analysis of the Chinese pharmacopoeias of the 20th century. Each titles is described in terms of authorship, contents, and socio-cultural and philosophical context.

Li Dai Zhong Yao Wen Xian Jing Hua 歷代中藥文獻精華 "The Essence of Chinese Materia Medica Literature Through The Ages" by Shang Zhijun 尙志鈞, Lin Qianliang 林乾良, and Zheng Jinsheng 郑金生. Publisher: Science and Technology Literature Publ. Co. 科學技術文獻出版社. First edition: 1989. 1 vol. 575 pp. 2 indexes: index to book titles and index to personal names.
The main text of this book has three sections: The first is an "Outline of Materia Medica", *Ben cao gai yao*本草概要. It relates the major steps in the development of Chinese materia medica from antiquity to the 20th century. The second section is on "Important Texts on Materia Medica", Ben cao yao ji本草要籍, and introduces 77 major *ben cao* 本草 works (plus an additional 14 titles in an appendix) in chronological order from antiquity to 1911. For each book is given the title, the author, the year of its appearance, the number of *juan*, its structure, its contents, its transmission, its availability, and its editions. The final section offers a "Grand Survey of Materia Medica [Literature]", Ben cao da xi 本草大系, listing, in chronological sequence of their appearance, approximately 1000 texts on Chinese materia medica published prior to 1911.

II.3. Further Selected Areas/Periods

Song Yi Qian Yi Ji Kao 宋以前醫籍考 "An Investigation of Medical Literature of Song times and before" by Okanishi Tameto 岡西爲人. Current publisher: Old Pavillon Book House 古亭書屋, Taibei. First edition: 1948 in Shenyang. 1 vol. 1460 pp. 2 indexes: stroke-number indexes to authors and titles.

This book lists altogether 1975 works written and published from the Han through the Song era. They are subdivided into four groups (classics, classic prescription works, materia medica, miscellaneous), and altogether 31 subgroups. Data provided, where applicable, for each text include: title, dynastic era, author, and bibliographical sources, as well as literal quotations of all references in these sources to the title discussed. Further: full quotations of prefaces and afterwords, as well as of author's biographies. Different editions are identified in detail. Occasionally, Okanishi added his own notes concerning authenticity and authorship of a work.

San Bai Zhong Yi Ji Lu 三百種醫籍錄 "A List of Three Hundred [Titles] from Medical Literature" by Jia Weicheng 賈維誠. Publisher: Heilongjiang Science and Technology Press 黑龍江科學技術出版社, Harbin. First edition: 1982. 1 vol. 412 pp. 2 indexes: stroke number indexes to authors and titles.
This is a selection of the three hundred most important titles from Chinese traditional medical literature, divided into four groups: classics, individual theoretical schools, materia medica, and texts for clinical application. For each title a summary of its contents is provided, as well as a characterization of the author, a list of current editions, and references in dynastic histories and catalogues of private libraries.

Hebei Yi Ji Kao 河北醫籍考 "An Investigation of Medical Literature from Hebei" by Guo Aichun 郭藹春 and Li Zixi 李紫溪. Publisher: Hebei People's Press, Shijiazhuang 河北人民出版社，石家莊. First edition: June 1979. 1 vol. 87 pp. No index.
A listing and characterization of texts from Chinese traditional medical literature written by authors from the province of Hebei. Guo Aichun and Li Zixi analysed 349 regional chronicles (the entire list of chonicles used is added as an appendix), 101 of which yielded data on medical works and their authors. This little book is valuable for its quotations from these chronicles. The texts are presented according to the following ten major groups: "On medical classics"; "The movement in the vessels and its diagnosis"; "Harm caused by cold"; "Pharmaceutics"; "Acupuncture-Moxibustion"; "Prescriptions"; "Case Histories"; "Nourishment of Life"; "Veterinary Medicine"; "Miscellaneous".

Zhong Yi Wai Ke Yi Ji Cun Yi Kao 中醫外科醫籍存佚考 "An Investigation of Extant and Lost Texts from the Branch of Chinese Medicine Concerned with External [Illnesses]" by Zhang Zanchen 張贊臣 and Yu Ying'ao 余瀛鰲. Publisher: People's Hygiene Press 人民衛生出版社, Beijing. First edition: April 1987. 1 vol. 113 pp. 2 stroke-number indexes.

This important little book is divided into five chapters with the following contents:

Ch. 1: a survey of the history of Chinese *wai ke* 外科, i.e. the branch of medicine concerned with illnesses in the external sections of the body. A general discussion of some of the more outstanding works on *wai ke* of the past two millennia.

Ch. 2: three lists of currently available medical book catalogues and bibliographies:
catalogues of public and private collections.
Bibliographies listed in literary sources
Annotated bibliographies

Ch. 3: corrections of errors and omissions regarding *wai ke* 外科listings in the *Zhong Guo Yi Ji Kao* 中國醫籍考.

Ch. 4: a chronological list of 231 wai ke titles from the Eastern Han until 1911, of 5 titles published after 1911, and of 103 titles published by Japanese authors. Each entry contains, where applicable, information on the number of *juan*, extant or lost, author, editions, general contents, and special contributions. The original sources from which these informations were taken are quoted.

Ch. 5: short biographies, including sources of information, of 237 personalities from the history of Chinese medicine who can be linked to *wai ke*.

The volume is concluded by an index of book titles, and by an index of names. The many important data provided in the individual descriptions and biographies are not indexed.

Zhong Yi Wen Xian Ci Dian 中醫文獻詞典, "Dictionary of Literature on Chinese Medicine" by Yu Ying'ao 余瀛鰲 and Li Jingwei 李經緯 (Eds.-in-Chief). Publisher: Beijing Science and Technology Publ. Co. 北京科學技術出版社. First edition: 2000. 1 vol. 732 pp. 2 indexes at the beginning of the book: Pinyin (Chinese phonetic alphabet) index to first characters of entries, Stroke-number index to first characters of entries.

This book has 6,100 entries on literature on Chinese Medicine and relevant periodicals published before 1989, ordered according to the number of strokes of the first character of each entry. Each publication is described according to nature of publication, number of *juan*, dynasty/era of publication, author, year of publication, major contents, and editions.

Zhong Yi Yi Ji Da Ci Dian 中醫醫籍大辭典, "Large Dictionary of Chinese Medicine Medical Literature" by Qiu Peiran (Ed.-in-Chief). Publisher:

Shanghai Science and Technology Press 上海科學技術出版社. First edition: 2002. 2 vols. 2194 pp. Two stroke-number indexes at the end of the book: Index to book titles, index to primary and secondary names of authors.
This is a reference book covering the entire literature on Chinese Medicine and Pharmaceutics published until the end of the 20th century. It lists more than 17,600 published works, and more then 4,700 lost titles. The titles are classified in accordance with their medical sub-disciplines. The first volume includes: A. *Nei Jing*, *Nan Jing* genre. B. Basic theory. C. *Shang Han Lun* and *Jin Gui Yao Lüe* genre. D. Diagnosis. E. Materia Medica. F. Formularies. G. General Clinical Medicine. H. Warmth Diseases. I. Internal Medicine. J. Gynecology. The second volume includes: K. Pediatrics. L. External Medicine. M. Traumatology. N. Ophthalmology. O. Otorhinolaryngology. P. Acupuncture. Q. Tuina Push-and-Pull-Massage. R. Nourishment of Life. S. Medical Case Histories. T. Historiography of Medicine. U. Writings of a General Nature. V. Others. W. Lost Titles. The entries in the group "Lost Titles" are ordered according to the number of strokes of their first character. All the others follow a chronological order in accordance with their year of publication. Each entry addresses the following data: title, serial number, abbreviated title, number of *juan* and volumes, author, date of compilation or publication, transmission through the ages, survey of contents, scholarly characteristics or value, editions. In some cases the libraries are named where the titles are kept.

II.4.Secondary Sources

Yi Xue Shi Lun Wen Zi Liao Suo Yin (1903-1978) 醫學史論文資料索引 "An Index to the Literature on Medical History". No impressum. Preface by Li Jingwei 李經緯, dated December 1982. 1 vol. 514 pp. 2 indexes: stroke-number indexes to authors and headings of publications.
This index includes references to 10,200 Chinese articles, from about 630 journals, on ancient, recent, and modern Chinese medical history, as well as on the history of medicine in countries other than China. The most comprehensive book of its kind available today.

Zhong Guo Yi Shi Wai Wen Wen Xian Suo Yin 中國醫史外文文獻索引 "Bibliography of Chinese Medical History in Foreign Languages, 1682-1965" by Wang Jimin 王吉民 and Fu Weikang 傅維康. Publisher: Shanghai Academy of Chinese Medicine, Medical History Museum 上海中醫學院醫史博物館. Authors' preface: January 1966. 1 vol. 274 pp. 2 indexes: alphabetical indexes to authors and general topics.

This listing contains 1412 references to English, German, French, Italian, Spanish, and Russion publications on the history of medicine in China, especially of the past one hundred years, with a Chinese translation of each title. The authors state, in English, in their preface: "This bibliography is divided into two main parts: I. Medicine in liberated areas and in New China. II. Medicine before the liberation. The first part enumerates the achievements in New China regarding the Party's medical directives, aims and policies; preventive medicine; sanitation and health; traditional treatment and drugs; medical education, research, etc. The second part describes the development of indigenous Chinese medicine prior to 1949; the history of its spread to Western countries, and its contribution, the introduction of Western medicine into China and its impact and effects."

Zhong Guo Yi Xue Wai Wen Zhu Shu Shu Mu 中國醫學外文著述書目 "Catalogue of Publications on Medicine in China in Foreign Languages 1656 – 1965" by Wang Jimin 王吉民 and Fu Weikang 傅維康. Publisher: Shanghai Academy of Chinese Medicine, Medical History Museum Shanghai. First edition: 1963. 1 vol. 104 pp. 1 index: alphabetical index to authors.
A listing of 433 publications in English, French, German, Russian, and Latin with titles translated into Chinese, and occasionally short descriptions of the contents in Chinese. The authors state, in English, in their preface: "This catalogue contains a list of works in foreign languages (Japanese not included) published during the past three hundred years. It deals with such subjects as general Chinese medicine; its spread to other countries and its practical applications; the introduction of western medical science into China, etc. The material is arranged according to subject matter, each entry according to date of publication, and the title is followed by its Chinese equivalent or a brief summary." The entries are grouped as follows: 1. General Medicine. 2. Medical History. 3. The Pulse. 4. Practical Medicine. 5. Acumoxatherapy. 6. Materia Medica. 7. Hygiene and Health. 8. Books and Periodicals. 9. Biography. 10. Miscellaneous.

III. Biographies

III.1. General

Zhong Guo Li Dai Yi Jia Zhuan Lu 中國歷代醫家傳錄 "Biographical Records of Chinese Physicians through the Ages" by He Shixi 何時希. Publisher: People's Hygiene Press 人民衛生出版社, Beijing. First edition: September 1991. 3 vols.: 581 pp./930 pp./974 pp. Two indexes: Stroke-number index of first characters of names referring to stroke number index of full names. 3 appendixes in vol. 3: (1) Listing of teacher-disciple relationships with stroke-number index. (2) A list of ancient texts and their authors still extant, ordered according to stroke-number of first character of title. (3) A list of secondary names of physicians and their identification, ordered according to stroke-number of first character of secondary names. (4) A list of all literary sources used to compile this dictionary, ordered according to stroke-number of first character of book titles.
Based on more than 3000 Chinese and foreign literary sources, this dictionary lists biographical records on more than 20,000 persons associated with the practice of medicine in China from remote antiquity to the first half of the 20th century. Entries include, where applicable, in addition to names, styles, and sobriquets, a person's medical specialty and dynastic era, place of origin, dates of life, writings, details/anecdotes from his life, and bio-bibliographical sources.

Zhong Yi Ren Ming Ci Dian 中醫人名辭典 "Biographical Dictionary of Chinese Medicine" by Li Yun 李雲 et al. Publisher: International Culture Publ. Co. 國際文化出版公司, Beijing. First edition: 1988. 1 vol. Two indexes: Stroke-number index of first characters of names referring to stroke number index of full names.
Based on ca. 600 literary sources, this dictionary lists approximately 10,500 medical personalities, many of which had not been taken into account by previous such reference works. For each person listed are noted, where applicable, his secondary names, life dates, dynasty, writings, and a brief biography, as well as teacher-disciple relationships, with the sources from which these data were taken added to each entry. Two indexes: Stroke-number index of first characters of names referring to stroke number index of full names. The information given is more detailed than in the *Zhong Guo Li Dai Yi Jia Zhuan Lu* 中國歷代醫家傳錄.

Zhong Yi Ren Wu Ci Dian 中醫人物詞典 "Dictionary of Personalities in Chinese Medicine" by Li Jingwei 李經緯 et al. Publisher: Shanghai Dictionaries and Reference Books Press 上海辭書出版社. First edition: 1987. 1 vol. Two indexes.
This dictionary contains more than 6200 biographies of authors, physicians, and other personalities from the history of Chinese medicine, including 20th century persons and outstanding representatives from various ethnic minorities. A first index lists style-names, sobriquets, and additional names, as well as teachers and students, and descendants. The second index refers to book titles mentioned in the biographical entries.

Zhong Guo Yi Xue Ren Ming Zhi 中國醫學人名誌 "Notes on the Names of Persons in Chinese Medicine" by Chen Bangxian 陳邦賢 and Yan Lingzhou 嚴菱洲. Publisher: Beijing People's Hygiene Press 北京人民衛生出版社. First edition: 1956. 1 vol. 248 pp. 1 index: stroke-number index of family names.
A listing of more than 2600 personalities – arranged according to the number of strokes of the family names – from the legendary beginnings of Chinese medicine through the entire imperial era to the early twentieth century. For each person the following data are provided, where applicable: name, dynastic period, place of origin, secondary names, writings, biographical sketch. For further details references to primary sources (local histories) are given.

Zhong Guo Li Dai Ming Yi Lu 中國歷代名醫錄 "List of Famous Chinese Physicians of All Ages" by Chen Julin 陳居霖 Publisher: The Institute of Present Day Chinese Medicine, Hong Kong 香港現代中醫藥學院. First edition: February 1955. 1 vol. 280 pp. 1 index: stroke-number index of family names.
A chronological listing of almost 2000 personalities from the legendary beginnings of Chinese medicine through the entire imperial age to the early 20th century. For each person, his/her name, secondary names, place of origin, publications, and a biographical sketch are provided. No sources are given for these data.

Zhong Guo Li Dai Ming Yi Zhuan 中國歷代名醫傳 "Biographical Records of Persons famous in Medicine in Chinese History" by Chen Menglai 陳夢賚. Publisher: Science Popularization Press 科學普及出版社, Beijing. First edition: January 1987. 1 vol. 12 + 476 pp. No index. Table of contents. Chronological list of all persons reviewed.

This book contains biographies of 213 persons who were either outstanding physicians or influenced the history of Chinese medicine in some other way, mainly through writings. The entries are ordered chronologically, beginning with Bian Que of the Zhou and ending with Tang Zonghai who died in 1918. In addition to birth and death, each entry provides, where applicable, data on the respective person's secondary names, geographic origin, affiliation with schools or tendencies, famous disciples and followers, noteworthy life events, civil service career, and judgments by earlier historiographers. The contents of influential writings are discussed and categorized. The book is useful as a starting point for further research because it gives the titles of literary sources for many of its statements. In a short preface, Chen Menglai offers a survey of the development of medical biographical works in the history of China beginning with Gan Bozong's 甘伯宗 *Ming Yi Zhuan* 名醫傳 of the Tang.

III.2. Selected Groups

Sichuan Yi Lin Ren Wu 四川醫林人物 "Sichuan Medical Personalities" by Chen Xianfu 陳先賦 and Lin Senrong 林森榮. Publisher: Sichuan People's Press Chengdu 四川人民出版社, 成都. First edition: 1981. 1 vol. 481 pp. + 18 pp. Table of contents. No index.
A chronological listing of 1071 Sichuanese who made themselves a name in medicine. For each person a short biography, including contributions to medicine as well as the major literary sources from which these biographical data were taken, are provided. The listing is ordered according to dynasties, beginning with the Eastern Han era and ending with the Qing dynasty. A list of 460 literary sources used to compile this book was added as an appendix.

IV. Miscellaneous

Zhong Guo Li Dai Yi Shi 中國歷代醫史 "Chinese Medical History through All Ages" by Medical History Committee of the Chinese Medical Literature Research Institute of Shanghai City. No impressum (no publisher, no date of publication). Date of preface: April 1957. 1 vol. 372 pp. No index.
A chronological account of major events and famous personalities throughout the history of medicine in China, based on an evaluation of more than 400 texts. After a short general introduction to the origins of various facets of Chinese medicine follow eleven historical periods, beginning with "antiquity", the two Han dynasties, and so on through the republican period. Each

period is divided into two major groups of data: 1. "Medical Policy", including data concerning administrative measures, and the general development of medicine during the period under review, and 2. "Famous Physicians", with shorter and longer references to the biographies of these people. For each entry the source from which it was taken is provided. This is the richest compilation of data on the history of medicine in China in the Chinese language. Its use is hampered by the absence of indexes. The names of the more than 4000 persons listed in the various chapters under "Famous Physicians" appear in the table of contents, partly following the order of the source materials, partly following the number of strokes of their family names.

Zhong Guo Yi Shi Nian Biao 中國醫史年表 "Chronological List of Events in Chinese Medical History" by Guo Aichun 郭靄春. Publisher: Heilongjiang People's Press 黑龍江人民出版社, Harbin. First edition: 1977. 1 vol. 343 pp. 2 indexes: stroke-number indexes to book titles and names of persons.
A chronological list of events in Chinese medical history beginning with remote, undatable antiquity. The final date given is 1911. Each page has seven columns: Year according to Western calendar. Chinese dynasty. Governmental Period. Year of Reign Period. Date of sixty years cycle. Event. Source.

Zhong Yi Chang Yong Gong Ju Shu Shou Ce 中醫常用工具書手冊 "Handbook of Chinese Medicine Reference Books/Dictionaries" by Li Jingwei 李經緯 et al. Publisher: Shanghai Science and Technology Press 上海科學技術出版社. First edition: 1988. 1 vol. 213 pp. Table of contents. 2 Indexes (appendix): Index to reference works in Chinese medicine and pharmacy ordered along subjects. Stroke-number index to book titles.
This small book is an indispensable guide to Chinese reference books available to users and researchers of Chinese medicine. Following a lengthy discourse on the meaning of "reference books" (*gong ju shu* 工具書), 195 such works are introduced in seven chapters: (1) General Dictionaries, (2) Pharmaceutical Dictionaries, (3) Handbooks (3.1.) Handbooks on all Clinical Specialties of Chinese Medicine, (3.2) Pharmaceutical Handbooks, (4) Bibliographies, Excerpts, Indexes, (5) Yearbooks, Encyclopedias, Classic Sources, (6) Illustrations, Chronologies, (7) Reference works for researching and cataloguing ancient Chinese medical texts.

General Glossary

礙	ài	to obstruct; to hinder 2.c
愛	ài	to love 3.f
艾	ài	moxa; common mugwort 10.d
安	ān	an interrogative; how? 1.f
安	ān	peace; tranquil 1.f
安	ān	to consider as comfortable 7.e
安	ān	to place 9.f
安泰	ān tài	peaceful; undisturbed 3.e
安慰	ān wèi	to comfort 10.d
案	àn	a law-case; a trial 2.f
按	àn	as for 5.b
按	àn	to feel (the vessels in order to examine the movement within them) 5.e
按	àn	according to 7.f
按	àn	examine; introductory particle to a commentary 9.a
按蹻	àn jiāo	pressing-lifting (a type of physical exercises) 7.e
八	bā	eight 1.c
八風	bā fēng	the eight winds (i.e. the winds from the eight cardinal points E, W, S, N, ES, EN, WS, WN) 7.d
八裏	bā lǐ	the eight internal (movements in the vessels; i.e. 微 *wéi* [feeble], 沉 *chén* [in the depth], 緩 *huǎn* [relaxed], 濇 *sè* [rough], 遲 *chí* [slow], 伏 *fú* [hidden], 濡 *rú*[soft], and 弱 *ruò* [weak]) 6.b

八脈	bā mài	the eight single conduit vessels; short for *qi jīng bā mài* 奇經八脈2.b
八正	bā zhèng	the eight cardinal [turning points] 1.c
八正	bā zhèng	the eight seasonal turning points (s.a. 1.c.) 3.b
拔	bá	to pluck up; to pull out 1.b
白	bái	white 2.b
白粉	bái fěn	White Powder 9.f
白華菜	bái huá cài	*baihuacai*, a drug prepared from Cleome gynandra L. 9.b
白珠	bái zhū	the white (section of the) eyeball 5.a
百	bǎi	hundred 2.a
百	bǎi	hundred; many; all 3.e
敗	bài	to destroy 4.c
敗	bài	to become eliminated; to vanish 6.e
敗瘡	bài chuāng	badly (healing) wounds 9.b
敗絮	bài xù	torn rags 7.c
拜謝	bài xiè	to thank 10.f
斑	bān	streak(-like skin rash) 6.f
斑猫	bān māo	*banmao*, a drug prepared from Mylabris phalerata Pall., and M. Cichorii L.; the cantharides flies 9.b
瘢	bān	illness with streak(-like rashes) 9.a
半	bàn	half 4.b
半夏	bàn xià	*banxia*, a drug prepared from Pinellia ternata (Thumb.) Breit. 9.e
傍	báng	to border on; by the side of 7.e
胞	bāo	the womb 2.b
胞	bāo	the bladder 2.f
胞	bāo	an eyelid 5.a
[心]胞絡	[xīn]bāo luò	the [heart] enclosing network 4.f
雹	báo	hail 7.b
褓	bǎo	a swaddling cloth 2.b
飽	bǎo	fullness 3.a
寶	bǎo	valuable; best 10.a

抱	bào	to hold in one's arms; to hatch, to encompass 2.a
暴	bào	violent 3.b
暴	bào	sudden 7.b
報刺	bào cì	retaliation piercing; i.e. method to treat pain changing its lcoation. A needle is inserted at a site of pain. The physician locates with his hand a second site of pain, withdraws the needle from the first and inserts it at the second site 10.c
抱朴子-內篇	bào pǔ zǐ nèi piān	*Bao pu zi nei pian*, the "Inner Section of the [Book Written by the] Master Embracing Purity"; a work by Gě Hóng 葛洪 281-341 9.f
悲	bēi	mourning 3.e
北	běi	north 2.d
背	bèi	the back 1.f
背	bèi	to turn one's back against; to stand in contrast to 3.e
輩	bèi	class; kind 7.c
倍	bèi	to double 8.c
焙	bèi	to dry over a fire in a pan 9.a
備	bèi	to provide; to prepare 1.f
備	bèi	to master completely 10.c
奔	bēn	to run; to be in a hurry 4.a
奔豚	bēn tún	running piglet (syndrom) 9.b
本	běn	a root 1.c
本	běn	basically; fundamental 1.f
本	běn	origin 3.c
本草	běn cǎo	"Materia medica"; here: short title of *Shen nong ben cao jing* 神農本草經; "Shennong's Classic on Materia Medica", a pharmaceutical classic compiled about the 1st c. CE 1.d
本草備要	běn cǎo bèi yào	*Ben cao bei yao*, a popular *materia medica* of the late 17th century, by Wāng Áng 汪昂 7.f

本草綱目	běn cǎo gāng mù	*Ben cao gang mu*, an encyclopedic materia medica of the 16th century, by Lǐ Shízhēn 李時珍 7.f
本經	běn jīng	the "Original Classic" (i.e. the *Shén nóng běn cǎo jīng* 神農本草經) 9.f
本症	běn zhèng	the typical patho-conditions accompanying a disease 5.d
鼻	bí	the nose 2.b
彼	bǐ	those 1.f
比	bǐ	to compare 8.d
畢	bì	to finish 1.b
必	bì	certainly; definitely; must 1.c
必須	bì xū	must 3.b
臂	bì	an arm 4.b
婢	bì	a female servant 5.c
閉	bì	to close; be closed 1.b
閉	bì	closure 6.d
弊	bì	narrow-mindedness 6.e
壁	bì	the wall of a house 7.c
避	bì	to avoid; to flee; to shun 7.d
痺	bì	the disease "blockage" 4.a
痹	bì	lame; paralyzed; limpness 4.c
痹	bì	closure; blockage 10.e
砭	biān	a pointed stone 1.c
邊	biān	a side 9.d
扁鵲	biǎn què	Bian Que, a legendary physician of the sixth or fifth c. BCE 1.f
變	biàn	to change; to transform 1.d
變化	biàn huà	variations 8.e
辯	biàn	to discuss; to distinguish 1.d
遍	biàn	everywhere 3.a
遍	biàn	a time; a turn 9.d
便	biàn	convenience; stool 2.d

便	biàn	particle indicating an immediate temporal sequence 5.a
便	biàn	urine and stools 5.c
便秘	biàn bì	constipation 6.f
辨證	biàn zhèng	to distinguish among patho-conditions (in order to apply a differential treatment) 8.f
辨證奇聞	biàn zhèng qí wén	*Bian zheng qi wen*, a medical treatise of the 17th century, by Chén Shìduò 陳士鐸
變蒸	biàn zhēng	the transformation and steaming (of newly-borns) 6.f
標	biāo	tip (of a disease); sign; secondary location of a disease 7.a
標本	biāo běn	tip and root 7.d
表	biǎo	outside; exterior 1.c
別	bié	to divide; to distinguish 1.d
別	bié	separate 2.c
別	bié	other 3.a
別錄	bié lù	*Bie lu*, short title of *Míng yī bié lù* 名醫別錄, the "Additional Notes of Renowned Physicians", a book (or individual notes) added by Táo Hóngjǐng to the *Shen nong ben cao* in 500 CE 9.c
癟	biě	shrivelled 4.c
濱	bīn	a beach 7.e
冰	bīng	to freeze 3.f
稟	bǐng	to receive from above; natural endowment 1.d
稟	bǐng	to receive supplies 2.c
稟質	bǐng zhì	natural disposition 8.b
餅酪	bǐng lào	cheese 9.c
幷	bìng	and; also 2.c
幷	bìng	together 4.f
幷	bìng	a particle adding emphasis if placed before a negative 10.b
病	bìng	illness; to be ill 1.a

病	bìng	to make ill; to cause an illness 3.b
病	bìng	disease 5.d
病機	bìng jī	the trigger of an illness; the movement of an illness (through the body); pathomechanism 8.c
病脈	bìng mài	(a movement in the) vessels (indicating an) illness 6.c
博	bó	extensive; broad 1.d
搏	bó	to seize 2.c
搏	bó	to accumulate (something which is normally dissipated); used here for 摶 *tuán*7.b
搏	bó	to beat 7.c
薄	bó	thin; poor; shabby 1.d
薄	bó	to strike 4.d
膊	bó	the upper arm; the shoulder 5.c
伯高	bó gāo	Bo Gao, one of the legendary advisers of Huang Di 2.c
伯有	bó yǒu	Bo You; another name of Liang Xiao, who was killed by Si Dai and returned as a demon to take revenge. The story is recorded in the Annals of the Spring and Autumn Period 3.c
博物志	bó wù zhì	*Bo wu zhi*, title of a collection of essays by Zhāng Huá 9.f
部	bù	a section 1.c
步	bù	a step; stride 3.f
布	bù	to spread 4.f
布	bù	a piece of cloth 9.c
補	bǔ	to supplement 4.b
不	bù	not 1.a
不待於	bù dái yú	not to depend on 5.e
不得	bù dé	cannot; must not 7.c
不爾	bù ěr	otherwise; if not so 8.c
不過	bù guò	only; but 5.b
不及	bù jí	insufficiency 6.d
不可不	bù kě bù	it is impossible not to; one must 5.d

不可勝舉	bù kě shèng jǔ	cannot all be named here one by one 5.d
不仁	bù rén	numb; insensitivity 4.a
才	cái	then; just then 10.f
纔	cái	only when 10.d
參	cān	to consider; to compare 1.d
參	cān	to take part; to be related 3.b
參	cān	to combine; to mix 6.e
參半	cān bàn	half and half 7.f
殘害	cán hài	to destroy; to injure 4.c
倉	cāng	hasty 1.e
蒼蒼	cāng cāng	ashen 10.e
蒼生	cāng shēng	the people 8.a
藏	cáng	to store 3.f
藏器	càng qì	Cangqi, personal name of Chén Càngqì 陳藏器, *materia medica* author 9.d
操	cāo	to hold; to lay into someone's hands; to burden on somebody 7.f
糙	cāo	coarse; raw 9.a
草	cǎo	grass; plant 2.a
草荄	cǎo gāi	*cao gai*: name of an herb or tree (?) 7.d
草蘇	cǎo sū	*cao su*: name of a drug (?); herbal leaves (?) 7.d
側身	cè shēn	to turn to the side; to turn half way round 10.d
參差	cēn cī	irregular; not uniform 10.b
曾	cēng	already; past 1.e
層	céng	a layer 9.f
差	chā	to differ; to miss 10.d
差無誤	chā wú wù	not the slightest mistake 9.e
察	chá	to investigate; to find out 5.b
柴胡	chái hú	*chaihu*, a drug prepared from Bupleurum chinense DC, and other Bupleurum herbs 8.e
瘥	chài	to recover; to get well 9.d
鑱	chán	chisel 1.f
纏	chán	to entwine 2.b
鑱鍼	chán zhēn	the chisel needle 10.a

產	chǎn	to give birth 2.d
長	cháng	profitable; excelling 1.d
長	cháng	long 2.f
長	cháng	to excel 7.f
長夏	cháng xià	late summer 4.a
長鍼	cháng zhēn	the long needle 10.a
常	cháng	normal; regular 1.d
常	cháng	regular; a rule 3.b
常	cháng	permanently; constantly; regularly 7.d
嘗	cháng	to taste; to try 1.e
嘗	cháng	indication of past tense 8.b
腸	cháng	the intestines 1.f
朝	cháo	the court 3.d
朝見	cháo jiàn	to have audience at the court 3.d
炒	chǎo	to stir-fry 9.e
坼	chè	to break open 3.f
齔	chēn	the period when the milk teeth are shed 2.b
辰	chén	one of the twelve divisions of daytime 2.a
辰州	chén zhōu	Chenzhou, name of a prefecture 9.f
臣	chén	your subject; used for "I" when addressing a superior 3.d
臣	chén	minister (drugs in a prescription) 8.a
臣	chén	civil servant; imperial subject 9.c
沈	chén	to sink down 2.c
沉	chén	in the depth (as a movement in the vessels) 5.f
沉	chén	deep 9.d
陳	chén	to spread out 3.f
陳方	chén fāng	age-old prescriptions 8.f
陳醬	chén jiàng	old bean sauce 9.c
陳壽	chén shòu	Chen Shou, editor of the *History of the Three Kingdoms* (233-297) 1.f
稱	chēng	name; designation 2.b
稱	chēng	to call; to name 4.c
成	chéng	to be fully developed; to complete 1.a

成	chéng	merit; good results 1.e
成	chéng	to become 2.b
成	chéng	to create 2.b
成	chéng	to constitute 3.e
成功	chéng gōng	to achieve success 1.e
乘	chéng	to seize; to avail oneself of 4.f
誠	chéng	sincerity 1.e
誠	chéng	truly 5.a
承	chéng	to contain; to collect 8.b
懲	chéng	to reprimand; to exhort 8.f
澄	chéng	to let settle 9.f
澄	chéng	clear 10.a
弛	chí	to relax 4.c
持	chí	to control 3.b
持	chí	to hold; to grasp 6.e
遲	chí	to be slow 4.d
尺	chǐ	the foot (-long section of the lower arm); i.e. a section stretching from the "gate" line near the wrist to the foot-marsh insertion hole near the elbow bend 5.c
豉	chǐ	salted beans 9.c
齒	chǐ	tooth 2.a
赤	chì	red 2.f
赤白	chì bái	red and white (colored stools) 9.b
赤水玄珠	chì shuǐ xuán zhū	*Chi shui xuan zhu*, a medical work of the 16th century, by Sūn Yīkuí 孫一奎
充	chōng	to fill; filled 3.b
充	chōng	to reach one's fullest extent 7.a
衝	chōng	a thoroughfare 2.d
衝	chōng	to pass through 4.c
衝脉	chōng mài	the through-way [conduit] vessel 2.f
衝門	chōng mén	the through-gates 2.d
重	chóng	to add 2.d
蟲	chóng	worms; insects; bugs 3.e

崇寧	chóng níng	the *chong ning* ("reverence of peace") reign period (CE 1102-1106) 2.f
重陽	chóng yáng	the doubling of yang (qi) 6.b
重陰	chóng yīn	the doubling of yin (qi) 6.b
抽	chōu	to pull open; to draw out 1.f
仇	chóu	to hate 3.c
愁	chóu	anxiety 5.f
出	chū	to go out; to leave 2.c
出	chū	to elapse; to pass 4.b
出	chū	to make leave; to eliminate 7.b
出候	chū hòu	appearance; manifestation 5.e
初	chū	the beginning 1.e
初	chū	initially 7.c
除	chú	to exclude; to remove 1.f
除…外	chú…wài	except for 6.e
畜	chù	domestic animal 9.b
處	chù	place 2.d
處	chù	to manage 6.a
觸	chù	to run against; to offend; to attack 3.c
觸	chù	to have contact with 4.c
觸	chù	to be affected by 4.e
觸冒	chù mào	to get into touch with, as with something potentially dangerous; to be affected 4.e
穿	chuān	to bore; to dig a hole 1.a
船廠	chuán chǎng	Chuanchang, a place-name 9.a
傳	chuán	to transmit 2.c
傳染	chuán rǎn	to be affected [by a disease] through transmission [from someone else] 4.c
喘	chuǎn	to pant 2.f
創	chuāng	wound 1.f
瘡	chuāng	a wound 3.e
瘡瘍	chuāng yáng	open sores 9.e
牀	chuáng	a bed 3.c
床	chuáng	a frame 8.b

吹	chuī	to praise; to brag 1.e
垂	chuí	to hang down; the scrotum 2.a
春	chūn	spring 3.f
春分	chūn fēn	spring equinox, in the middle of the second month 4.e
唇	chún	the lips 2.d
純	chún	pure 8.a
輟	chuò	to rest 7.c
雌	cí	female 1.c
雌黃	cí huáng	auripigment 9.f
此	cǐ	these 3.a
此則疑彼	cǐ zé yí bǐ	to consider this (which is near) as a rule and doubt that (which is distant) 6.e
此之謂也	cǐ zhī wèi yě	this expresses the meaning of that [what was said above] 1.a
次	cì	next 2.b
次	cì	a series 2.c
次次	cì cì	time and again; continuously 9.f
次第	cì dì	sequence; in order 5.d
次第之序	cì dì zhī xù	a sequential order 5.b
刺	cì	a thorn 1.b
刺	cì	to pierce 1.c
聰耳	cōng ěr	to sharpen one's hearing 9.a
從	cóng	to follow; to comply with 1.a
從	cóng	to originate from; to start from 1.d
從容	cóng róng	to approach naturally 1.c
從事	cóng shì	to perform one's duties 7.f
從事	cóng shì	to deal with 8.b
叢	cóng	crowded; clump of herbs 10.d
腠理	còu lǐ	skin structures 3.b
粗	cū	rough 7.c
卒	cù	suddenly; urgent 1.e
卒然	cù rán	suddenly 4.b
促	cù	hurried (movement in the vessels) 6.c

醋	cù	vinegar 9.f
脆	cuì	fragile 7.c
悴	cuì	sad distressed 9.c
焠刺	cuì cì	cauterization piercing [with a heated needle] 10.c
焠鍼	cuì zhēn	cauterizing needle 10.d
存	cún	to be in existence; to exist 1.e
存乎其人	cún hū qí rén	to be up to a suitable person 8.e
寸	cùn	inch 2.e
寸	cùn	the inch (section of the wrists where the movement in the vessels can be felt) 6.b
寸白蟲	cùn bái chóng	tape worm 9.b
寸口	cùn kǒu	the inch-opening; a location at the wrists where the movement in the vessels can be felt 5.b
撮	cuō	to gather; to pick 6.b
搓	cuō	to rub between the hands 10.b
錯	cuò	mistake 5.a
措手	cuò shǒu	to set the hand to 10.f
答	dá	to answer 3.b
達	dá	to apprehend; to penetrate 1.e
達	dá	to reach to; to pass through 4.b
大	dà	great; extensive 1.e
大	dà	strong; serious 4.b
大便	dà biàn	stools 6.c
大腸	dà cháng	the large intestine 2.b
大抵	dà dǐ	generally speaking 6.f
大都	dà dū	for the most part 8.b
大黃	dà huáng	*dahuang*, a drug prepared from Rheum palmatum L. (and other Rheum plants) 8.f
大略	dà lüè	general rule 7.a
大名	dà míng	name of a prefecture 2.f
大氣	dà qì	the important qi (refers here to the qi of the universe that enter the body through inhalation) 2.c
大小便閉	dà xiǎo biàn bì	constipation of stools and urine 6.d

大寫刺	dà xiè cì	piercing to induce drainage of large [quantities of pus or blood] 10.c
大要	dà yào	*Da yao*, "Great Essential", an antique text, now lost 10.a
大鍼	dà zhēn	the large needle 10.a
大指	dà zhǐ	the thumb 6.a
大眥	dà zì	the inner canthus 5.a
逮	dǎi	to reach; to be sufficient 8.b
代	dài	to substitute; to act on behalf of 4.f
代	dài	intermittent (movement in the vessels) 5.e
待	dài	to wait for 1.e
待	dài	must 7.c
帶	dài	belt; to carry with; connected with 9.f
迨	dài	until 2.b
殆	dài	dangerous 10.a
單	dān	singular (movement in the vessels) 6.f
丹	dān	a small ball (formed to contain all the ingredients of a prescription) 8.e
丹田	dān tián	the cinnabar field; an anatomically nonverifiable area in the body conceptualized in the context of alchemistic-macrobiotic reasoning 2.f
單行	dān xíng	(drugs which prefer) to act alone 8.c
膽	dǎn	the gallbladder 2.b
癉瘧	dǎn nüè	the solitary (heat-)*nüe*, i.e. solitary (heat-) malaria 9.e
但	dàn	but 3.a
但	dàn	only 6.f
淡	dàn	light, in color 6.f
淡	dàn	weak in flavor; bland 7.b
啖	dàn	to eat; to bite 9.c
膻中	dàn zhōng	the *dan zhong* (insertion point) 2.e
當	dāng	ought; should 1.f
當	dāng	exactly 2.d
當	dāng	to bear 2.f

當	dāng	appropriate; fitting 3.a
當歸	dāng guī	*danggui*; a drug prepared from Angelica sinensis (Oliv.) Diels 9.e
蕩	dàng	to excite; to agitate 8.a
蕩漾	dàng yàng	the rippling of water 8.a
導	dǎo	to lead 2.e
導引	dǎo yǐn	guiding-pulling (a type of physical exercises) 7.e
禱	dǎo	to pray 3.a
到	dào	to reach 8.e
道	dào	a way; a path 1.c
道	dào	a doctrine 1.d
盜	dào	robber 2.f
盜汗	dào hàn	robber sweat; night sweat 9.d
倒行逆施	dào xíng nì shī	to move contrary (to all rules) 5.d
得	dé	to acquire 1.b
得	dé	ought; should 1.e
得	dé	to achieve; to be able 3.a
得非	dé fēi	is is not that …? 1.e
燈草	dēng cǎo	reed used for lamp wicks 10.d
登厠	dēng cè	to mount a privy 4.c
燈火	dēng huǒ	the flame of a lamp 10.d
等	děng	sign of plural 3.c
等	děng	equal 8.d
低	dī	to hang down 10.d
鍉鍼	dī zhēn	the arrowhead needle 10.a
滌	dí	to wash 1.f
抵	dǐ	to arrive 2.f
骶骨	dǐ gǔ	the sacrum 4.d
帝	dì	Di; thearch (mythical); emperor (secular) 3.b
第	dì	order; sequences; (with numbers: first, second, third, etc.) 7.b
地	dì	the earth 1.c
地	dì	a field; an arena 8.f

癲疾	diān jí	the falling sickness 9.b
點	diǎn	to nod 5.c
點	diǎn	a dot 9.a
點	diǎn	eye-drops; to drop (a liquid into the eyes) 9.c
點	diǎn	to light 10.d
電	diàn	lightning 2.a
調	diào	to move; to transfer 4.f
調	diào	to investigate 5.e
錠	dìng	an ingot; a cake 8.a
定	dìng	to identify; to determine 5.a
定	dìng	to fix; to keep in a position 9.a
定	dìng	ingot, used here for 錠 *dìng* 9.f
定粉	dìng fěn	Ingot Powder (i. e. powder pressed into the shape of an ingot) 9.f
東垣	dōng yuán	Dongyuan, style-name of Lǐ Gǎo李杲 (1180-1251); author of medical texts 5.a
東醫寶鑒	dōng yī bǎo jiàn	*Dong yi bao jian*, a Korean treatise on medicine of the early 17th century, by Xǔ Jùn 許浚 7.f
冬	dōng	winter 2.a
冬至	dōng zhì	winter solstice 3.f
動	dòng	to move; to take action 1.e
動	dòng	to set in motion; to excite 3.e
動	dòng	excited (movement in the vessels) 6.c
動履	dòng lǚ	daily activities 1.e
動脈	dòng mài	moving vessel 6.a
斗	dǒu	a peck 2.f
鬪	dòu	to fight; battle 1.a
豆	dòu	a bean 6.c
痘	dòu	pox (in modern medical literature: small pox) 6.f
痘科	dòu kē	the branch of medicine concerned with pox 9.a
都	dū	all; the whole 3.a
督脈	dū mài	the supervisor vessel 2.d
毒	dú	poison; toxic 1.c

讀	dú	to study; to read 1.d
獨	dú	only; alone 3.a
獨	dú	alone; isolated 4.f
睹	dǔ	to observe 3.c
肚	dù	the belly 6.b
肚	dù	the stomach; the entrails 9.b
度	dù	degree 8.c
度	dù	to measure; standard 8.c
度	dù	rule 10.e
度量	dù liàng	capacity 3.e
端	duān	a point of departure; a principle 1.d
端	duān	beginning; final cause 3.a
端	duān	one aspect; one end 5.b
短	duǎn	short 2.f
短刺	duǎn cì	short piercing; i.e. deep insertion of a needle until it comes close to a bone 10.c
斷	duàn	to break off; to cut off 1.f
斷	duàn	to decide; to conclude 5.c
斷	duàn	definitely 7.f
對	duì	to reply 7.d
對	duì	to direct against; to confront 8.f
對語	duì yǔ	conversation; dialogue 4.c
頓	dùn	a time; a turn 8.a
頓服	dùn fú	to take in one dose; to ingest together 8.a
多	duō	many 1.e
多	duō	frequent 5.c
奪	duó	to take away 3.f
墮	duò	to fall 4.c
墮胎	duò tāi	to cause an abortion 9.f
痾	ē	ailment 3.e
額	é	the forehead 6.a
惡	è	vicious; bad; malevolent 2.f
惡	è	vice 4.c
遏	è	to check; to prevent 8.c

而	ér	and; and yet 1.a
而已	ér yǐ	and nothing else 1.d
兒	ér	son; boy 4.c
耳	ěr	a final particle 1.f
耳	ěr	ear 2.b
爾	ěr	only 3.a
餌	ěr	cake 10.f
二	èr	two 2.a
發	fā	to rise; to erupt; to develop 1.d
發	fā	to stimulate (heat or perspiration) 8.b
發	fā	to send out; to eliminate; to emit 10.a
發背	fā bèi	to develop on one's back (as a sore) 10.d
發明	fā míng	explanation 9.d
發熱	fā rè	to stimulate heat 8.d
發熱	fā rè	to develop heat (as a body); fits of heat; fever 9.a
發散	fā sàn	to stimulate dispersion; to dissipate 7.b
發泄	fā xiè	to stimulate discharge 8.d
發針	fā zhēn	to withdraw the needle 10.e
罰	fá	to punish 3.f
乏	fá	to be in want of 6.e
法	fǎ	method 4.b
法	fǎ	pattern 5.d
法場	fǎ chǎng	the place of execution 2.f
髮	fà	the hair on the head 2.b
凡	fán	all 1.f
蕃	fán	opulence 3.f
煩	fán	vexed 4.f
煩	fán	uneasiness; vexation 8.b
反	fǎn	to oppose 1.a
反	fǎn	to turn over 1.e
反	fǎn	in contrast 4.f
反	fǎn	short for 反治 *fǎn zhì*: a treatment in contrast to (what one should expect; i.e. a treatment which

		disregards misleading symptoms and is directed against the true nature of an illness) 8.d
反胃	fǎn wèi	a stomach that turns back (the food it receives) 4.b
反掌	fǎn zhǎng	to turn the hand; very easily done 1.e
泛	fàn	superficial;superficiality 8.e
泛濫	fàn làn	to overflow 7.a
犯	fàn	to invade; to offend; to attack 3.c
范曄	fàn yè	Fan Ye, compiler of the *History of the Eastern Han Dynasty* (died 445) 1.f
方	fāng	direction; region 1.d
方	fāng	prescription; recipe 1.d
方	fāng	method 1.e
方	fāng	just in this moment; just then 1.e
方	fāng	square 2.a
方書	fāng shū	title of a book; possibly referring to a text compiled by Xú Dùzhēn 徐杜真 of the Yuan era 5.a
方向	fāng xiàng	direction 4.c
防	fáng	to protect from 1.e
防	fáng	to prevent 6.f
放	fàng	to loosen; to let go 10.a
非	fēi	to be not; to be wrong; to regard as wrong; condemn 1.b
非	fēi	(is) not 1.d
非節	fēi jié	unseasonable; out of season 4.e
非…不…	fēi…bù…	if .. is not, then …does not 1.d
飛	fēi	to fly 2.d
飛門	fēi mén	the flying gate 2.d
肥	féi	fat 7.e
沸	fèi	to bubble up; to boil 1.f
肺	fèi	the lung 2.b
分	fēn	a part 1.c
分	fēn	to divide; to distinguish 1.d

分	fēn	to divide; to separate 2.b
分	fēn	section; one tenth of an inch; fen 2.e
分崩	fēn bēng	to fall apart; to disintegrate 8.b
分刺	fēn cì	piercing of the partings [of the flesh] 10.c
分間	fēn jiān	the region of the partings [of the flesh] 10.a
分兩	fēn liǎng	candareens and taels; quantities 8.f
分氣	fēn qì	the qi in the partings [of the flesh] 10.a
分肉	fēn ròu	the flesh under the skin 4.c
紛紜	fēn yún	perturbation 9.a
粉錫	fěn xī	Powdered Tin (i.e. white lead; lead carbonate) 9.f
糞	fèn	feces 9.f
膹瞋	fèn zhēn	swollen 4.c
賁門	fén mén	the big gate 2.d
封	fēng	to seal up 9.f
風	fēng	fame; reputation 1.e
風	fēng	wind 2.a
風府	fēng fǔ	the wind palace 4.d
風關	fēng guān	the wind-gate(-section; i.e. the section between the base fold, adjoining the palm, and the second fold on the inside of the index finger) 6.f
風爐	fēng lú	a wind-stove (i.e. a stove that is fanned by the natural flow of wind air, and that does not need a bellows 9.f
風癇	fēng xián	convulsions (caused by) wind 6.f
豐裕	fēng yù	rich; wealthy 8.b
鋒鍼	fēng zhēn	the lance-point needle 10.a
馮氏錦囊	féng shì jǐn náng	*Feng shi jin nang*, a medical work of the 17th century, by Féng Chǔzhán 馮楚瞻 7.f
縫	féng	to seam; to sew 1.f
縫	fèng	seam; slit 9.f
奉	fèng	to receive; to pay tribute to; to support 3.e
否	foǔ	if not 3.c
否	foǔ	or not 5.c
夫	fū	now 1.a

夫	fū	husband 2.a
傅	fū	to apply (an ointment) 1.f
膚	fū	the skin 3.b
弗	fú	not 3.b
伏	fú	to hide; hidden 3.f
伏熱	fú rè	deep-lying heat 9.b
浮	fú	to float; surface 4.b
浮刺	fú cì	surface piercing; i.e. a slanted superficial insertion 10.c
桴鼓	fú gǔ	drumstick and drum [need to come together to produce a sound] 5.e
符水	fú shuǐ	amulet [dissolved in] water 10.f
服	fú	to ingest (pharmaceutical substances); to take (medicine) 1.f
服	fú	to yield 7.d
福	fú	happiness; prosperity 7.f
府	fǔ	a "palace" processing unit in the body, i.e. gall bladder, small intestine, triple burner, stomach, large intestine, urinary bladder 1.c
府	fǔ	collecting point 2.e
府	fǔ	a prefecture 2.f
拊摩	fǔ mó	to pat 10.f
腑	fǔ	to have a strong odor 7.e
腐	fǔ	rotten; to spoil 2.e
腐	fǔ	foul 5.f
父	fù	father 2.b
富	fù	wealthy 1.c
副	fù	to assist 1.c
復	fù	to return; again 1.d
復	fù	additional 5.a
復	fù	to restore 7.a
復	fù	to recover 7.b
腹	fù	the abdomen 1.f
附	fù	to attribute; to add to 1.f

附	fù	to attach 9.d
附會	fù huì	to add and to assemble; farfetched 8.e
附子	fù zǐ	*fuzi*, a drug prepared from Aconitum carmichaeli Debx. 9.a
附著	fùzhuó	possession (by demons) 3.e
負	fù	to succumb 4.f
婦	fù	woman 5.c
覆	fù	turnover 6.d
茯苓	fù líng	*fuling*, a drug prepared from Poria cocos (Schw.) Wolf 9.a
蓋	gài	initial particle: namely; for; now; the fact is … 1.d
蓋	gài	to cover 2.f
甘	gān	sweet 2.c
甘草	gān cǎo	*gancao*, a drug prepared from Glycyrrhiza uralensis Fisch. and other Glycyrrhiza herbs 8.a
肝	gān	the liver 2.b
乾	gān	dry 4.a
疳	gān	the *gan*-illness 6.f
敢	gǎn	to dare 1.e
感	gǎn	to affect; to touch 2.b
感冒	gǎn mạo	to be affected by adverse (climatic qi) 4.c
肛	gāng	the rectum 2.d
肛門	gāng mén	the rectum-gate 2.d
剛	gāng	hard 7.e
綱領	gāng lǐng	a pervasive principle 5.b
綱目	gāng mù	abbreviated title of the *Běn cǎo gāng mù* ("Materia Medica Arranged According to Drug Descriptions and Technical Aspects") compiled by Lǐ Shí-zhēn 李時珍 (1518-1593) 9.f
高	gāo	high 2.a
膏	gāo	ointment 1.f
膏	gāo	below the heart 3.a
膏粱	gāo liáng	rich; wealthy (lit.: fat meat and fine millet) 7.c
告	gào	to announce 7.f

歌	gē	song; to sing 5.f
疙瘩	gē da	knots 4.c
格	gé	to resist; to obstruct 1.a
格	gé	to come or go to; to reach 1.e
格	gé	to investigate 8.a
割	gé	to cut 1.f
隔	gé	to separate; to wrap 9.a
隔	gé	to push aside 10.f
膈	gé	the diaphragm 2.e
膈	gé	blockage 4.b
合	gé	one tenth of a Chinese pint 9.c
蛤粉	gé fěn	powdered oyster shells 9.f
葛根	gé gēn	*gegen*, a drug prepared from Pueraria lobata (Willd.) Ohwi 8.e
葛根湯	gé gēn tāng	"decoction with *gegen* (i.e. the roots of Pueraria lobata (Willd.) Ohwi)" 5.a
格拒	géjù	to meet with obstruction; to ward off 6.d
各	gè	each; every; all 1.c
箇	gè	classifier 2.f
箇箇	gè gè	one by one; each 2.f
根	gēn	origin; root 2.d
跟	gēn	the heel 6.a
亘	gèn	to revolve 6.e
更	gèng	more; furthermore 1.d
更	gèng	to change; alternately 4.d
更	gèng	even more 7.b
工	gōng	a practitioner 1.f
攻	gōng	to attack 7.b
恭	gōng	Gong, abbreviated taboo version of the name of Sū Jìng 蘇敬, co-author of the *Táng běn cǎo* 唐本草 9.f
公	gōng	a gentleman; Sir; Mr. 10.f
公子彭生	gōng zǐ	Gongzi Pengsheng; name of a courtier of Qi

	péng shēng	who was executed in 693 BCE and is said to have reappeared as a pig-shaped demon 3.c
功能	gōng néng	effects 8.e
弓弦	gōng xián	a bow-string 6.c
鈎	gōu	hook(-like movement in the vessels) 5.e
鈎	gōu	hook; sickle; to take on a hook; to pull 9.d
溝	gōu	a ditch 9.f
苟	gǒu	if 4.f
覯	gòu	to encounter 7.c
孤	gū	solitary 6.d
孤虛	gū xū	lucky and unlucky (days of the calendar) 4.c
古	gǔ	ancient 1.f
谷	gǔ	valley 2.a
骨	gǔ	bone 2.a
骨蒸	gǔ zhēng	bone-steaming 9.b
穀	gǔ	grain 2.c
鼓	gǔ	drum 4.a
鼓	gǔ	to chatter, as jaws or teeth 4.d
鼓舞	gǔ wǔ	to stimulate 7.c
臌	gǔ	bloating 4.b
蠱	gǔ	the *gu*(-spirit) 4.c
蠱毒	gǔ dú	the poison of *gu* 8.c
汩	gǔ	to throw into disorder 8.b
故	gù	cause; reason 1.d
故	gù	fact 10.f
顧	gù	used here for 故 *gù*; therefore 1.e
固	gù	definitely 1.f
固	gù	firm; strong 3.c
固	gù	to strengthen 7.b
固冷	gù lěng	constipation resulting from cold 7.b
痼	gù	chronic illness 10.a
寡	guǎ	a term of depreciation used by princes of themselves 3.d
寡	guǎ	few 8.f

寡婦	guǎ fù	a widow 5.c
乖	guāi	perversion; error 9.f
官	guān	officer; official 2.f
官粉	guān fěn	Superior Powder 9.f
棺	guān	a coffin 9.d
關	guān	a pass; to close; to be closely linked 1.e
關	guān	a gate 2.d
關	guān	the gate (section of the wrists where the movement in the vessels can be felt) 6.b
關	guān	the gate(-line separating the inch and the foot sections at the wrist) 6.d
關	guān	the gate(-sections of the index fingers of small children) 6.f
關於	guān yú	to be related to; to result from 3.a
關元	guān yuán	the *guan yuan* (needle insertion point; located three inches below the navel) 2.d
觀	guān	to observe 7.d
管	guǎn	a tube 2.f
貫	guàn	to go through; to connect 7.a
光	guāng	to shine 3.f
光	guāng	bare; shiny 9.a
光粉	guāng fěn	Radiant Powder 9.f
廣	guǎng	extensive; broad 3.a
歸	guī	to return; to turn to; to end up somewhere 4.f
歸	guī	to be counted as ...; to belong to ... 7.b
歸	guī	short for *danggui*, a drug prepared from Angelica sinensis (Oliv.) Diels 9.e
鬼	guǐ	demon 3.a
貴	guì	high-class; noble 1.c
貴	guì	to value 6.e
桂枝	guì zhī	*guizhi*, a drug prepared from Cinnamomum cassia Presl. 8.e
鯀	gǔn	Gun, father of the legendary Yǔ the Great 7.b
郭	guō	a rim 3.b

虢	Guó	name of an ancient feudal state 1.f
膕	guó	the hollow behind the knee 2.a
國家	guó jiā	country; the state 1.e
果	guǒ	really 5.b
果子	guǒ zǐ	fruits; berry 7.f
裹	guǒ	to wrap 2.f
過	guò	to exceed 2.b
過	guò	error 3.c
過	guò	to pass by; to pass through 3.d
骸	hái	the human bones 2.b
海	hǎi	sea; ocean 2.c
海陽	Hǎiyáng	Haiyang, a place name in today's Guangzhou 9.e
害	hài	to injure; injury 1.e
害	hài	harm 6.e
酣	hān	intoxicated; merry 7.c
寒	hán	cold 1.d
寒熱往來	hán rè wǎng lái	alternative fits of cold and heat 9.e
頷	hán	the jaws 4.d
含	hán	to retain in one's mouth 8.a
悍	hàn	fierce; violent 4.c
汗空	hàn kōng	a sweat opening 4.d
杭州	háng zhōu	Hangzhou, name of a prefecture 9.f
毫	háo	fine; minute 2.a
毫	háo	an intensive; especially before negatives 8.f
毫鍼	háo zhēn	the hair needle 10.a
好	hào	to love 1.f
耗	hào	to destroy; to diminish 4.f
合	hé	to join; to pair 1.d
合	hé	together 2.c
合	hé	a confluence (generic name for all final insertion points on the conduit-streams in the extremities) 10.b

合和	hé hé	to combine (drugs in a) balanced (prescription) 8.c
和	hé	harmony with 3.b
和	hé	pleasant 4.e
和	hé	to mix; to blend 6.d
涸	hé	dried up; exhausted 6.e
何	hé	what? 1.d
何	hé	how? 7.b
何	hé	specific 8.e
何啻千萬	hé chì qiān wàn	a countless multitude (lit.: how could it be only thousands of myriads?) 5.d
何其多也	hé qí duō yě	what could be more numerous; innumerable 7.b
何以	hé yǐ	by what means; how 5.b
闔	hé	to close 10.b
褐	hè	serge; rough clothing; [garments of] hair 7.e
黑	hēi	black 2.f
黑珠	hēi zhū	the dark (section of the) eyeball 5.a
痕	hén	a scar; mark 10.f
脝	hēng	fat; bloated 4.b
横	héng	to harbor; to carry 8.f
横	héng	sideways; to all sides; laterally 9.a
横	héng	bulging 10.e
横連	héng lián	to attach horizontally 4.d
横鶩	héng wù	to behave as wild as a duck 7.b
洪	hóng	vast 4.f
洪水	hóng shuǐ	a great flood 7.b
紅	hóng	red 10.d
弘景	hóng jǐng	Hongjing, abbreviated name of Táo Hóngjǐng 陶弘景 (456-536), Daoist and author of materia medicas 9.f
喉管	hóu guǎn	the wind-pipe 2.f
喉嚨	hóu lóng	the wind-pipe 2.c
喉嚨	hóu lóng	the throat 2.f
後	hòu	after 1.a

後	hòu	afterwards; later 1.d
後	hòu	behind
候	hòu	sign of a disease 5.b
候	hòu	to examine 6.a
候	hòu	indicator 1.c
候	hòu	to wait 10.b
厚	hòu	thick; substantial; generous 1.d
厚	hòu	strongly developed (quality of a drug) 8.a
乎	hū	interrogative 1.a
乎	hū	in; at (used for 於 *yú* and 于 *yú*) 1.e
呼	hū	to exhale 2.c
呼	hū	to shout; to call 5.f
胡粉	hú fěn	Foreign Powder 9.f
糊	hú	paste 9.f
狐臭	hú xiù	fox odor (from under the arm-pits) 9.f
虎	hǔ	tiger 3.e
虎口	hǔ kǒu	(the width of an opened) tiger mouth; i.e. the distance between the tip of one's thumb and the tip of one's index finger if spread apart from one hand 6.f
戶	hù	door 2.d
戶門	hù mén	the door-gate 2.d
護	hù	to protect; to preserve 3.e
互	hù	mutually; reciprocal 6.e
互相	hù xiāng	vice versa 8.d
瓠	hù	a gourd 9.c
花	huā	flower 2.b
華	huá	to bloom 3.f
華	huá	excellent; rich [food] 7.e
華	huá	flowers 8.c
華蓋	huá gài	a canopy 2.f
華英	huá yīng	beauty; splendor 3.f
滑	huá	smooth 5.c
化	huà	to transform 1.d

化	huà	to digest 6.f
畫	huà	to draw a picture; picture 2.f
華佗	huà tuó	Hua Tuo, physician and medical author (110-207) 1.f
踝	huái	the ankle 6.a
壞	huài	ruined 1.e
環	huán	a ring; to encircle 3.e
還	huán	to return 10.f
桓侯	huán hōu	Marquis Huan 3.d
緩	huǎn	slow 1.d
緩	huǎn	relaxed 3.b
緩	huǎn	to temper 3.f
患	huàn	to suffer; suffering 1.e
豢	huàn	to feed 7.c
豢養	huàn yǎng	to nourish 8.b
換	huàn	to remove 10.d
患人	huàn rén	a patient 5.b
肓	huāng	above the diaphragm 3.a
惶恐	huáng kǒng	to fear; to be frightened 10.c
黃丹	huáng dān	Yellow Balls (i.e. minium; lead tetroxide) 9.f
黃帝	huáng dì	Huang Di, The Yellow Thearch; legendary ruler whose dialogues with his advisers constitute major parts of the classical Chinese medical texts 2.c
黃連	huáng lián	*huanglian*, a drug prepared from Coptis chinensis Franch. (and other Coptis plants) 9.e
黃芩	huáng qín	*huangqing*, a drug prepared from Scutellaria baicalensis Georgi 9.e
黃庭	huáng tíng	the "yellow court"; a Daoist term referring to the center of the body, and to the navel 2.d
黃庭經	huáng tíng jīng	*Huang ting jing*, the "Classic of the Yellow Court"; in its nuclear parts a late Han text on human meditative physiology 2.d
灰	huī	ashes 9.d

恢刺	huī cì	broad piercing; i.e. piercing next to a cramped or painful sinew. The needle is moved back and forth to widen the opening at the insertion point 10.c
廻避	huí bì	to turn away 10.d
毀	huǐ	to destroy 1.f
會	huì	to combine; to bring together 1.d
會	huì	to meet; to associate with 1.f
會厭	huì yàn	the epiglottis 2.d
晦	huì	obscure
穢	huì	foul; spoiled 1.f
恚	huì	range 5.f
喙	huì	a beak; a snout 10.a
昏	hūn	confused; irregular 3.a
昏憒	hūn kuì	dazed; confused 5.c
魂	hún	the *hun*-soul (believed to continue existing after a person's physical death) 2.b
活	huó	alive; to keep alive 1.f
火鍼	huǒ zhēn	the fire needle 10.d
或	huò	sometimes, in some cases, someone 1.b
或	huò	or else; perhaps 1.e
或	huò	occasionally; in some cases 4.a
或	huò	whether 5.c
或時	huò shí	occasionally 6.f
禍	huò	calamity; to cause misery 3.c
惑	huò	to doubt 3.c
霍	huò	violent (intestinal disturbance); short for 霍亂 *huòluàn* (often interpreted now as cholera) 9.b
肌	jī	the flesh under the skin 1.f
饑	jī	hunger 3.a
鷄	jī	chicken; fowl 3.f
鷄子白	jī zǐ bái	egg-white 9.f
機	jī	trigger; mechanics; movement 7.c

機關	jī guān	the (sections where the bones) move and have their joints 10.a
積	jī	to gather; to store up 1.f
積	jī	accumulation 6.b
積年	jī nián	many years 9.d
積曲	jī qū	to have [many] bends [inside]; coiled 2.f
積鬱	jī yù	accumulation 4.c
及	jí	to reach; and 1.e
脊	jí	the spine; the back 2.f
極	jí	very 2.f
急	jí	urgent; fast 1.d
急	jí	tense; taut 3.b
急	jí	to hurry 8.b
疾	jí	illness 1.b
疾	jí	fast 3.b
集	jí	to collect; to gather 3.c
亟	jí	fast; quickly 3.f
吉	jí	auspicious 4.c
吉凶	jí xiōng	good or bad fortune 7.f
即	jí	instantly; immediately 4.e
極	jí	to treat exhaustively 3.e
極	jí	thorough; (to reach a) final (conclusion) 5.e
奇	jí	uneven (as numbers) 8.a
己	jǐ	self 2.b
幾	jǐ	subtle; hidden; some 1.e
幾	jǐ	how many? 5.a
幾	jǐ	minute 5.b
幾分	jǐ fēn	what percentage; how much of it 8.f
紀	jì	a skein; to regulate; a principle 1.c
際	jì	a time; while 1.e
忌	jì	to avoid 1.e
記	jì	to record; record 1.f
既	jì	after 1.f
既	jì	if; when 2.d

既	jì	already 4.b
既	jì	to supply with; to nourish 2.c
計	jì	to count 2.c
計	jì	to plan; to scheme 2.f
繫	jì	to bind; to be attached to 3.e
繼	jì	to follow 4.c
寄	jì	to entrust to 7.f
劑	jì	a formula; a prescription 7.b
劑	jì	a dose (of drugs) 8.b
季	jì	a season 9.b
悸	jì	palpitations 9.a
濟	jì	to complete 9.f
記	jì	to record; to mark 10.d
既而	jì ér	afterwards 1.f
加	jiā	to add; to apply 1.e
家	jiā	a specialist 5.a
家	jiā	a house; a family 7.f
佳	jiā	excellent; good 10.d
頰	jiá	a cheek 6.a
假	jiǎ	to receive 2.b
假令	jiǎ lìng	suppose; if, for example, ...; take, for example, … 5.f
架	jià	shelf 7.f
湔	jiān	to wash 1.f
尖	jiān	pointed 2.f
堅	jiān	firm; hard 3.b
間	jiān	space between 2.d
間	jiān	to divide; to distinguish 6.b
肩	jiān	shoulder 2.a
肩	jiān	to shoulder 7.f
煎	jiān	to decoct 9.a
兼	jiān	to unite; additional; joint 5.d
兼病	jiān bìng	additional disease 5.d

兼症	jiān zhèng	adjunct patho-conditions accompanying a disease 5.d
減	jiǎn	to diminish; to reduce 3.b
減	jiǎn	to be reduced; to fall short of 6.d
賤	jiàn	low; common 1.c
見	jiàn	to see 1.d
見	jiàn	view; perspective 3.c
漸	jiàn	gradually 3.a
薦	jiàn	[garments of] grasses 7.e
健	jiàn	to strengthen 9.b
件	jiàn	item; thing 9.c
劍	jiàn	a double-edged sword 10.a
間	jiàn	among; in; occasionally 1.e
間日	jiàn rì	to skip a day 4.d
間有	jiàn yǒu	if occasionally 5.b
將	jiāng	a particle indicating future; here: or (connecting two questions) 3.b
將	jiāng	to intend 3.e
將	jiāng	to take into one's hands; particle preceding an object 8.f
將	jiāng	a general 10.d
漿	jiāng	broth; liquid 8.b
講	jiǎng	to investigate
降	jiàng	to descend 8.a
交	jiāo	to interact; to change; to deliver 1.d
交	jiāo	to exchange; to communicate; to join 1.e
交	jiāo	to meet each other; to exchange 2.b
交馳	jiāo chí	to move as fast as a horse 7.b
交錯	jiāo cuò	interlocking; intertwined 10.b
焦	jiāo	a burner 2.c
焦	jiāo	burnt (breath odor) 5.f
膠固	jiāo gù	firm 7.c
撟	jiǎo	to stretch 1.f
撟引	jiǎo yǐn	massage 1.f

絞	jiǎo	to twist; to squeeze 9.c
脚氣	jiǎo qì	(evil) qi (which have moved down into the) legs. This term is used in modern medicine to refer to the disease of beri-beri. In Chinese traditional medicine, the term included a wide range of different syndromes. 9.b
教	jiào	teachings 1.d
校	jiào	used here for 較 *jiào*: obvious; clear 7.c
攪	jiào	to stir up 9.f
較	jiào	to compare 10.d
叫呼	jiào hū	to shout 3.e
皆	jiē	all 1.e
痎	jiē	*jie*, an ancient term for a disease unidentifiable today 3.f
竭	jiē	to exhaust; exhausted 4.b
階	jiē	class; standard 7.b
結	jié	to tie knots; to bind 1.b
結	jié	to clot; clotting 1.f
結	jié	to unite 2.b
結	jié	to finish 2.d
結固	jié gù	conglomeration 6.c
捷徑	jié jìng	a short-cut 8.f
捷效	jié xiào	to be successful 8.e
結實	jié shí	firm 9.a
節	jié	section
節	jié	season 4.e
截	jié	to cut 9.f
解	jiě	to untie 1.b
解	jiě	to separate 2.b
解	jiě	to resolve 3.c
解	jiě	to loosen 4.e
解	jiě	to dissolve 8.a
解錫	jiě xī	Dissolved Tin 9.f
借	jiè	to borrow; to depend upon 2.f

界	jiè	a boundary; a border 9.e
疥癬	jiè xuǎn	itching skin diseases, consisting of either eruptive, scattered, small patches (*jiè* 疥), or noneruptive, large patches (*xuǎn* 癬) 9.f
斤	jīn	a catty 9.f
今	jīn	now 1.b
筋	jīn	the sinews 1.f
金	jīn	metal 3.e
金	jīn	gold 7.e
金瘡	jīn chuāng	wounds caused by metal weapons; sword wounds 9.b
金匱方	jīn guì fāng	*Jin gui fang*, short title of *Jīn guì yù hán yào luè fāng lùn* 金匱玉函要略方論, the "Concise Discussion of Important Prescriptions from the Golden Coffer and Jade Sheath", by Zhāng Jī 張機 (142-220?) 9.c
金陵	jīn líng	Jinling, a place name 9.f
津	jīn	body liquid 8.a
津液	jīn yè	liquid 2.c
謹	jǐn	attentive; carefully 1.e
緊	jǐn	tight (movement in the vessels) 6.c
僅	jǐn	merely 8.e
盡	jìn	entirely; all; wholly 1.e
盡	jìn	to exhaust 3.e
近	jìn	to approach 5.b
近	jìn	to be close to; to accompany 7.a
近世	jìn shì	in recent times 8.b
竟	jìn	finally; in the end 8.e
進	jìn	to advance 8.f
進	jìn	to give (a drug to a patient) 9.a
禁	jìn	to prohibit 9.e
晉景公	jìn jǐng gōng	Duke Jing of Jin 3.a
經	jīng	a warp; to pass through; invariable rule; a standard 1.c

經	jīng	classic (scripture; containing standards of knowledge) 1.c
經	jīng	a conduit 1.d
經	jīng	a big river; stream 2.a
經	jīng	daily pursuits 3.e
經	jīng	a stream (generic name for all fourth insertion points on the twelve conduit-streams in the extremities) 10.b
經刺	jīng cì	piercing of conduits; i.e. piercing of the conduit primarily affected by a disease 10.c
經紀	jīng jì	ordering principle; invariable rule 1.c
精	jīng	subtleties 1.d
精	jīng	semen; essence 2.b
精	jīng	essence; essential 2.c
精	jīng	pure 3.b
精	jīng	to be versed in; to be an expert 5.b
經營	jīng yíng	to engage in 7.c
井	jǐng	a well 1.a
井	jǐng	a well (generic name for all first insertion points on the twelve conduit-streams in the extremities) 10.b
景岳全書	jǐng yuè quán shū	*Jing yue quan shu*, the medical writings of Zhāng Jǐngyuè 張景岳 of the 17th century 7.f
莖	jìng	stalk; the penis 2.a
淨	jìng	pure; clean 2.f
驚	jìng	to startle; be terrified 3.c
驚	jìng	fright; terror 3.e
脛	jìng	the shinbone 5.f
徑	jìng	a short-cut; direct 6.d
徑庭	jìng tíng	a narrow track and a wide hall; very unlike 6.e
靜	jìng	quiet 10.a
敬	jìng	to revere 10.f
究	jiū	to examine into 1.e
究心	jiū xīn	to conduct thorough inquiries 1.e

久	jiǔ	a long time 1.b
灸	jiǔ	to cauterize, mostly by burning moxa 1.c
酒	jiǔ	wine 1.f
九	jiǔ	nine 1.c
九變	jiǔ biàn	the nine variations (in the method of piercing) 10.c
九候	jiǔ hòu	the nine indicators (where the movement in the vessels can be felt) 1.c
九鍼	jiǔ zhēn	the nine [types of] needles [used in acupuncture] 7.e
就	jiù	to approach; to seek 3.f
舊	jiù	formerly; before 9.f
救	jiù	to aid; help 7.f
救誤	jiù wù	to save from the mistakes [committed by someone else] 7.f
僦貸季	jiù dài jì	Jiu Daiji, legendary physician of ancient times 7.d
居	jū	to dwell; to rest 1.d
居	jū	to be 2.f
拘攣	jū luán	cramps 7.b
舉	jǔ	to raise; to recommend 1.d
舉	jǔ	an activity; something one "takes up" 5.a
聚	jù	to gather 1.f
具	jù	prepared 2.b
具	jù	tool; agent 3.c
具	jù	to have 7.b
俱	jù	all; every 2.d
俱	jù	together with 3.f
句	jù	a sentence 6.e
劇	jù	troublesome; distressing 4.c
劇	jù	a crisis 6.c
劇	jù	to add to; to increase 7.f
據	jù	to hold; according to; evidence 3.c
據	jù	to occupy; to take possession 7.c

據	jù	according to 9.e
遽	jù	suddenly; immediately 10.f
巨刺	jù cì	grand piercing; i.e. piercing a site on the right side of the patient if the illness is located on the left, and vice versa 10.c
巨陽	jù yáng	the great-yang (conduit) 4.d
卷	juǎn	to roll up 9.f
倦	juàn	fatigued; weary 5.f
眷慕	juàn mù	to think [of someone] with sentimental affection 7.d
决	jué	to clear a water-way; to open 1.b
决	jué	decidedly; before a negative adds strong emphasis 1.f
决	jué	to decide 6.a
覺	jué	to perceive; to feel 1.f
抉	jué	to take out; to tear out 1.f
絕	jué	to cut off 4.b
厥	jué	a personal pronoun; he, his, theirs 1.e
厥	jué	receding [qi] 3.f
厥病篇	jué bìng piān	the treatise Jue bing ("Recession Diseases") of the *Líng shū* 靈樞 10.b
厥冷	jué lěng	cold (hands and feet) due to ceasing (yang) 6.d
厥陰	jué yīn	the ceasing-yin (conduits) 9.e
均	jūn	all 3.c
君	jūn	gentleman; noble 2.f
君	jūn	ruler; term to address a superior 3.d
君	jūn	ruler (drug in a prescription) 8.a
君子	jūn zǐ	the noble man; the gentleman 4.e
䐃	jùn	lump; accumulation of flesh 2.a
開	kāi	to open 2.f
揩摩	kāi mó	to rub 10.a
堪克	kān kè	able for 8.b

坎陷	kǎn xiàn	the "cave at the bottom" (where all liquids gather); identified here as a designation of the kidneys 8.b
看	kàn	to examine; to look at 5.c
康子	kāng zǐ	Kang Zi, a statesman, contemporary of Confucius 1.e
考	kǎo	to examine 2.d
考	kǎo	thoughtful attention 8.f
咳	ké	to cough 4.a
客	kè	visitor; guest 3.d
客	kè	to reside 7.b
渴	kě	to be thirsty; thirst 1.a
可	kě	can; be able 1.b
可否	kě foǔ	what is right and what is wrong; what can be and what cannot be 6.e
尅	kè	to destroy 4.b
尅化	kè huà	to digest 4.b
肯	kěn	to consent; to be willing 6.e
空	kōng	empty 3.b
空鬆	kōng sōng	hollow and loose; soft 9.a
恐	kǒng	to fear 3.d
孔	kǒng	hole 10.d
口	kǒu	the mouth 2.b
口	kǒu	opening 2.c
寇	kòu	bandit 2.f
刳	kū	to cut open 1.f
哭	kū	to wail 5.f
枯槁	kū gǎo	to wither; to dry out 4.b
苦	kǔ	bitter 2.c
酷烈	kù liè	fierce 4.c
塊	kuài	lump; piece 2.f
駃	kuài	fast; swift 6.c
寬	kuān	broad; extensive 10.b
狂	kuáng	mad; reckless 1.e

況	kuàng	further; moreover 2.d
虧	kuī	deficiency; fault 3.c
揆度	kuí duó	to consider; to estimate 4.f
饋	kuì	to offer food to a superior 1.e
匱	kuì	failing; deficient; exhausted 7.c
潰	kuì	to scatter; to disperse 10.d
憒憒	kuì kuì	confused 3.c
坤	kūn	the earth; female 2.b
困	kùn	difficult; critical 6.e
闊大	kuò dà	capacious 10.d
臘月	là yuè	the twelfth lunar month 9.b
來	lái	to receive 2.f
來	lái	to come 3.a
賴	lài	to rely upon; to need 3.c
闌	lán	a barrier 2.d
闌門	lán mén	the screen-gate 2.d
懶	lǎn	unwilling; lazy 5.c
攬	lǎn	to seize 7.b
爛	làn	to decay; rotten 4.c
爛	làn	brightness (of eyes) 9.d
狼	láng	wolf 3.e
醪	láo	the lees of wine; wine 3.d
牢	láo	firm (movement in the vessels) 6.f
癆	láo	wasting; consumption 7.f
勞	láo	taxation 3.a
勞	láo	exhausting 5.a
勞	láo	wasting 9.b
勞復	láo fù	recurrence (of an illness) due to (physical) taxation 9.f
勞役	láo yì	to toil; to indulge in exhausting labor 7.c
勞勩	láo yì	to toil 8.b
老	lǎo	old; aged 1.d
樂	lè	joy; to rejoice 1.f

樂	lè	to enjoy something; to be happy about something 7.b
雷	léi	thunder 2.a
羸	léi	emaciated 8.b
類	lèi	class; sort; kind 3.c
類	lèi	similar 4.b
類推	lèi tuī	to conclude by analogy 5.d
累	lèi	to tie; to bind; entanglement 7.d
淚	lèi	tears 9.c
冷	lěng	cool; cold 3.a
離	lí	to part; to separate 2.d
離	lí	to leave; to turn one's back to 7.d
離魂	lí hún	departure of one's *hun*(-soul) 9.a
藜藿	lí huò	coarse food; common vegetables 7.c
藜蘆	lí lú	*lilu*, a drug prepared from Veratrum nigrum L. 9.a
裏	lǐ	inside; interior 1.c
醴	lǐ	sweet wine 1.f
理	lǐ	to structure; to arrange; an order; structure 1.c
理	lǐ	principle; structure 1.d
理	lǐ	to manage; to order 5.b
理	lǐ	the [skin] structures; short for: 腠理 *còu lǐ* 7.e
理	lǐ	to regulate 8.f
李幾道	Lǐ Jīdào	name of an otherwise unknown physician 10.f
李子豫	lǐ zǐ yù	Li Ziyu; name of a legendary healer of the Zhou era 3.a
癘	lì	a serious illness affecting many 3.a
力	lì	strength 3.a
力食	lì shí	to toil physically to make a living 7.c
力作	lì zuò	to exert one's strength 7.c
例	lì	precedent; example 3.a
利	lì	gain; profit 3.d
利	lì	free passage 4.c
利	lì	dysentery 9.b

利用	lì yòng	to employ 7.c
慄	lì	to tremble; to shiver 4.d
厲	lì	to grind; to destroy 4.e
痢	lì	dysentery 5.d
立	lì	to establish 1.d
立	lì	to stand; to exist 4.f
立	lì	immediately 9.c
立方	lì fāng	to compose a prescription 7.f
連	lián	at once 10.f
練	liàn	to practice 7.b
梁	liáng	a family name 2.f
涼	liáng	cool; fresh 4.e
良	liáng	good 5.d
良久	liáng jiǔ	quite a long time 9.c
量	liáng	to measure 10.b
兩	liǎng	two; a pair 2.a
兩	liǎng	a tael 9.f
療	liáo	to heal; to cure 3.a
遼東	liáo dōng	Liaodong, name of a region; Manchuria 9.a
列	liè	to arrange in order 2.a
冽	liè	biting cold 4.e
烈	liè	violent; fierce 8.b
裂	liè	to rip open; to open 1.f
劣	liè	want of strength; weakness 9.b
林	lín	forest 2.a
淋漓	lín lí	to drip 4.c
淋瀝	lín lì	strangurious drip 9.a
臨	lín	just before 2.f
臨	lín	in the face of 7.c
臨時	lín shí	when the time has come 10.d
臨診	lín zhěn	clinical diagnosis 7.c
臨證指南	lín zhèng zhǐ nán	*Lin zheng zhi nan*, a medical treatise of the 18th century, by Yè Guì 葉桂 7.f
陵	líng	earthen mound 7.e

苓	líng	the pharmaceutical drug *fúlíng* 茯苓, prepared from Poria cocos Wolf 8.b
靈	líng	spirits 3.a
靈	líng	abbreviated title of the *Líng shū*靈樞, one of the books constituting the corpus 黃帝內經 *Huang Di nei jing*10.b
靈樞	líng shū	*Ling shu*, abbreviation of the *Huang Di nei jing ling shu*, "Huang Di's Inner Classic, Magic Pivot" 2.d
令	lìng	[monthly] commands [i.e. ancient rules guiding appropriate behavior in conformity with the seasons]; to cause; to let 1.d
令	lìng	an order 4.f
流	liú	to flow; to spread 3.a
留	liú	to keep; to remain 3.b
留心	liú xīn	to focus attention 5.a
瘤	liú	tumor 8.c
劉復真	liú fù zhēn	Liu Fuzhen, honorary style-name of Liú Kāi 劉開, author of a book on pulse-lore of the 14th century 6.b
硫黃	liú huáng	sulphur 9.f
流言	liú yán	to speak (about something) at various occasions 7.b
六	liù	six 1.c
六合	liù hé	the six [cardinal points] uniting [the world] (i.e. East, West, South, North, Above, Below); the world 7.d
聾	lōng	deaf; hard of hearing 5.c
癃	lóng	protuberance ill; blockages (in the path of urine and other body liquids) 9.b
隆	lóng	abundant 10.b
籠統	lóng tǒng	general 8.f
漏器	lòu qì	a funnel 8.b
爐	lú	stove; furnace 9.f

蘆頭	lú tóu	the stalk on top (of the ginseng root) 9.a
魯	lǔ	stupid 3.c
露	lù	dew 2.b
路	lù	road; way; path 2.e
履	lǚ	to walk; to proceed 1.e
膂	lǚ	the spinal column 4.d
律	lǜ	the yang sounds among the twelve pitch-pipes 2.a
慮	lǜ	to consider 5.f
攣	luán	cramp 7.e
攣縮	luán suō	bent and shrunk; cramps 9.b
卵	luǎn	testicles 9.b
卵	luǎn	egg 10.a
亂	luàn	disorder; chaos 1.a
亂	luàn	disturbance; confused 3.a
略	lüè	summary; outline 1.d
略	lüè	a little; minor 8.b
論語	lún yǔ	*Lun yu*, the *Confucian Analects* 1.e
論	lùn	to discuss; discourse 1.f
論	lùn	to sentence 2.f
論	lùn	statement 5.a
論	lùn	argument; view 6.e
論	lùn	to take into consideration 8.f
羅	luó	net; spread out 2.f
落	luò	to fall; to lose 4.c
絡	luò	a network (vessel) 1.d
絡刺	luò cì	piercing of network [vessels]; i.e. piercing of small vessels in the region directly below the skin to drain blood 10.c
麻	má	numb; numbness 1.f
麻痹	má bì	numbness 7.b
麻油	má yóu	hemp oil 10.d
馬蹄	mǎ tí	the hoof of a horse 2.f
埋	mái	to bury 9.d

衇(脉, 脈)	mài	the blood vessels; the vessels 1.f
脉	mài	a vessel; a blood vessel; a movement in the vessels 1.d
脉（=脈）	mài	the [movement in the] vessels 4.f
脉度篇	mài dù piān	the treatise “Mai du” (of the *Ling shu*) 6.d
脈經	mài jīng	*Mài jīng* 脈經; "Classic on [Movements in] the Vessels”. Classic on vessel diagnosis by Wang Shuhe 王叔和 of the 3rd c. CE 1.d
滿	mǎn	full; entire 2.b
滿	mǎn	swollen 4.b
慢	màn	neglectful 1.e
漫	màn	ubiquitous 6.e
漫	màn	to overflow; everywhere 8.b
慢	màn	slow; chronic 9.a
毛	máo	body hair 2.a
毛	máo	hair(-like movement in the vessels) 5.e
毛刺	máo cì	piercing [of the skin as cautiously as if with a] hair 10.c
毛際	máo jì	the (upper) border-line of the (pubic) hair 6.a
氂	máo	a yak’s tail 10.a
冒	mào	risky; false; to neglect what is right 3.e
毷落	mào luò	used here for 毻落 *tuò luò*, to shed feathers or fur 4.c
眉	méi	the eyebrows 4.c
每	měi	each 4.d
美	měi	delicious; beautiful 7.e
昧	mèi	obscure; dark 3.c
寐	mèi	to sleep 5.c
門	mén	gate; door 2.d
捫	mén	to feel; to lay the hand on 2.d
悶	mèn	pressing (sensation in one’s chest) 5.c
悗	mèn	frightened 10.e
懵	mēng	ignorant 5.a
夢	mèng	dream 9.a

彌	mí	very; especially 9.f
米粉	mǐ fěn	rice flour 9.b
泌	mì	to gush forth 2.c
密	mì	close; sealed 4.e
蜜	mì	honey 9.b
覓	mì	to search for 9.d
免	miǎn	to avoid 1.e
免	miǎn	to expel 3.c
勉强	miǎn qiáng	to force; to compel 4.b
面	miàn	the face 6.b
妙	miào	subtle; subtlety 6.e
憫	mǐn	to pity; to grieve 8.a
明	míng	clear; to understand 1.c
明	míng	brilliance; brilliant 1.e
蓂	míng	a creeping plant 2.a
名	míng	name; to name 2.c
名醫	míng yī	renowned physician 7.f
命	mìng	life; fate 1.d
命	mìng	to order 2.f
命	mìng	used for 名 *míng*; to name 5.e
命關	mìng guān	the life-gate(-section; i.e. the uppermost of the three sections of the inside of the index finger) 6.f
命門	mìng mén	the gate of life 2.d
膜	mó	membrane 2.f
末	mò	an end 5.b
末	mò	powder 8.a
莫不	mò bù	no one not; all 7.c
末流	mò liú	mediocre [physicians] 8.b
墨	mò	ink 10.d
墨子	mò zǐ	Mozi, Master Mo; the philosopher Mò Dì 墨翟 9.f
謀	móu	to devise; a plan 7.c
母	mǔ	mother 2.b

牡	mǔ	male 9.e
目	mù	eye 2.a
木	mù	wood; tree 2.a
募	mù	membrane (used here for 膜 *mò*) 2.a
暮世	mù shì	later generations 7.d
募原	mù yuán	the membrane plain (alternative writing: 膜原) 4.d
那	nǎ	what? Which? 7.f
納	nà	to receive; to ingest; to consume (food) 4.b
納	nà	to insert [a needle] 10.b
捺	nà	to press heavily downwards 10.d
乃	nǎi	then 1.f
乃	nǎi	namely; that is to say 8.a
奈何	nài hé	how can one? How is it? 2.c
男	nán	male 2.b
南	nán	the South 5.a
難	nán	difficult; hard 7.a
難	nàn	difficulty; here: short title for *Nan jing* 難經, "Classic of Difficult Issues", a medical classic compiled about the 1st or 2nd c. CE 1.d
難經	nàn jīng	*Nan jing*; the "Classic of Difficult Issues" of the 1st c. CE 3.c
腦	nǎo	the brain 9.b
內	nèi	inner 1.a
內	nèi	to take in 2.e
內	nèi	among 2.f
內關	nèi guān	internal closure 6.d
內經	nèi jīng	*Nei jing*, abbreviation of *Huang Di nei jing*, "Huang Di's Inner Classic" 2.d
內外經	nèi wài jīng	short for *Nei jing* ("Inner Classic") and *Wai jing* ("Outer Classic"), referring to ancient writings listed in the bibliographical section of the History of the Han dynasty 4.f
內格	nèigé	inner obstruction 1.a

能	néng	to be able; can 1.d
泥	ní	mud 7.b
泥	ní	narrow-minded 8.e
溺	nì	to drown 3.e
匿	nì	to shut in 3.f
擬	nì	to make propositions 6.e
逆	nì	to oppose 1.a
逆從	nì cóng	(therapies relying on drugs with a nature) opposite to or identical with (the nature of a patient's symptoms) 8.d
年	nián	a year; age 1.c
釀	niáng	to cause 1.e
釀成	niáng chéng	to bring about 1.e
尿	niào	urine 2.c
溺	niào	urine 2.d
凝	níng	to congeal; to freeze; to coagulate 2.b
寧	níng	tranquil 3.f
寧古臺	níng gŭ tái	Ninggutai, a place-name 9.a
牛肉	niú ròu	beef 9.b
膿	nóng	pus 4.c
濃	nóng	viscous; strong 8.b
努肉	nŭ ròu	flesh(-like) growths (in one's eyes). Also written: 胬肉 9.c
怒	nù	anger; rage 2.a
女	nǚ	female; woman 2.a
女菀	nǚ wǎn	*nüwan*, a drug prepared from Aster fastigiatus Fisch. 9.e
暖	nuǎn	warm; mild 4.e
瘧	nüè	malaria 3.f
歐希範	ōu xī fàn	Ou Xifan; name of a criminal 2.f
偶	ǒu	unexpectedly 1.e
嘔	ǒu	to vomit 4.a
偶	ǒu	accidental 4.c
偶	ǒu	a pair; even (as numbers) 8.a

偶刺	ǒu cì	paired piercing; i.e. piercing of two sites of pain on the back and front of a patient 10.c
排	pái	to arrange; arranged 2.f
排	pái	to open up 10.a
派	pài	to send; to order someone to do something 8.f
盤	pán	to coil up; to wind around 2.f
傍	páng	side; side-wise 2.e
傍刺	páng cì	side-wise piercing; i.e. piercing to the side of a needle already inserted 10.c
龐安常	páng ān cháng	Pang Anchang, style-name of Páng Ānshí 龐安時 10.f
膀胱	páng guāng	the bladder 2.b
脬	pāo	a bladder; a balloon 2.f
配合	pèi hé	to join (drugs) together (in a prescription) 8.c
胚	pī	embryo 2.b
砒	pī	arsenic 8.e
被髮	pī fà	the hair hanging dishevelled down the back 3.f
鈹鍼	pī zhēn	the sword needle 10.a
皮	pí	the skin 1.f
皮膚	pí fū	the skin 3.b
脾	pí	the spleen 2.b
疲	pí	tired; weary; exhausted 3.e
痞	pǐ	obstruction; blocked (qi in the chest) 5.d
譬	pì	to compare; to be comparable 1.a
僻	pì	secluded; remote 9.d
篇	piān	a book; a section of a book 2.d
偏	piān	onesided; unilateral 6.c
偏勝	piān shèng	to be unilaterally dominant 8.b
駢	pián	joined together 4.c
片	piàn	a strip 9.f
貧	pín	poor 1.c
頻	pín	repeatedly 10.d
品	pǐn	class; rank 1.c
品	pǐn	thing 8.a

品	pǐn	a substance 8.b
平	píng	peaceful; even 1.e
平	píng	normal 1.f
平	píng	balance 3.f
平	píng	equally; both 4.b
平	píng	flat 7.e
平	píng	balanced (thermo-qualities of pharmaceutical drugs) 9.c
平昔	píng xī	in former times; beforehand 1.e
憑	píng	to rely on 1.e
憑	píng	to avail oneself of 3.c
瓶	píng	a jar 9.f
屏絕	píng jué	to put aside; to do away with 8.b
頗	pō	very 4.f
頗	pō	somewhat; a little 7.b
破	pò	to break 1.f
魄	pò	the *po*-soul (believed to cease to exist after a person's physical death) 2.b
魄門	pò mén	the *po*-gate 2.d
仆	pū	to fall to the ground; to collapse 10.e
僕	pú	a servant 5.c
欺	qī	to cheat 1.f
妻	qī	wife 2.a
七	qī	seven 1.d
七表	qī biǎo	the seven external (movements in the vessels; i.e. 浮 *fú* [at the surface], 芤 *kōu* [hollow], 滑 *huá* [smooth], 實 *shí* [replete], 弦 *xián* [string-like], 緊 *jǐn* [tight], and 洪 *hóng* [vast]) 6.b
七竅	qī qiào	the seven orifices 10.c
七情	qī qíng	seven natures (of behavior shown by drugs in their interactions) 8.c
其	qí	this; a demonstrative and possessive pronoun 1.b
奇	qí	strange; rare 1.f
奇邪	qí xié	irregular qi 10.e

祈	qí	to pray 3.a
歧	qí	a fork; forked 6.a
歧伯	qí bó	Qi Bo, legendary informant of Huang Di on medicine 4.d
岐伯	qí bó	alternative writing to 歧伯 Qí Bó 5.e
臍	qí	the navel 2.d
齊	qí	to fast (used for 齋 *zhāi*) 1.e
齊	qí	the navel 2.e
齊	qí	the state of Qi 3.d
齊	qí	all alike 4.b
齊	qí	regular; uniform 10.b
齊刺	qí cì	combination piercing; i.e. the insertion of one needle each to the left and right of a needle inserted directly into an affected area 10.c
期	qí	a period; a fixed time 6.c
耆	qí	the pharmaceutical drug *huángqí* 黃耆, prepared from Astragalus membranaceus Fisch. and others 8.b
鬐	qí	a mane 9.b
旗燄	qí yàn	blazing flag 2.f
起	qǐ	to rise 1.d
起	qǐ	to raise 1.f
起伏	qǐ fú	emergence and disappearance 7.c
泣	qì	tears 5.f
棄	qì	to discard; to abandon 9.d
氣	qì	qi; vapor; breath; finest matter (forming the entire world and circulating in the body) 1.d
氣關	qì guān	the qi-gate(-section; i.e. the middle section of the inside of the index finger) 6.f
氣街	qì jiē	the qi street; *qi jie* (insertion point) 2.e
氣門	qì mén	the qi-gate 2.d
千	qiān	thousand 2.b
千古	qiān gǔ	ancient times 8.f

千金方	qiān jīn fāng	*Qian jin fang*, short title of *Bèi jí qiān jīn fāng* 備急千金要方, the "Important Prescriptions Worth Thousands in Gold, Prepared for Use in Urgent Need" by Sūn Sīmiǎo 孫思邈 (581-682?) 9.c
遷	qiān	to shift 1.d
鉛	qiān	lead (metal); grey 9.a
鉛丹	qiān dān	Lead Balls (i.e. minium; lead tetroxide) 9.f
鉛粉	qiān fěn	Lead Powder 9.f
鉛華	qiān huá	Lead Shine 9.f
乾	qián	heaven; male 2.b
前	qián	former; earlier 1.d
前	qián	in front of; prior to; before 2.d
淺	qiǎn	shallow; near the surface 3.b
遣	qiǎn	to banish; to send away 9.d
欠	qiàn	to yawn 4.d
强	qiáng	strong 2.d
强	qiáng	definitely 7.f
强力	qiáng lì	to force oneself; to exert one's strength 5.f
襁	qiǎng	the cloth in which children are carried on the back 2.b
蕎麥	qiáo mài	buckwheat 9.b
竅	qiào	hole; opening; orifice 2.a
誚	qiào	to blame; to ridicule 6.b
且	qiě	moreover 1.d
怯	qiè	to be afraid; timidity 1.c
妾	qiè	a female servant; a concubine 5.c
切	qiè	particle used to add emphasis before a negative 10.d
切脈	qiè mài	to press the vessels 5.b
親	qīn	to approach; to be near to 6.e
親	qīn	relatives 7.f
侵	qīn	to intrude 8.b
親戚	qīn qì	relatives 10.f
擒	qín	to arrest 2.f

禽獸	qín shòu	animals 7.d
青	qīng	blue 4.b
圊	qīng	to visit a privy 4.c
清	qīng	clear 2.c
清	qīng	cool 7.f
輕	qīng	minor; light 3.a
輕	qīng	light-minded 5.a
輕身	qīng shēn	to take the material weight from the body 8.c
輕視	qīng shì	to consider as unimportant; to hold in disdain 5.b
輕調	qīng tiáo	to regulate (a health problem by means of) light (drugs) 8.a
情	qíng	emotion; affect 1.d
情	qíng	facts; condition; feelings; emotions 3.c
請	qǐng	to ask 1.e
窮	qióng	exhausted 1.d
窮	qióng	to investigate thoroughly 3.c
窮思極想	qióng sī jí xiǎng	thorough considerations and farreaching thoughts 8.f
秋	qiū	autumn 3.f
秋毫	qiū háo	autumn down 10.a
求	qiú	to seek after 1.e
求	qiú	to take into account 8.e
曲	qū	crooked; bent 2.f
曲	qū	a bend; a curve 10.b
祛	qū	to drive off 3.a
屈	qū	to crouch; to bend down 4.a
屈	qū	to bother 10.f
驅	qū	to expel 7.a
趨筋	qū jīn	the running sinews muscles (a term referring to m. satorius and m. quadriceps femoris in the upper thighs) 6.a
取	qǔ	to take hold of; to take away 1.b
取	qǔ	to select [a hole for piercing] 10.b

去	qù	to remove 1.f
去	qù	to leave 3.d
泉	quán	spring 2.a
全	quán	all 2.d
全	quán	entirely; completely 4.b
全	quán	to cure 5.e
權	quán	authority; responsibility 7.f
權	quán	Quan, abbreviated name of Zhēn Quán 甄權, 7th century author of the *Yào xìng běn cǎo* 藥性本草 9.f
缺	quē	deficiency; to be lacking 1.d
缺盆	quē pén	the broken basin (i.e. the supraclavicular fossa) 4.d
瘸	qué	lame; deformation 4.c
確	què	correct 5.a
雀	què	small birds 9.c
羣	qún	all 1.d
群	qún	a multitude 2.f
然	rán	to be like this 1.d
然	rán	however 1.e
然	rán	particle added to an adjective to indicate adverbial use 8.f
然後	ránhòu	thereafter; this way 1.d
擾	rǎo	to disturb 3.f
繞	rào	to wind around 4.b
熱	rè	hot; heat 1.d
人	rén	human 3.a
人參	rén shēn	*renshen*, ginseng; a drug prepared from Panax ginseng C.A. Meyer 9.a
仁	rén	the attitude of humaneness 5.a
稔	rěn	to be familiar with 1.e
刃	rèn	a sword 10.a
任	rèn	to tolerate; to stand 4.f
任	rèn	responsibility; burden 7.f

任脉	rèn mài	the controller [conduit] vessel 2.f
妊娠	rèn shèn	pregnant 9.a
姙孕	rèn yùn	pregnant 10.f
認作	rèn zuò	to identify as 4.f
仍	réng	yet; still 4.b
日	rì	a day 1.e
日	rì	the sun 2.a
日	rì	day by day; each day 8.b
日華子	rì huá zǐ	Rihuazi, according to Li Shizhen the sobriquet of a man called Da Ming 大明, Tang dynasty author of the *Rìhuázǐ běn cǎo* 日華子本草 9.c
日久	rì jiǔ	for a long time 7.b
容	róng	to contain 2.f
容	róng	to take in; to harvest; to gather 3.f
容	róng	to allow; to tolerate 9.e
容易	róng yì	easy 5.b
榮	róng	used for 營 *yíng*, (military) camp 3.c
榮	róng	to flourish 3.f
鎔化	róng huà	to smelt 9.f
融會	róng huì	a comprehensive understanding 6.e
柔	róu	soft 7.c
肉	ròu	flesh 2.a
肉	ròu	meat 9.b
儒	rú	Confucian 1.d
如	rú	just as; like 1.e
濡	rú	soft (movement in the vessels) 5.f
乳	rǔ	the breasts 2.e
乳	rǔ	milk 7.e
乳癎	rǔ xián	convulsions (in children that are still) breast(-fed) 6.f
乳汁	rǔ zhī	(human) milk sap 9.b
入	rù	to enter; into 2.c
軟	ruǎn	soft; to soften 8.d

銳[骨]	ruì(-gǔ)	the pointed (bone); i.e. the exterior tip of the ulna in the wrists 6.a
潤	rùn	to moisten 8.a
若	ruò	if; when 1.f
弱	ruò	weak 2.d
焫	ruò	to burn 7.e
塞	sāi	to stop up 3.c
三	sān	three 1.e
三部	sān bù	three sections 6.a
三部	sān bù	the three sections (at the wrists where the movement in the vessels can be felt; i.e. the inch, the gate, and the foot section) 6.b
三蟲	sān chóng	the three worms (which inhabit the human body and may cause illness) 9.f
三關	sān guān	the three gate(-sections of the index fingers of small children) 6.f
三候	sān hòu	three indicators 6.a
三候	sān hòu	the three indicator (levels in each section at the wrists where the movement in the vessels can be felt; i.e. at the surface, in the center, and in the depth) 6.b
三焦	sān jiāo	the triple burner 2.b
散	sǎn	powder 1.f
散	sǎn	diffuse 7.b
散	sàn	to disperse; to distribute 4.c
散	sàn	dispersed (movement in the vessels) 5.f
桑榆	sāng yú	old age (lit.: mulberry and elm – trees whose tops are lit by the rays of the evening sun) 7.a
桑榆之收	sāng yú zhī shōu	the harvest of old age 7.a
臊	sāo	fetid 5.f
掃	sǎo	a broom; to brush 9.f
色	sè	color; complexion 1.d
濇	sè	rough 5.e
澀	sè	rough 4.a

澀	sè	astringent 8.a
塞	sè	speckled 9.a
殺	shā	to kill 1.f
沙	shā	sand 7.e
沙	shā	crumbly; in crumbs 9.f
痧	shā	illness with sand(-like skin eruptions) 9.a
山	shān	mountain 2.a
刪繁方	shān fán fāng	*Shan fan fang*, prescription collection written by Xiè Shìtài 9.d
善	shàn	good; to be good in; to be an expert in 1.b
善醫	shàn yī	to be well versed in medicine; medical expert 7.a
傷	shāng	harm; to harm 1.d
傷寒	shāng hán	harm caused by cold 4.e
傷暑	shāng shǔ	to be harmed by summer-heat 5.f
賞	shǎng	to reward; to praise 3.f
尙	shàng	still 1.e
上	shàng	upper 2.c
上	shàng	superior 5.e
上胞	shàng bāo	the upper eyelid 5.a
上古	shàng gǔ	high antiquity 10.b
上脘	shàng wǎn	the upper (opening of the stomach) duct 7.b
燒	shāo	to burn 9.d
燒	shāo	to heat 10.d
稍	shāo	a little 1.f
韶州	sháo zhōu	Shaozhou, name of a prefecture 9.f
少	shǎo	few 3.c
少略	shǎo lüè	to diminish; to leave out 1.d
少	shào	young 1.c
少保	shào bǎo	Junior Guardian (of the heir apparent); honorary title conferred upon high officials 2.f
少腹	shào fù	the lower abdomen 5.a

少火	shào huǒ	the small fire (supposedly burning in the kidneys and being responsible for the maintenance of all physiological processes) 8.b
少師	shào shī	Shaoshi; one of the legendary advisers of Huang Di 3.b
少陽	shào yáng	the minor-yang (conduit) 8.e
少陰	shào yīn	the minor-yin (conduit) 9.b
舌	shé	the tongue 3.e
蛇	shé	snake 9.c
舍	shě	to release; to bestow 1.f
舍	shě	to reside; to settle; to lodge 4.d
捨	shě	to reject; to determine 5.a
攝	shè	to assist; to preserve 1.e
設	shè	to establish; to arrange 1.f
射	shè	to shoot; to spurt 10.c
身	shēn	the body 1.e
深	shēn	deep 2.a
深	shēn	intense; very 3.a
深鑒	shēn jiàn	to be deeply concerned 6.e
呻	shēn	to groan 5.f
伸	shēn	to stretch 4.d
參	shēn	the pharmaceutical drug *rénshēn* 人參, i.e. ginseng, prepared from Panax Ginseng C.A. Meyer 8.b
神	shén	spirit 1.e
神	shén	spirit(-like); miraculous 9.c
神明	shén míng	spirit brilliance 7.d
神農	shén nóng	Shen Nong, name of the legendary founder of Chinese materia medica; the "Divine Husbandman" 8.a
審	shěn	to conduct an examination; to investigate 1.c
審	shěn	to examine; truly; really 1.f
沈僧翼	shěn sēng yì	Shen Sengyi, name of an otherwise unknown patient 9.d

慎	shèn	to act with care 1.e
腎	shèn	the kidneys 2.b
甚	shèn	very 3.c
甚	shèn	serious 7.b
滲	shèn	to leak; to drain 7.b
滲泄	shèn xiè	discharging through leakage (i.e. perspiration) 8.d
升	shēng	to ascend 4.f
升	shēng	one Chinese pint (a measurement of changing quantities in the course of the dynasties) 9.c
聲	shēng	voice; sound 2.a
生	shēng	life 1.a
生	shēng	to give life to 1.f
生	shēng	to live 1.f
生	shēng	to grow 2.b
生	shēng	to generate 2.b
生	shēng	fresh (drugs) 8.a
生薑	shēng jiāng	*shengjiang*, fresh ginger; a drug repared from Zingiber officinale Rosc. (mostly written: 生姜) 8.a
盛	shèng	abundant; flourishing 3.b
勝	shèng	to overcome
勝	shèng	to dominate 4.f
勝	shèng	superior 8.b
聖惠方	shèng huì fāng	*Sheng hui fang*, short title of *Tài píng shèng huì fāng* 太平聖惠方, the "Prescriptions of the Grand Peace [Reign Period Compiled] under Imperial Auspices", a prescription collection of CE 992 9.c
聖人	shèng rén	a sage 1.a
施	shī	to act; to do; used to strengthen the verb which it precedes 1.d
施	shī	to discharge 2.d
施	shī	to bestow 2.f

施行	shī xíng	to provide with 2.f
施用	shī yòng	to put into use; to make use of 4.b
濕	shī	humidity; dampness 3.a
濕	shī	damp 7.e
師	shī	a teacher 6.e
尸蟲	shī chóng	corpse worms (i.e. the three worms inhabiting the human body) 9.f
尸疰	shī zhù	corpse possession, i.e. possession by the *hun*-soul of an alien corpse 9.d
失	shī	to lose; to fail 5.e
失	shī	loss 10.b
失度	shī dù	out of proportion 4.c
失節	shī jié	to lose rhythm; irregular 4.f
失據	shī jù	to lose one's orientation (for instance, due to fright) 10.c
拾遺	shī yí	*Shi yi*, short title of *Běn cǎo shī yí* 本草拾遺, "Additions to the *Materia Medica*" by Chén Càngqì 陳藏器 (early 8th century) 9.d
十	shí	ten 2.a
十	shí	to increase tenfold 8.c
十二節	shí èr ji	the twelve limb-sections; i.e. hands, lower arms, upper arms, feet, lower legs, upper legs 2.a
十二節	shí èr jié	the twelve sections (of the method of piercing) 10.c
石	shí	a stone 1.c
石	shí	stone(-like movement in the vessels) 5.e
石蛔	shí huí	stone(-like) roundworms 9.d
石室秘錄	shí shì mì lù	*Shi shi mi lu*, a medical treatise of the 17th century, by Chén Shìduò 陳士鐸 7.f
時	shí	a season 1.c
時	shí	time 1.f
時	shí	occasionally 6.c
時行氣	shí xíng qì	seasonally prevalent (harmful) qi 4.e

時醫	shí yī	physicians (who follow only the trends of their own) time 7.f
時珍	shí zhēn	Shizhen, personal name of Lǐ Shízhēn 李時珍 (1518-1593), author of the *Běn cǎo gāng mù* 本草綱目 9.d
食	shí	food 2.f
食	shí	to eat; to take in 8.c
食復	shí fù	recurrence (of an illness) due to (inappropriate) eating 9.f
食壓	shí yā	to press (drugs down in the body) by means of food 8.a
實	shí	repletion 1.d
實	shí	really 1.d
實	shí	substance; substantial 4.f
實	shí	to replenish 4.f
識	shí	to know 1.d
蝕	shí	to "eat-away" 9.b
史	shǐ	history; historical accounts 3.c
矢	shǐ	ordure; droppings 4.b
使	shǐ	to send; to let 1.d
使	shǐ	to cause 1.f
使	shǐ	aide (drugs in a prescription) 8.c
使	shǐ	messenger (drug in a prescription) 8.d
始	shǐ	the beginning 1.c
始	shǐ	to begin 2.b
始	shǐ	only if ..., then ... 7.b
屎	shǐ	excrement 9.c
是	shì	this; that 1.a
是	shì	to be; is; are 2.d
是	shì	in fact 3.a
是故	shì gù	hence 1.a
是以	shì yǐ	therefore; same as 以是 *yǐ shì* 3.d
士	shì	scholar 3.c
士	shì	a person 7.c

示	shì	to proclaim; to instruct 1.d
世	shì	an age 1.e
世間	shì jiān	in the world 7.b
世人	shì rén	mankind; all the people 5.a
室	shì	dwelling 3.c
室女	shì nǚ	an unmarried girl 5.c
視	shì	to look 2.f
適	shì	to happen; just now 2.f
適	shì	to suit; proper 3.b
適	shì	to adapt oneself to 4.f
適	shì	to follow; to go to 5.a
嗜	shì	to long for; to lust after 5.c
勢	shì	strength 1.e
勢	shì	a feature 7.e
事	shì	an affair 1.c
事	shì	to employ; to resort to 8.b
事事	shì shì	everything; in every respect 3.c
拭	shì	to wipe (the eyes) 9.d
試	shì	to examine 10.f
釋	shì	to explain 1.e
釋名	shì míng	*Shi ming*, "Explanation of Names"; title of a Han dynasty book on terminology 9.f
收	shōu	to contract (as one's limbs) 5.f
收	shōu	to take in; to gather; to contract 7.e
收	shōu	to pull together (what is relaxed) 8.d
收斂	shōu liàn	to collect 3.f
首	shǒu	numerary adjunct for prescriptions 8.f
首	shǒu	first 9.c
首	shǒu	chief 2.f
首惡	shǒu è	chief culprit 2.f
手	shǒu	hand 2.a
手少陰	shǒu shào yīn	the hand-minor-yin (region) 6.a
手太陰	shǒu tài yīn	the hand-major-yin (region) 6.a
手心	shǒu xīn	the center of the hand; palm 4.b

手陽明	shǒu yáng míng	the hand-yang-brilliance (region) 6.a
守	shǒu	to guard; to protect 3.a
守	shǒu	to focus on 6.e
受	shòu	to receive; to absorb 1.e
壽	shòu	longevity 1.f
瘦	shòu	thin; emaciated 3.a
授	shòu	to transmit 6.e
書	shū	books; writing 1.d s
書載	shū zài	recorded in the literature 9.e
殊	shū	really 1.e
殊	shū	different 4.b
殊不	shū bù	definitely not; not at all 5.b
疏	shū	lax; separated; open 4.d
疏理	shū lǐ	open skin structures 7.e 7.e
舒	shū	to expand; to dissipate 8.b
腧	shū	transport (acupuncture insertion point) 10.a
腧穴	shū xuè	transport point (where a needle is inserted in acupuncture to affect the passage of qi) 2.d
輸	shū	to transport 4.c
輸	shū	transporter (generic name for all third insertion points on the twelve conduit-streams in the extremities) 10.b
輸刺	shū cì	piercing of transport [holes]; i.e. piercing of the five insertion points “well” through “confluence” in the distal extremities 10.c
輸刺	shū cì	transport piercing; i.e. fast and deep insertion and withdrawal of a needle 10.c
叔和	shū hé	Shuhe, style-name of Wáng Xī 王熙 (3rd c.), author of the *Mài jīng* 脈經 6.e
樞要	shū yào	of central importance; essential 6.b
熟	shú	cooked; to process 2.e
熟	shú	mature 7.b
孰	shú	who? 8.e
黍粟	shǔ sù	millet 8.c

暑	shǔ	summer-heat 3.a
屬	shǔ	to belong to 2.b
屬	shǔ	to go to 10.a
蜀本	shǔ běn	*Shu ben*, short title of *Shǔ chóng guǎng yīng gōng běn cǎo* 蜀重廣英公本草, the “Shu Materia Medica” compiled between 934 and 965 9.c
術	shù	art; technique; skills 1.b
漱	shù	to rinse out 1.f
數	shù	to enumerate 1.d
數	shù	numerous 3.c
數	shù	a number 6.a
數	shù	short for 度數 *dù shù*: a pattern 10.e
庶	shù	it is to be hoped; possibly 6.b
庶子	shù zǐ	tutor to the heir apparent 1.f
樹	shù	a tree 6.e
竪	shù	to set up; to establish 10.b
束手無策	shù shǒu wú cè	hands tied and without plan; helpless 7.f
衰	shuāi	to decay; weak 3.c
率	shuài	standard 6.f
霜降	shuāng jiàng	“frost’s descent”, a solar term denoting the middle of the ninth month 4.e
水	shuǐ	water 2.a
水粉	shuǐ fěn	Water Powder 9.f
水缸	shuǐ gāng	a large open-mouthed water jar 9.f
睡	shuì	to sleep 8.a
順	shùn	to be appropriate; to act appropriately 1.a
說	shuō	to explain; an explanation; a statement; a doctrine 1.b
說	shuō	to say 2.d
說明	shuō míng	to explain 7.f
數	shuò	often; again and again 3.e
數	shuò	frequent (movement in the vessels) 6.b
斯	sī	this 1.e
司	sī	to control 2.d

思	sī	to think; to ponder 3.c
私	sī	secret 3.f
死	sǐ	death 1.a
四	sì	four 1.c
四大	sì dà	the four elements (constituting the body) 8.b
似	sì	like; resembling 1.d
似	sì	it seems 3.c
俟	sì	to wait; when 7.f
俟	sì	as soon as 10.b
送	sòng	to send 2.f
溲	sōu	to urinate 7.b
嗽	sòu	to cough 2.f
蘇恭	sū gōng	Su Gong, taboo version of the name of Sū Jìng 蘇敬 (fl. 657), co-author of the *Táng běn cǎo* 唐本草 9.f
酥酪	sū lào	curd 9.c
俗	sú	vulgar; common 2.d
素	sù	pure; basic; here: short title for *Huang Di nei jing, Su wen* 黃帝內經素問, "Huang Di's Inner Classic, Basic Questions", a medical classic first compiled probably during the Han dynasty but lost in the original version and recompiled between the Han and Tang dynasties 1.d
素	sù	originally 4.c
素	sù	congenital; all along 5.c
素	sù	vegetarian 5.c
素	sù	abbreviated title of the *Sù wèn* 素問, one of the books constituting the *Huang Di nei jing* corpus 10.b
素稱	sù chēng	commonly called 7.f
速	sù	hurried 1.e
速	sù	quickly 7.b
宿食	sù shí	food remaining (in the stomach without being digested) 6.f

酸	suān	sour 2.c
痠	suān	aching of the limbs 4.c
雖	suī	even if; although 1.b
隨	suí	to follow; in accordance with 3.a
遂	suí	to follow; consequently 1.f
遂	suí	to proceed to 3.a
遂	suí	to extend 6.d
髓	suǐ	marrow 3.d
歲	suì	year 2.a
祟	suì	curse by evil spirits 6.f
孫	sūn	grandchild; tertiary 2.b
飧	sūn	a meal; food 3.f
損	sǔn	to injure; to damage 1.f
縮	suō	to shrink 4.c
縮	suō	to draw in 10.f
鎖	suǒ	a lock; to lock 2.d
索	suǒ	a large rope; to bind 6.c
所	suǒ	(preceding a verb; usually replacing its object:) that which; whom; etc. 1.c
所以	suǒ yǐ	that which (someone) takes; that which (someone) relies on 1.f
所以	suǒ yǐ	therefore 4.b
所以然者	suǒ yǐ rán zhě	this being so; consequently 7.a
所在	suǒ zài	location 5.a
他	tā	other; another 4.c
撻	tà	to flog 9.b
胎	tāi	the fetus 2.b
胎前	tāi qián	pregnancy 9.e
胎元	tāi yuán	the fetus 2.d
太倉	tài cāng	the big granary; the stomach 2.d
太過	tài guò	great excess 6.d
太史公	tài shǐ gōng	lit.: Great Historiographer. Title of Sīmǎ Qiān 司馬遷 (145 - ca. 80 BCE), the compiler of the *Shǐ jì* 史記 1.f

太陽經	tài yáng jīng	the major-yang conduit 5.a
痰	tán	phlegm 3.c
譚	tán	to boast; claim 5.a
談	tán	ta talk; rhetoric 8.e
湯	tāng	hot liquid; decoction 1.f
湯	tāng	hot water; hot baths 3.d
湯液	tāng yè	*Tang ye*, abbreviated title of the *Tāng yè běn cǎo* 湯液本草 by Wáng Hàogǔ 王好古of the 13th century 9.f
唐本	táng běn	*Tang ben*, short title of *Táng xīn xiǔ běn cǎo* 唐新修本草, the "Newly Revised Edition of the *Materia Medica* of the Tang Dynasty", published in 659 9.c
溏泄	táng xiè	turbid diarrhea 9.e
桃	táo	the peach 2.b
逃	táo	to flee; to escape 3.d
陶隱居	táo yǐn jū	Tao Yinju, sobriquet of Táo Hóngjǐng 陶弘景 (412-536), Daoist and author of a *materia medica* 9.c
討論	tǎo lùn	to debate; to discuss 6.e
套語	tào yǔ	conventional phrases 8.f
特	tè	alone; only 8.b
疼	téng	pain 4.a
涕	tī	snivel 5.f
體	tǐ	the body 2.f
體	tǐ	the essentials 6.b
天	tiān	heaven 1.c
天下	tiān xià	under heaven; the world; the empire 6.e
添	tiān	to add to; to increase 6.f
恬憺	tián dàn	peaceful and tranquil 7.d
髫	tiáo	the tufts of hair on the head of little children 2.b
調	tiáo	to adjust 4.e
條	tiáo	a section; a paragraph 7.b

庭	tíng	court; hall 3.f
挺	tǐng	rather; rigid 7.c
挺	tǐng	a stick 10.a
通	tōng	to penetrate; to understand 1.d
通	tōng	throughout 3.a
通	tōng	passage 8.b
通	tōng	to make passable 9.a
通治	tōng zhì	cure-all 8.e
同	tóng	identical; alike 1.d
同身寸	tóng shēn cùn	[individually] standardized body inch 10.b
同一	tóng yī	the same 2.f
桐城	tóng chéng	the city of Tong in Anhui province 10.f
童	tóng	boy 2.b
僮	tóng	a boy; a servant 5.c
統	tǒng	all; general 7.b
筒	tǒng	a tube 9.f
痛	tòng	pain 4.a
頭	tóu	the head 2.a
頭角	tóu jiǎo	the temples 6.a
投	tóu	to add (to a prescription) 8.a
凸	tū	protruding 4.b
圖	tú	to plan; to seek; to envisage 5.b
徒	tú	only 6.e
徒	tú	a follower 7.b
荼毒	tú dú	poison 4.c
土	tǔ	soil 4.b
吐	tù	to vomit 4.b
吐	tù	to spit 8.b
吐藥	tù yào	drugs causing vomiting; emetics 8.c
推	tuī	to draw conclusions; to continue a line of thought 5.a
推	tuī	to investigate 6.e
推	tuī	to push 10.b
退	tuì	to withdraw 3.d

吞	tūn	to swallow 8.a
豚	tún	a sucking pig; piglet 9.b
脫	tuō	to escape; to leave 3.c
脫	tuō	to loose; loss 7.b
脫	tuō	to get lost; to go asunder 8.a
脫下	tuō xià	to sink down (of the surface of a structure); to shrink 7.b
脫瀉	tuō xiè	loss (of qi) through drainage; diarrhea 8.b
脫衣	tuō yī	to undress 8.a
駝	tuó	camel 9.c
唾	tuò	spittle 5.f
瓦粉	wǎ fěn	Brick Powder 9.f
外	wài	outside; extra 2.d
外格	wài gé	external obstruction 6.d
外關	wài guān	external closure 6.d
外科	wài kē	the branch of medicine concerned with external illnesses, including impact and other traumatic injuries, surgery, bone-setting, and skin diseases 9.a
完	wán	to finish; to complete 1.f
丸	wán	a pill 3.a
頑	wán	heavy; clumsy 4.a
頑固	wán gù	obstinate 4.c
晚	wǎn	late 1.a
脘	wǎn.	a duct in the body 2.e
挽	wǎn	to save; to rescue 8.b
挽回	wǎn huí	to bring back (health) 5.d
萬	wàn	ten thousand; myriad 2.b
萬病回春	wàn bìng huí chūn	*Wan bing hui chun*, a popular collection of prescriptions of the late 17th century, by Gōng Tíngxián 龔廷賢 7.f
萬物	wàn wù	the myriad things; everything 8.a
亡	wáng	to perish 1.e
亡	wáng	to lose 8.b

王	wáng	king; royal 1.f
王叔和	wáng shū hé	Wang Shuhe, style-name of Wáng Xī 王熙 (210-285), author of the *Mài jīng* 脉經, the classic of pulse-lore 6.b
王晏	Wáng Yàn	name of an otherwise unknown person 9.d
王宗正	wáng zōng zhèng	Wang Zongzheng, a 12th c. author of medical texts 6.e
罔	wǎng	to have not; there is no ... 1.e
罔不	wǎng bù	there is nothing which not ..; in all cases; always 1.e
往	wǎng	to proceed to 6.c
往	wǎng	formerly; in the past 7.d
往來寒熱	wǎng lái hán rè	alternating fits of cold and heat 5.d
往往	wǎng wǎng	often 7.a
魍魎	wǎng liǎng	sprites 9.d
旺	wàng	to prosper; to be present in abundance 8.b
妄	wàng	wildly; incoherently; disorderly 1.d
妄	wàng	absurd; foolish; false 5.a
妄	wàng	used for 忘 *wàng*: to forget 10.a
望	wàng	to look at (from a distance) 3.d
望	wàng	to look forward to; to hope 6.e
望聞-問切	wàng wén-wèn qiè	the four diagnostic approaches: to look (at a patient's complexion), to smell (his breath) and listen (to the pitch of his voice), to ask (him about his condition), and to press (his vessels to feel the movement within them) 5.b
危險	wēi xiǎn	dangerous 9.a
微	wēi	subtle; minute 1.d
微	wēi	weak; minor 1.e
微	wēi	feeble (movement in the vessels) 6.c
惟	wéi	only; here; initial particle 1.e
爲	wéi	to be; to represent 1.a
爲	wéi	to manage; to cure 1.f
爲	wéi	to do 5.e

爲度	wéi dù	take as measure; take as limit; until 9.f
爲用	wéi yòng	function 8.d
維持	wéi chí	to maintain 7.a
違逆	wéi nì	to oppose 3.e
委	wěi	to commission; to engage someone; to give up 1.e
痿	wěi	limpness 3.f
萎	wěi	to wither; to dry out 4.a
尾	wěi	tail; end 6.c
痏	wěi	the wound [where a needle was inserted] 10.b
未	wèi	not yet 1.a
謂	wèi	to say; to call; to express the meaning of 1.a
謂	wèi	to say; that is to say 1.e
胃	wèi	the stomach 1.f
味	wèi	flavor 2.c
衛	wèi	protective; to guard 2.a
謂	wèi	that is to say 3.a
位	wèi	position 4.f
畏	wèi	to die a violent death 3.e
畏	wèi	to fear 5.d
味	wèi	a (pharmaceutical) substance 8.f
溫	wēn	warm 3.b
溫	wēn	used for 蘊 *yùn*: to accumulate; to collect 10.a
瘟疫	wēn yì	warmth epidemics 9.a
聞	wén	reputation 1.e
聞	wén	to hear 2.c
聞	wén	to smell 4.c
文	wén	literature; text 6.e
文理浩繁	wén lǐ hào fán	complicated textual structure 6.b
文人學士	wén rén xué shì	literati and learned scholars 8.f
紋	wén	(skin-)lines 6.f
蚊虻	wén méng	mosquito 10.a
問	wèn	to inquire 1.c
踒	wō	to slip; to sprain 3.e
我	wǒ	I; myself 8.f

臥	wò	to lie down 2.a
握	wò	to hold fast; to grasp 6.b
污	wū	filthy; soiled 1.b
吾	wū	I; me 1.f
烏梅	wū méi	black plums 9.b
無	wú	to be without; to have not 1.d
無常	wú cháng	abnormal 6.c
無忌	wú jì	reckless 1.e
無論	wú lùn	no matter; regardless of 8.b
無奈之何	wú nài zhī hé	nothing can be done 3.d
無窮	wú qióng	inexhaustible 1.d
無事	wú shì	nothing to worry about; no problems 1.f
無以	wú yǐ	there is nothing to rely on to ...; there is no way to ... 1.d
五	wǔ	five 1.b
五痺	wǔ bì	the five blocks (i.e. of skin, flesh, sinews, bones, and vessels) 7.d
五方	wǔ fāng	the five cardinal points, including North, South, West, East, and Center 1.d
五疳	wǔ gān	the five types of *gan*-illness 9.e
五經	wǔ jīng	the five conduits 4.f
五癆	wǔ láo	the five types of consumption 9.e
五靈脂	wǔ líng zhī	*wulingzhi*, a drug prepared from the droppings of Trogopterus xanthipes Milne-Edwards 9.a
五癃	wǔ lóng	the five protuberance ills; the five blockages (in the paths of liquids through the body) 9.b
五邪	wǔ xié	the five evils 5.f
五行	wǔ xíng	the five agents; five interrelated categories of all phenomena in existence 3.e
侮	wǔ	to insult; to attack 3.c
忤	wǔ	hostile 3.e
忤	wǔ	to irritate 10.b
勿	wù	a negative; not; do not 3.f
悟	wù	to apprehend 2.d

悟入	wù rù	to enter into a perfect understanding of reality 6.e
惡	wù	to hate; to have an aversion 5.d
物	wù	matter; substance 2.f
物	wù	a thing; an entity 7.b
務	wù	obligation; [to consider] necessary 8.b
誤	wù	to be mistaken 3.c
誤	wù	to commit a mistake 8.b
誤	wù	mistake 9.f
霧	wù	fog; mist 2.c
夕	xī	evening 7.d
吸	xī	to inhale 2.c
昔	xī	formerly
悉	xī	all 4.f
錫	xī	tin 9.f
惜	xī	to pity 10.f
膝	xī	knee 2.a
吸門	xī mén	the inhalation-gate 2.d
西戎	xī róng	the Xirong, Western tribes 9.c
息	xí	breath; to breathe 6.c
息	xí	to rest; to stop 6.e
襲	xí	to inherit; heritage 4.c
襲	xí	to appropriate; to clad oneself with 8.f
席	xí	a mat 9.d
洗	xǐ	to wash; to cleanse 1.f
喜	xǐ	joy 2.a
喜	xǐ	to enjoy; to prefer 2.c
喜	xǐ	to tend to 3.e
係	xì	to belong to; to depend on 1.e
系	xì	link; connection 2.b
細	xì	fine; emaciated 4.b
細	xì	fine (movement in the vessels) 6.f
暇	xiá	leisure 1.e
夏	xià	summer 2.a

下	xià	downwards 2.c
下	xià	below 2.d
下	xià	to descend 2.e
下	xià	to purge 4.b
下	xià	inferior 5.e
下	xià	to lower 10.d
下胞	xià bāo	the lower eyelid 5.a
下焦	xià jiāo	the lower [section of the triple] burner 4.f
下藥	xià yào	drugs causing defecation; laxatives; purgatives 8.c
先	xiān	before; at first 1.d
先	xiān	first; foremost 1.f
先論	xiān lùn	previously mentioned 7.b
先生	xiān sheng	Mister 7.f
先天	xiān tiān	previous to one's existence; transmitted by one's parents 2.d
賢	xián	virtuous; exemplary (man) 1.d
弦	xián	string(-like movement in the vessels) 5.e
弦	xián	a string 10.a
涎	xián	saliva 4.b
癇	xián	convulsions 9.b
鹹	xián	salty 2.c
咸	xián	all: in all cases 9.e
閒人	xián rén	unaffected people 4.c
嫌疑	xián yí	suspicion; doubt 7.d
鮮	xiǎn	rare; few; seldom 5.b
顯	xiǎn	evident; obvious 8.e
險	xiǎn	dangerous 9.a
灑淅	xiǎn xī	shivering 6.c
洒洒	xiǎn xiǎn	to shiver 5.f
綫	xiàn	a thread 4.b
陷	xiàn	a fold 2.e
陷	xiàn	to sink 6.c
陷	xiàn	to penetrate into; to insert 10.a

現	xiàn	to manifest; become apparent 3.c
現成	xiàn chéng	ready-made (as of medications) 8.e
香	xiāng	aromatic 5.f
相	xiāng	reciprocal; each other 1.d
相反	xiāng fǎn	(drugs which) are opposed to each other (in their effects) 8.c
相殺	xiāng shā	(drugs which) kill each other's (effects) 8.c
相勝	xiāng shèng	the mutual destruction (among the five agents) 5.e
相生	xiāng shēng	the mutual generation (among the five agents) 5.e
相使	xiāng shǐ	(drugs which) reinforce each other (in their effects) 8.c
相推	xiāng tuī	to look at and conclude; to study 2.f
相畏	xiāng wèi	(drugs which) fear each other (i.e. suppress each other's effects) 8.c
相惡	xiāng wù	(drugs which) hate each other (i.e.; depotentiate each other) 8.c
相須	xiāng xū	(drugs which) depend on each other (in their effects) 8.c
相與	xiāng yǔ	together 10.f
詳	xiáng	detail 2.f
想	xiǎng	to think 8.f
向	xiàng	towards; in favor of 7.f
象	xiàng	image; reflection 4.b
項	xiàng	the neck 4.d
相	xiàng	to observe; to look at 7.a
相	xiàng	a minister 4.f
相	xiàng	to examine with one's eyes 10.e
相火	xiàng huǒ	the minister fire 4.f
消	xiāo	to wane 1.d
消	xiāo	to disperse 8.b
消	xiāo	to digest 8.c

消息	xiāo xí	ebb and flow; to act within the limits of one's assessment 10.d
削成	xiāo chéng	to cut into 9.f
曉	xiǎo	to know 2.e
小	xiǎo	small 2.a
小	xiǎo	minor (movement in the vessels) 5.e
小	xiǎo	short for 小便 *xiǎo biàn*, to urinate 7.b
小便	xiǎo biàn	urine 4.a
小腸	xiǎo cháng	the small intestine 2.b
小兒	xiǎo ér	small children 6.f
小腹	xiǎo fù	the lower abdomen 5.f
小節	xiǎo jié	small section; i.e. the end sections of fingers and toes 2.a
小人	xiǎo rén	petty person 2.f
小眥	xiǎo zì	the outer canthus 5.a
效	xiào	effect 4.b
效	xiào	success 5.b
脅	xié	the ribs 2.f
邪	xié	evil; abnormal 3.a
挾	xié	to carry; to include 9.a
泄	xiè	to discharge 2.d
泄	xiè	to flow away 3.f
瀉	xiè	to drain 4.f
洩	xiè	to leak 9.b
蟹	xiè	a crab 9.f
寫	xiè	used here for 瀉 *xiè*, to drain 10.e
懈惰	xiè duò	idle; lame 4.a
謝士泰	xiè shì tài	Xie Shitai, a 6th-7th century author of medical works 9.d
洩瀉	xiè xiè	to drain off; to purge 4.b
泄瀉	xiè xiè	diarrhea 5.d
心	xīn	the heart; the mind 1.e
[心]胞絡	[xīn]bāo luò	the [heart] enclosing network 4.f
辛	xīn	acrid 2.c

辛苦	xīn kǔ	tired; suffering 4.e
信	xìn	to believe; confidence 7.f
星	xīng	star 2.a
興	xīng	to rise 3.f
腥	xīng	fishy 5.f
星曆	xīng lì	the sidereal calendar 4.c
形	xíng	physical appearance 1.e
形	xíng	to take shape 3.e
形像	xíng xiǎng	figure; form 2.b
行	xíng	to move 2.c
刑	xíng	punishment 1.f
刑	xíng	the death-penalty; execution 2.f
行	xíng	to pass on; to carry out 4.f
滎	xíng	a brook (generic name for all second insertion points on the twelve conduit-streams in the extremities) 10.b
幸	xìng	lucky; fortunate 1.f
性	xìng	nature; disposition 3.e
性	xìng	thermo-quality of a pharmaceutical drug 8.b
凶	xiōng	inauspicious 4.c
兇兇	xiōng xiōng	to behave aggressively 7.d
胸	xiōng	the breast; the chest 2.c
胸	xiōng	the mind 8.f
兄弟	xiōng dì	elder brother and younger brother 8.c
雄	xióng	male 1.c
秀	xiù	blossoming; luxuriance 3.f
臭	xiù	odor 5.f
須	xū	necessary; must 1.d
虛	xū	depletion; depleted 1.d
虛	xū	to deplete 4.f
虛	xū	void (of meaning); meaningless 8.f
虛	xū	to loosen 9.b
虛心	xū xīn	open-minded; without prejudice 6.e
鬚	xū	whiskers 9.a

徐	xú	Xu, name of a district 2.f
徐	xú	slow; sedate 3.b
徐嗣伯	xú sì bó	Xu Sibo, physician and author of prescription works of the 5th century 9.d
詡	xǔ	to brag; to boast 8.f
許	xǔ	place; to allow 2.e
許	xǔ	perhaps; it may be 6.e
許	xǔ	about 10.d
許諾	xǔ nuò	to promise 10.f
蓄	xù	to collect 4.d
序	xù	series; order 4.e
緒	xù	the end of a ball of thread 5.d
續	xù	to succeed to; to follow 6.c
宣	xuān	to spread 8.c
旋	xuán	to come back; to move in a circle 9.e
懸蹄	xuán tí	the (rear) suspended toes (of artiodactyles) 9.b
薛氏醫案	xuē shì yī àn	*Xue shi yi an*, a collection of medical case histories of the 16th century, by Xuē Jǐ 薛己 7.f
學	xué	to study 1.d
學問	xué wèn	scholarship 8.f
學士	xué shì	a scholar 6.e
血	xuě	blood 1.d
血絡	xuě luò	the blood [vessel] network 10.c
血脈	xuě mài	the blood vessels 3.d
血室	xuě shì	the blood-chamber (of women; i.e. the womb) 9.e
雪	xuě	snow; here: to whiten; to cleanse 1.b
穴	xuè	hole (insertion point for needles in acupuncture) 2.b
循	xún	to follow; because 1.f
尋	xún	to search for 3.e
尋	xún	subsequently 10.d
詢	xún	to inquire about 5.c
壓	yā	to be killed by a falling wall 3.e

牙	yá	tooth 2.a
焉	yān	final affirmative 3.e
湮	yān	to submerge; to drown 7.b
言	yán	to speak; to state 1.b
嚴	yán	strict; severe 4.e
延	yán	to extend 5.b
延年	yán nián	to prolong the years of life 8.c
衍義	yán yì	*Yan yi*, short title of *Běn cǎo yán yì* 本草衍義, the "Expanded Interpretation of *Materia Medica*" by Kǒu Zōng-shì 寇宗 奭 of 1116 9.c
鹽	yán	salt 7.e
研	yán	to rub; to grind (in a mortar) 9.c
炎	yán	a flame; to flame 9.e
眼	yǎn	eye 2.f
驗	yàn	to examine; to experience; success 1.f
厭	yàn	to be wearied with; satiated 3.f
晏	yàn	late 4.d
燕	yàn	(the state of) Yan (in the far north) 5.a
楊	yáng	the willow tree 3.a
揚刺	yáng cì	scattered piercing; i.e. the insertion of four needles around a first needle 10.c
陽結	yáng jié	clottings of yang (qi) 6.c
陽明	yáng míng	the yang-brilliance (conduit) 4.d
楊宗	yáng zōng	Yang Zong; name of a bandit 2.f
羊矢	yáng shǐ	sheep droppings (a term referring to the inguinal lymphatic glands palpable in the groins) 6.a
養	yǎng	to support; to nourish 1.e
癢	yǎng	to itch 4.c
恙	yàng	illness; indisposition 10.f
夭	yāo	to die young 1.f
腰	yāo	the lower back 4.d
腰痛	yāo tòng	lumbar pain 10.c
搖	yáo	to shake; to agitate 6.c
要	yào	important; essential point 5.b

藥	yào	pharmaceutical drug; to employ drugs 1.a
藥蠱	yào gŭ	drug poisoning 8.b
藥品	yào pĭn	(pharmaceutical) drugs 8.a
藥性	yào xìng	*Yao xing*, abbreviated title of the *Yào xìng běn căo* 藥性本草 ascribed to Zhēn Quán 甄權 of the 7th century 9.f
耶	yé	a final interrogative particle 1.e
也	yě	final particle 1.b
也	yě	is 1.d
也	yě	also 4.d
野	yě	field 6.a
液	yè	juices; extract 1.f
腋	yè	armpit 2.a
夜	yè	night; darkness 2.a
葉	yè	a lobe 2.f
葉	yè	a leaf 5.e
謁	yè	to visit 10.f
一	yī	one 1.d
衣	yī	clothes; to dress 7.e
依阿兩可	yī ē liăng kě	to flatter with ambiguous statements 7.f
醫	yī	medicine 1.d
醫方集解	yī fāng jí jiě	*Yi fang ji jie*, a popular collection of prescriptions of the late 17th century, by Wāng Áng 汪昂 7.f
醫籍	yī jí	medical literature 6.e
醫學	yī xué	the medical teachings 5.b
醫藥	yī yào	medication 8.b
貽累	yí lèi	to involve 3.c
怡然	yí rán	happy; harmonious 3.e
邑	yí	a city; town 2.a
移	yí	to change residence; to move 4.a
宜	yí	suitable; fitting 1.d
宜	yí	ought; should 4.b
疑	yí	to doubt; to suspect 6.e

倚仗	yǐ zhàng	to rely on; to trust 9.a
已	yǐ	already 1.a
已	yǐ	finished 1.d
已	yǐ	to come to an end; to heal 4.a
已	yǐ	extremely; intensive particle 4.e
已上	yǐ shàng	identical with 以上 *yǐ shàng*, "ascending from here"; "here and above" 7.a
以	yǐ	so as to; in order to; thereby 1.c
以	yǐ	or 2.e
以	yǐ	and 6.d
以次	yǐ cì	consecutively; step by step 2.c
以上	yǐ shàng	... and above 6.f
以爲	yǐ wéi	to hold; to believe 1.f
以下	yǐ xià	… and below 6.f
以至	yǐ zhì	until; up to 2.b
矣	yǐ	a final particle 1.c
矣	yǐ	particle indicating completion of a development 2.b
一	yì	another 2.e
一	yì	all 6.e
一	yì	as soon as 10.d
一或	yì huò	in case; if 5.d
一直	yì zhí	in straight lines 10.b
亦	yì	also; likewise 1.a
亦	yì	both 8.a
異	yì	different 1.c
異	yì	strange 9.a
易	yì	to change; here: short title for *Yì jīng* 易經, "Book of Changes" 1.d
易	yì	easy 2.b
逸	yì	indulgence; idleness 3.a
疫	yì	epidemic 3.a
役	yì	to indulge in; to employ 3.e
意	yì	a thought 1.e

意	yì	meaning 3.e
意會	yì huì	to reach a comprehensive understanding 6.b
嗌	yì	the throat 4.a
噫	yì	to belch 4.a
益	yì	to benefit 3.a
益	yì	more; to increase 4.d
溢	yì	to flow out 4.f
溢	yì	overflow 6.d
議	yì	to deliberate; to propose 5.a
抑	yì	or; or if 5.c
藝	yì	skill 10.f
義	yì	moral standards; moral behavior; principle; meaning; interpretation 1.d
義理	yì lǐ	moral standards; moral order; principles 1.d
因	yīn	hence; consequently 1.f
因	yīn	to follow 1.f
因	yīn	cause 3.a
因	yīn	because of 3.a
因	yīn	used here for 由 *yóu*, "originating from" 10.e
音	yīn	sound; tone 2.a
陰	yīn	shade 7.d
陰刺	yīn cì	yin piercing; i.e. piercing of the foot-minor-yin conduit on both it right and left course 10.c
陰毒	yīn dú	poisoning by (the presence of purely) yin (qi and the absence of yang qi) 9.a
陰結	yīn jié	clottings of yin (qi) 6.c
陰陽	yīn yáng	yin and yang, the two categories of all phenomena. The term yin yang refers here to natural law in general; it stands for the processes of generation and decline, of balance and mutual interdependence of virtually all aspects of existence 1.a
陰陽大論	yīn yáng dà lùn	Yin yang da lun, Comprehensive Treatise on Yin and Yang; a larger treatise no longer extant, with

		some passages surviving as quotes in the present text and in the *Huang Di nei jing su wen* 4.e
淫	yín	excess; excessive 3.e
吟	yín	to moan 10.f
飲	yǐn	to drink; beverages 3.e
引	yǐn	to pull 1.f
引	yǐn	to pull/conduct (qi into a specific conduit) 5.a
引	yǐn	short for 導引 *dǎo yǐn* ; (a qi) conducting (therapy); gymnastics 7.c
引經藥	yǐn jīng yào	drugs conducting/pulling (qi) into specific conduits 5.a
隱	yǐn	hidden 1.e
隱忍	yǐn rěn	to bear secretly 7.c
隱隱	yǐn yǐn	scarcely visible 6.f
膺	yīng	to oppose 6.e
瑩	yíng	bright; pure 2.f
營	yíng	camp [qi] 2.c
營	yíng	to circulate 6.d
盈	yíng	full; overflowing 8.b
迎	yíng	to move against 10.b
影響	yǐng xiǎng	shadow and echo 5.e
影響	yǐng xiǎng	effect; trace 8.e
應	yìng	to correspond 2.a
應	yìng	to respond 3.d
硬	yìng	hard 6.c
硬	yìng	rigid 8.f
庸	yōng	ordinary; common 1.f
庸醫	yōng yī	common physician 7.f
壅	yōng	to stop up; to obstruct 6.f
擁	yōng	to block; to obstruct 9.b
癰疽	yōng jū	welling and deep-seated abscesses 9.e
癰瘍	yōng yáng	welling abscess 7.e
勇	yǒng	brave; courage 1.c
湧	yǒng	to [make] gush forth; to induce vomiting 7.b

湧泄	yǒng xiè	discharging through gushing forth (i.e. vomiting) 8.d
用	yòng	to use 1.b
用	yòng	application; tool 3.a
用	yòng	usage 8.d
用事	yòng shì	to perform functions 4.b
憂	yōu	grief 3.e
憂思	yōu sì	concern 3.e
猶	yóu	like; similar to 1.a
猶	yóu	still 1.b
幽門	yōu mén	the dark gate 2.d
尤	yóu	more; particularly; especially 1.d
尤在	yóu zài	the most important is ... 5.d
由	yóu	origin 1.f
由	yóu	from 2.b
由來	yóu lái	origin 3.a
遊	yóu	to travel; to arrive 2.b
猶	yóu	to compare 3.c
猶	yóu	especially 5.b
疣	yóu	swelling 9.d
有	yǒu	to have 1.b
有	yǒu	it may be that 5.f
牖	yǒu	window 3.e
友	yǒu	friend 7.f
幼	yòu	young; immature 1.d
右	yòu	right 2.b
又	yòu	again; in turn; moreover 2.d
瘀	yū	to stagnate 4.c
瘀血	yū xuě	stagnating blood 4.b
於	yú	with reference to 1.c
於	yú	at 1.e
於	yú	in; into 2.c
於	yú	indicating passive: by/from someone or something 2.c

於是	yú shī	thereupon; then 9.d
余	yú	I; myself 3.b
于	yú	in; at; with 4.b
愚	yú	stupid 1.e
愚	yú	ignoramus. Here, a term of self-depreciation: I; myself 6.b
魚	yú	fish 3.a
魚	yú	the fish(-line separating the palm from the wrist) 6.d
魚腹	yú fù	the fish-belly (a term referring to a protuberance palpable in the upper thighs between the musculus sartorius and the musculus quadriceps femoris) 6.a
魚際	yú jì	the fish-border (which separates the palm from the wrist) 6.d
魚子	yú zǐ	fish roe 9.b
逾	yú	to exceed; to pass 7.f
餘	yú	superabundance 4.f
餘	yú	the remaining 8.e
隅	yú	an angle; an edge 10.a
與 (A)- 不若 (B)	yú .. bù ruò	(A) is not as good as (B); in comparsion to (A) it is better that (B) 1.f
俞跗	yú fū	Yu Fu, a legendary physician 1.f
禹錫	yǔ xī	Yuxi, personal name of Zhǎng Yǔxī 掌禹錫 (992-1068), civil servant and commentator of the *Shu materia medica* 9.c
予	yú	I; myself 7.b
予	yǔ	to grant; to give 3.f
雨	yǔ	rain 2.a
與	yǔ	to take part in; together with; to give 1.e
與	yǔ	and 1.f
與	yǔ	with 2.c
與	yǔ	final interrogative particle 5.b
與乎其中	yǔ hū qí zhōng	[this] is part of them; [this] one of them 1.e

語	yǔ	to converse; language 5.f
禹	yǔ	the legendary emperor Yǔ 9.f
愈	yù	to heal 1.f
愈	yù	very (愈 ... 愈…: the more … the more) 5.a
愈	yù	better 7.f
遇	yù	to meet 3.b
禦	yù	to resist; to ward off 3.c
禦	yù	to oppress 8.a
欲	yù	to desire; tò wish 3.d
浴	yù	to wash; to bathe 4.d
豫	yù	beforehand 7.a
裕	yù	abundant 7.c
鬱	yù	obstruction 7.c
鬱發	yù fā	to set free 3.e
域	yù	region 7.e
玉	yù	jade 7.e
玉堂	yù táng	the *yu tang* (insertion point) 2.e
預	yù	beforehand 7.f
嫗	yù	an old woman 9.d
宛陳	yù chén	long-term accumulation 10.a
冤譴	yuān qiǎn	innocently blamed for some wrong 3.c
元	yuán	origin; original 2.d
元氣	yuán qì	to original qi 4.f
芫青	yuán qīng	*yuanqing*, a drug prepared from the beetle Lytta caraganae Pallas 9.b
原	yuán	a source; an origin 5.c
原	yuán	originally; basically 8.b
源	yuán	a source 3.a
緣	yuán	to affect 7.d
緣	yuán	a hem 9.d
緣	yuán	because 9.e
圓	yuán	round 2.a
員利鍼	yuán lì zhēn	the round-sharp needle 10.a
員鍼	yuán zhēn	the round needle 10.a

遠	yuǎn	long; distant 5.a
遠道刺	yuǎn dào cì	piercing from a distance; i.e. piercing at a point far away from the affected area 10.c
願	yuàn	to desire; to wish 2.c
怨	yuàn	resentment 7.f
約	yuē	concise 1.d
曰	yuē	to say; it is said 1.e
月	yuè	month 1.f
月	yuè	the moon 2.a
悅	yuè	pleased; happy 3.d
噦	yuè	to belch 9.a
月郭空	yuè guō kōng	new moon 3.b
月經	yuè jīng	a (woman's) monthly period 9.c
月水	yuè shuǐ	the monthly water; menstrual blood 5.c
越	yuè	to exceed 6.d
越人	yuè rén	Yueren, personal name of Bian Que 1.f
鑰	yuè; yào	a key 2.d
云	yún	to say 1.e
勻	yún	even; uniform 6.f
殞滅	yǔn miè	to die; to perish 6.e
孕	yùn	to be pregnant 2.b
熨	yùn	to iron; to apply hot pressure 3.d
運	yùn	to revolve; time period 1.d
運	yùn	to move 4.b
運氣	yùn qì	moving qi 4.f
雜	zá	mixed; confused 4.a
雜	zá	diverse 7.e
雜亂無紀	zá luàn wú jì	no order whatsoever 5.d
哉	zāi	an exclamation 2.b
在	zài	at; in; with reference to 1.e
在	zài	to depend on 4.b
暫	zàn	for a time 8.b

贊刺	zàn cì	supportive piercing; i.e. shallow piercing to drain blood and support the dispersion of pain and swellings 10.c
藏	zàng	a "depot" storage unit in the body, i.e. liver, heart, spleen, lung, and kidneys 1.b
糟粕	zāo pò	waste; dregs 2.c
早	zǎo	early 3.f
蚤	zǎo	early 8.a
燥	zào	dry; dryness 3.e
造	zào	to produce 9.f
造化	zào huà	to create 4.c
造化	zào huà	the process of creation 6.e
皂莢	zào jiá	*zaojia*, a drug prepared from Gleditsia sinensis Lam. 9.e
皂角	zào jiǎo	*zaojiao*, a drug prepared from Gleditsia sinensis Lam. 9.a
則	zé	a particle indicating consequence or result; translated here as "then … results" 1.a
則	zé	a rule 6.e
擇	zé	to select 1.e
澤	zé	smooth; slippery 9.c
賊	zèi	robber 9.e
賊風	zèi fēng	the robber wind 3.b
增	zēng	to add to; to increase 1.f
甑	zèng	a steamer 9.f
齋	zhāi	to abstain; to fast 5.c
宅	zhái	to reside; lodging 3.a
粘	zhān	to adhere; to stick to 2.f
譫言	zhān yán	to speak incoherently 5.f
斬	zhǎn	to cut in two 9.d
盞	zhǎn	small bowl; numerical for lamps 10.d
戰	zhàn	war 1.e
蘸	zhàn	to dip into 10.d
張	zhāng	a classifier of flat objects 2.f

張蒼	zhāng cāng	Zhang Cang, statesman of the Qin-Han era; lived 256-152 9.c
張華	zhāng huá	Zhang Hua, scholar and statesman of the 3rd c. CE 9.f
張潔古	zhāng jié gŭ	Zhang Jiegu, style Yuánsù 元素, 12th c., was one of the theoreticians of the Song-Jin-Yuan era contributing to the development of a pharmacology of systematic correspondence. 8.e
張景聲	zhāng jĭng shēng	Zhang Jingsheng, name of an otherwise unknown patient 9.d
張世賢	zhāng shì xián	Zhang Shixian, a renowned 16th c. medical author and editor of the *Nàn jīng* 6.d
長	zhăng	to grow; senior 1.c
長幼	zhăng yòu	old and young 4.e
掌	zhăng	the palm of the hand 1.e
脹	zhàng	to swell up 4.a
召	zhāo	to call; to summon 3.c
朝	zhāo	morning 7.d
螫	zhē	poison; poisonous 9.f
哲	zhé	wise 3.e
折	zhé	to break in two 3.e
折	zhé	broken; a curve 10.b
者	zhě	those who 1.b
者	zhě	that which 1.f
者	zhě	a particle indicating that the preceding word is to be read as a noun 2.c
真	zhēn	pure; genuine 9.f
真氣	zhēn qì	true qi; i.e. man's congenital qì 5.a
真藏	zhēn zàng	the true (qi of a) depot 6.d
針	zhēn	a needle 1.b
針灸	zhēn jiŭ	acupuncture and moxibustion 5.a
鍼	zhēn	needle; to insert a needle 10.d
鍼頭	zhēn tóu	the point of a needle 10.d
甄權	zhēn quán	Zhen Quan, 7th century pharmaceutical author 9.f

斟酌	zhēn zhuó	to consider 8.c
診	zhěn	to examine; diagnosis 1.c
疹	zhěn	pustules; eruptions 6.f
枕	zhěn	a head-rest; a pillow 9.d
鎮	zhèn	to settle; to press down 8.a
鴆	zhèn	the Zhen-bird 8.e
陣	zhèn	battle order 10.d
震亨	zhèn hēng	Zhenheng, abbreviated name of Zhū Zhènhēng 朱震亨(1281-1358), scholar and medical author, best known under his sobriquet Zhū Dānxī 朱丹溪 9.f
正月	zhēng yuè	first month of the year 4.e
爭	zhēng	struggle 4.d
徵	zhēng	evidence 8.e
蒸髓	zhēng suǐ	(heat) steaming from the marrow (of one's bones). Equivalent to 骨蒸 *gǔ zhēng* in 9.b 8.b
正	zhèng	proper; regular 3.a
正	zhèng	short for 正治 *zhèng zhì*: regular treatment (i.e. a treatment directed against the nature of an illness as it is apparent from its symptoms) 8.d
正	zhèng	exactly 9.e
正	zhèng	to correct 9.f
正方	zhèng fāng	prescription for a [manual] correction [treatment] 4.a
正經	zhèng jīng	the regular conduits 5.f
正脈	zhèng mài	a regular (movement in the) vessels 6.b
症	zhèng	illness; evidence of disease 3.e
症	zhèng	a pathological condition; patho-condition 4.b
證	zhèng	evidence; symptoms 1.d
之	zhī	pronoun, referring here to the laws of yin and yang 1.a
之	zhī	a possessive pronoun 1.b
之	zhī	to arrive at; to go to 4.c
支(肢)	zhī	a branch 1.f

支	zhī	to prop up 8.b
支解	zhī jiě	dismemberment 1.f
肢	zhī	limb 2.a
枝	zhī	a branch 7.d
汁	zhī	juice; sap 2.c
知	zhī	to know; to be aware of 1.c
知	zhī	to administer 2.f
脂	zhī	fat 2.f
脂	zhī	lard 9.b
直	zhí	only; merely 1.e
直	zhí	exactly 2.e
直	zhí	directly 4.c
直	zhí	straight 10.a
直針刺	zhí zhēn cì	direct piercing; i.e. piercing into a lifted skin-fold without damaging the flesh 10.c
植	zhí	to plant 3.a
執	zhí	to hold 3.c
執一而論	zhí yī ér lùn	to treat all alike 7.a
只	zhǐ	only 10.b
止	zhǐ	to halt; to stop 4.b
旨	zhǐ	meaning 5.b
指	zhǐ	finger; toe 2.a
指	zhǐ	to refer; to point to 2.d
趾	zhǐ	the toes 4.c
祇	zhǐ	only 8.b
紙	zhǐ	paper 9.a
治	zhì	order; to put in order; to regulate. This term is applied to the treatment or management of both individual and social crisis. The present paragraph combines both these meanings 1.a
至	zhì	to reach; to arrive at 1.d
至	zhì	extremely; very 1.d
至	zhì	until 4.e
至	zhì	accomplished 5.b

至	zhì	as for; as far as 9.e
至寶丹	zhì bǎo dān	the "extremely precious balls"; a formula recommended to treat a great number of illnesses with sudden onset 8.e
至人	zhì rén	someone who has reached highest perfection; a sage 4.f
至數	zhì shù	the perfect numbers 6.a
至陰	zhì yīn	the *zhi yin* ("extreme yin") (insertion point) 2.d
至於	zhì yú	as for 3.c
制	zhì	to restrain; to control 7.b
制	zhì	laws; regulations 8.d
制	zhì	to formulate (a prescription), identical with 製 8.f
制	zhì	design [of the needles] 10.c
製	zhì	to make; to construct 1.d
製	zhì	to compound; to formulate (a prescription) 8.a
滯	zhì	to obstruct 2.c
致	zhì	to cause; to result in 3.a
致	zhì	to make [something] reach [a certain destination] 7.b
緻	zhì	fine; dense 3.b
緻理	zhì lǐ	to have tight [skin] structures 7.e
志	zhì	the mind 3.e
志	zhì	Zhi, personal name of Mǎ Zhì 馬志 (fl. 975), co-author of the *Kāi bǎo běn cǎo* 開寶本草 9.f
志意	zhì yì	thought 3.e
質	zhì	substance; matter. Here: disposition 4.c
智	zhì	wisdom; knowledge 9.a
痔	zhì	piles 9.b
置	zhì	to place; to arrange 9.f
中	zhōng	middle 1.e
中	zhōng	in 2.c
中	zhōng	amidst; surrounded by 3.a
中	zhōng	the center (of the body) 4.b
中央	zhōng yāng	center 7.e

終	zhōng	end 2.e
終身	zhōng shēn	an entire lifetime 8.f
種	zhǒng	seed; many; numerous 3.a
種	zhǒng	species; kind 4.b
種種	zhǒng zhǒng	all kinds; all types 4.b
腫	zhǒng	to swell; a swelling 4.b
冢	zhǒng	tomb 9.d
踵	zhǒng	to follow; to imitate 9.f
中	zhòng	to hit; to strike 3.b
中風	zhòng fēng	to be struck by wind 5.f
中惡	zhòng è	to be struck by the malevolent 6.f
中濕	zhòng shī	to be struck by dampness 5.f
中窾	zhòng kuǎn	to hit the mark 8.b
仲景	zhòng jǐng	Zhongjing, style-name of Zhāng Jī 張機, 142-220 (?), author of the prescription work *Shāng hán zá bìng lùn* 傷寒雜病論, "On Harm Caused by Cold and Various [Other] Diseases" 9.e
衆	zhòng	all; the whole of 7.e
重	zhòng	important 1.d
重	zhòng	grave 3.a
重	zhòng	to treat as important; to emphasize 7.c
重	zhòng	heavy 7.f
重	zhòng	pronounced (quality of a drug) 8.a
重	zhòng	to value 10.b
州	zhōu	district 2.a
晝	zhòu	daytime; daylight 2.a
紂	zhòu	(King) Zhou, the last ruler of the Yin dynasty, 12th c. BCE 9.f
皺	zhòu	wrinkled 2.f
珠	zhū	a pearl 6.c
諸	zhū	all; every 2.f
諸	zhū	fusion of *zhī yú* 之於; "in it"; "to it" 7.b
猪	zhū	a hog 9.b
誅	zhū	to eradicate; to eliminate 10.a

朱新仲	zhū xīn zhòng	Zhu Xinzhong, style-name of Zhū Yi 朱翌 (1097-1167), a Song era official and literatus 10.f
朱震亨	zhū zhèn hēng	Zhu Zhenheng, scholar and medical author (1281-1358) 9.f
朱紫	zhū zǐ	(a hierarchy of different ranks characterized by) red and purple (seals); hierarchy 7.f
茱萸	zhū yú	*zhuyu*, a drug prepared from Evodia rutaecarpa (Juss.) Benth. 9.b
术	zhú	the pharmaceutical drug *báizhú* 白术, prepared from Atractylodes macrocephala Koidzumi 8.b
主	zhǔ	to master 1.c
主	zhǔ	to rule; to govern 4.f
主	zhǔ	to be responsible, as a conduit or depot, for the condition of an external organ or section of the body 5.a
煮	zhǔ	to boil; to decoct 9.d
屬意	zhǔ yì	to focus one's attention on 10.a
注	zhù	to flow 3.e
著	zhù	to manifest 1.e
著	zhù	to write, as a book 4.f
著	zhù	to stick to; to adhere 10.e
註	zhù	to comment; commentary 6.d
助	zhù	to assist; to support 7.c
疰	zhù	possession (by demons) 3.e
鑄	zhù	to cast metals 1.a
筯	zhù	chopstick 10.e
祝由	zhù yóu	to invoke the origin (a term used to denote therapeutic exorcism) 7.d
耑	zhuān	only; exclusively; identical with 專 *zhuān* 8.e
專	zhuān	especially; in particular 5.d
專長	zhuān cháng	special expertise; special abilities 8.e
轉	zhuǎn	to revolve; to turn over 2.b
轉	zhuǎn	in turn; in addition; on top of 8.b
轉	zhuǎn	to change basically 8.f

轉	zhuǎn	to twirl [a needle after insertion] 10.b
傳	zhuàn	a biography 1.f
壯	zhuàng	strong; robust 2.b
壯	zhuàng	to strengthen; to fill 3.c
狀	zhuàng	appearance; form 2.f
錐	zhuī	a pointed weapon, used here in the sense of "weapon" in general 1.a
椎	zhuī	vertebra; backbone section 2.d
墜	zhuì	to bring down; to make fall down 9.f
準	zhǔn	to weigh; to compare 5.b
著	zhuó	to be attached to 4.d
酌	zhuó	to deliberate; to think about 5.b
灼	zhuó	to cauterize 10.d
濁	zhuó	turbid 2.c
濁	zhuó	thick 10.e
恣	zī	to throw off restraint 1.e
恣意	zī yì	at random; careless 1.e
資	zī	to help; to provide; to nourish 2.c
滋	zī	to nourish; to supply 2.c
滋	zī	more; very 9.e
子	zǐ	the Master 1.e
子	zǐ	noun-ending 2.a
子	zǐ	child 2.a
子	zǐ	spot 2.f
紫	zǐ	dark red; purplish 2.f
紫金錠	zǐ jīn dìng	the "dark-red golden ingot", a formula recommended to cure all possible eye afflictions 8.e
紫石英	zǐ shí yīng	*zishiying*, a mineral drug; fluorite 9.a
字	zì	a word 5.b
眥	zì	the corner of an eye; canthus 5.a
自	zì	from; from itself; naturally 1.e
自	zì	self 1.e
自	zì	since; because 2.d
自 ..而後	zì .. ér hòu	from (a certain point of time) on 1.e

自病	zì bìng	to fall ill by itself (as of a regular conduit, in contrast to an illness transmitted from another depot or conduit) 5.f
自汗	zì hàn	to sweat without apparent external reason, such as hot weather, thick clothing, etc. 5.d
自然	zì rán	naturally; by itself 10.d
自作孽	zì zuò niè	misfortune brought upon one by oneself 3.c
宗	zōng	the most important 6.b
縱	zòng	to be indulgent; to give oneself to 5.c
縱	zòng	even if 8.b
總	zǒng	to sum up; all 3.e
走	zǒu	to depart; to go 2.c
走	zǒu	to move 7.b
奏功	zòu gōng	to have the intended effect 5.d
卒	zú	finally; eventually; as a result 1.e
卒	zú	completely; in all details 5.e
足	zú	foot 2.a
足	zú	enough 2.a
足厥陰	zú jué yīn	the foot-ceasing-yin (location) 6.a
足少陰	zú shào yīn	the foot-minor-yin (location) 6.a
足太陰	zú tài yīn	the foot-major-yin (location) 6.a
祖	zǔ	ancestor; grandfather 10.f
阻截	zǔ jié	to obstruct 9.a
祖宗	zǔ zōng	ancestors 3.c
最	zuì	very; most; extreme 1.e
醉	zuì	intoxicated; drunk 1.f
佐	zuǒ	assistant (drugs in a prescription) 8.c
左	zuǒ	left 2.b
左右	zuǒ yòu	those to the left and right; an entourage 3.d
作	zuò	to do 2.f
作	zuò	to make; to be 2.f
作	zuò	to be active 4.d
作	zuò	to act; to be active 7.d
坐	zuò	to sit 5.f
鑿鑿可徵	zuò zuò kě zhēng	indisputable evidence 3.c

Forgotten Traditions of Ancient Chinese Medicine

the *I Hsu Yuan Liu Lun* by Hsu Ta-chun

Translated by Paul U. Unschuld

Here is a text for scholars, for students of Chinese language and culture, and for those clinicians (particularly herbalists) who recognize a relationship between their clinical skill and their understanding of Chinese thought. The author, Hsu Ta-Chun, wrote in the 18th century immediately prior to the introduction of Western science and medicine to China. He achieved recognition and influenced the history of medicine because the medicine he championed was pristine in logic and method. In any period, or any culture, Hsu would have been a remarkable thinker. A literate, broadly skilled scholar, he practiced medicine as an expression of personal and social responsibility. Even with his articulate and profound attachment to classical ideas, he was able to recognize progress in medicine, while retaining an ability to critically examine popular ideas and modern physicians. He could both recognize others for their accomplishments, and scathe with uncompromising prose those whom he felt corrupted the art of medicine. He was a conservative who understood the practical necessities of patient care.

In his extensive prologue Dr. Unschuld includes a detailed analysis of Hsu's work. We learn that Chinese medicine does differ from Western medicine, offering a holistic view of disease and the human who suffers. However, we also learn that Hsu and his European contemporaries would not have regarded one another as strangers. Hsu's 100 essays are broad and fascinating. The scope of these essays gives us a view of Chinese medicine that is whole and inclusive. His discussions of illness, pathoconditions, formulas, and substances are often more lucid than the explanations offered by modern texts. Some are of particular interest to historians, philologists, and philosophers; others are of direct interest to clinicians. By speaking his opinions clearly and reporting on an art with which he was deeply intimate, Hsu has bequeathed us a richly detailed vision of Chinese medicine at its height. The essays read well and demonstrate that rigorous scholarship can draw back the curtains of time, language, and preconceived notion to reveal the mind and thought of an exceptional individual. By carefully selecting terms that are suitable for the variety of circumstances in which a Chinese character is used, Unschuld helps us to refine our understanding of important Chinese concepts.